W9-CES-129

Contributors

Piero Anversa, MD
Professor of Medicine
New York Medical College
Department of Medicine
Vosburgh Pavilion
Valhalla, New York

Alberto A. Diaz-Arias, MD
Assistant Professor
Department of Pathology
University of Missouri-Columbia
Columbia, Missouri

Jill E. Bishop, PhD
Division of Cardiopulmonary
    Biochemistry
Department of Medicine
University College London
The Rayne Institute
London, United Kingdom

Christian G. Brilla, MD, PhD
Associate Professor of Medicine
Philipps University of Marburg
Center of Internal Medicine
Division of Cardiology
Marburg, F.R.G.

François Cambien, MD
Director, INSERM SC7
Paris, France

Scott E. Campbell, PhD
Assistant Professor of Medicine
Director, Cardiac Structure Lab
Department of Internal Medicine
Division of Cardiology
University of Missouri-Columbia
Columbia, Missouri

Dr. Ir. Jack P.M. Cleutjens, PhD
Department of Pathology
Cardiovascular Research Institute
    Maastricht (CARIM)
University of Limburg
Maastricht, The Netherlands

Dr. Mat J.A.P. Daemen, MD, PhD
Department of Pathology
Cardiovascular Research Institute
    Maastricht (CARIM)
University of Limburg
Maastricht, The Netherlands

A. Martin Gerdes, PhD
Professor and Chairman
Department of Anatomy and Structural
    Biology
School of Medicine
University of South Dakota
Vermillion, South Dakota

Eduarto Guarda, MD
Profesor Auxiliar de Medicina
Departamento de Enfermedades
    Cardiovasculares
Universidad Católica de Chile
Santiago, Chile

Ramareddy V. Guntaka, PhD
Professor
Department of Molecular Microbiology
    and Immunology
School of Medicine
University of Missouri-Columbia
Columbia, Missouri

Jeffrey R. Henegar, MA
Senior Research Specialist
University of Missouri
Division of Cardiology
Columbia, Missouri

G. Scott Herron, PhD, MD
Assistant Professor of Medicine
Department of Dermatology
Stanford University School of Medicine
Stanford, California

Matthias Herzum
Department of Internal Medicine and
    Cardiology
Philipps University-Marburg
Marburg, Germany

Günter Hufnagel
Department of Internal Medicine and
  Cardiology
Philipps University-Marburg
Marburg, Germany

Joseph S. Janicki, PhD
Professor of Medicine and Physiology
Cardiology 1E65
University of Missouri
Columbia, Missouri

Jagan C. Kandala
Research Associate Professor
Department of Molecular Microbiology
  and Immunology
School of Medicine
University of Missouri-Columbia
Columbia, Missouri

C. Chandrasekharan Kartha, MD
Division of Cellular and Molecular
  Cardiology
Sree Chitra Tirunal Institute for
Medical Sciences & Technology
Kerala, India

Shogo Katsuda, MD
Professor
Department of Pathology
Kanazawa Medical University
Ishikawa, Japan

Laxmansa C. Katwa, PhD
Assistant Professor of Medicine
Division of Cardiology,
Department of Internal Medicine
University of Missouri-Columbia
Columbia, Missouri

Attila Kovacs, MD
Instructor
Department of Medicine
School of Medicine
University of Missouri-Columbia
Columbia, Missouri

Geoffrey J. Laurent, PhD, FRCPath
Professor
Division of Cardiopulmonary
  Biochemistry
and Centre for Respiratory Research
University College London Medical
  School
London, United Kingdom

Bernhard Maisch
Chairman of the Department of Internal
  Medicine and Cardiology
Philipps University-Marburg
Marburg, Germany

Leonard G. Meggs, MD
Associate Professor of Medicine
New York Medical College
Department of Medicine
Vosburgh Pavilion
Valhalla, New York

Paul R. Meyers, PhD, MD, FACC
Associate Professor of Medicine
Division of Cardiology
Vanderbilt University
Nashville, Tennessee

Isao Nakanishi, MD, PhD
Professor
Department of Pathology, School of
  Medicine
Kanazawa University
Ishikawa, Japan

Hanumanth K. Reddy, MD
Assistant Professor of Medicine
Assistant Director-Clinical Cardiology
University of Missouri-Columbia
Columbia, Missouri

Ute Schönian
Department of Internal Medicine and
  Cardiology
Philipps University-Marburg
Marburg, Germany

Dr. Jos F.M. Smits, PhD
Department of Pharmacology
Cardiovascular Research Institute
  Maastricht (CARIM)
University of Limburg
Maastricht, The Netherlands

Florent Soubrier, MD, PhD
INSERM U36
College de France
Paris, France

Francis G. Spinale, MS, MD, PhD
Associate Professor of Surgery and
  Physiology
Division of Cardiothoracic Surgery
Medical University of South Carolina
Charleston, South Carolina

Ronald J. Stoney
Professor Emeritus, Department of
 Surgery
Division of Vascular Surgery
President, Pacific Vascular Research
 Foundation
University of California-San Francisco
San Francisco, California

Yao Sun, MD, PhD
Assistant Professor of Medicine
Division of Cardiology,
Department of Internal Medicine
University of Missouri Health Sciences
 Center
Columbia, Missouri

Suresh C. Tyagi, PhD
Assistant Professor of Medicine and
 Biochemistry
University of Missouri-Columbia
Medical Sciences Building
Columbia, Missouri

Elaine N. Unemori, PhD
Group Leader Cell Biology
Connective Therapeutics, Inc.
Palo Alto, California

Karl T. Weber, MD
Professor and Chairman
Department of Internal Medicine
University of Missouri Health Sciences
 Center
Columbia, Missouri

Peter Whittaker, PhD
Director of Microscopy
The Heart Institute
Good Samaritan Hospital &
Assistant Professor of Research Medicine
University of Southern California
Los Angeles, California

Preface

*And when the body of knowledge changes, so do
we. Each change brings with it new attitudes and
institutions created by new knowledge.*

(James Burke, *The Day the Universe Changed,*
Little, Brown & Co., London, 1985)

Cardiovascular disease is a worldwide health problem of major proportions. It directly causes large numbers of morbid and mortal events, and indirectly impacts economics and productivity. New insights are desperately needed if we are to develop preventive strategies and effective remedies. Can we find order amid the chaos? Is there common ground which might provide insights?

Inflammation and wound healing are fundamental properties of all vascularized tissues, and this includes the heart and vasculature. Through inflammation and repair, injuries are contained and wounds healed. What can prove lifesaving on one hand, can become harmful on the other when invoked in the absence of injury or when continued unabated.

Atherosclerotic disease, hypertension, cardiomyopathies, and valvular heart disease—the most prevalent expressions of cardiovascular disease—represent examples of wound healing gone awry.

In response to cell injury, or following invasion by foreign chemical, bacterial toxin, or protein, tissues initiate a cascade of responses designed to first contain assault and then heal violated tissue. Characterized as exudative, inflammatory, fibroplastic and fibrogenic phases of healing, this complex process can be orchestrated by polypeptides (or cytokines and growth factors), locally generated peptides and/or circulating hormones. The nature of the response depends on the exciting stimulus.

Understanding this process would likely permit us to prevent distortions in cardiovascular structure that ultimately impair tissue function.

In Wound Healing and Cardiovascular Disease, an international group of clinicians and biomedical scientists, interested in abnormal cardiovascular structure and organ failure, have compiled their perspectives on inflammation and wound healing in cardiovascular disease. Two broad topics are featured. These include: a) Expressions of Wound Healing, such as myocardial infarction and rupture, chronic ischemic heart disease, the dilated failing heart, myocarditis, endomyocardial fibrosis, and coronary restenosis following revascularization; and b) Regulatory Aspects of Wound Healing, which addresses the regulation of collagen turnover and collagen degradation in the diseased heart, aorta and atherosclerotic lesion; the association between circulating peptide and steroid hormones and myocardial fibrosis, the role of locally produced peptides in promoting tissue repair, the potential association between angiotension I-converting enzyme gene polymorphism and cardiovascular risk, and the regulation of fibrillar collagen gene expression.

It is my belief that there is indeed order to the chaos. It is time to search for common pathophysiological mechanisms of disease. Wound healing, with its inflammatory and reparative components, is a property common to vascularized tissue. It therefore is an appropriate point at which to begin.—K.T.W.

Library of Congress Cataloging-in-Publication Data

Wound healing in cardiovascular disease / edited by Karl T. Weber.
        p.   cm.
    Includes bibliographical references and index.
    ISBN 0-87993-620-7
    1. Cardiovascular system—Pathophysiology.   2. Wound healing.
 I. Weber, Karl T.
    [DNLM: 1. Wound Healing.   2. Cardiovascular Diseases.   WO 185
 W93835 1995]
    RC669.9.W68   1995
    616.1′0473—dc20
    DNLM/DLC
    for Library of Congress   95-12157
                                                                        CIP

Copyright 1995
Futura Publishing Company, Inc.

Published by
Futura Publishing Company, Inc.
135 Bedford Road
Armonk, NY   10504-0418

LC#95-12157
ISBN#: 0-87993-620-7

Printed in the United States of America.

This book is printed on acid-free paper.

Wound Healing
in Cardiovascular Disease

Edited by

Karl T. Weber, MD

Professor and Chairman
Department of Internal Medicine
University of Missouri Health Sciences Center
Columbia, Missouri

Futura Publishing
Company, Inc.
Armonk, NY

Table of Contents

Chapter 1

Inflammation and Healing in the Heart

Karl T. Weber, M.D.

Introduction

Inflammation and healing are fundamental properties of the arterial and venous vasculature that serve to contain tissue injury and invasion by foreign agents or toxins. An inflammatory response, which begins within minutes to hours in involved vessels, occurs when tissue is disrupted by such diverse pathophysiological outcomes as parenchymal cell necrosis, microbial infection, chemical toxin, foreign material, or antigen-antibody complex. Involved vessels release chemical mediators that promote their dilatation and augment their permeability. This exudative phase of inflammation, characterized by tissue edema, is followed by a series of responses that include: an activation of polypeptide regulatory molecules (e.g., cytokines), inflammatory cell invasion (e. g., polymorphonuclear leukocytes, then macrophages), fibroblast proliferation (fibroplasia), and new blood vessel formation (i.e., angiogenesis). Collectively, these responses account for and constitute granulation tissue. A fibrogenic phase of repair, with fibrous tissue formation, follows as granulation tissue is gradually resorbed. At sites of parenchymal cell necrosis, the appearance of connective tissue (or scarring) restores structural integrity to tissue and therefore represents a *reparative fibrosis*. In the absence of cell loss, the accumulation of fibrillar collagen represents a *reactive fibrosis* that can seal off toxins or foreign material. Such a reactive fibrosis also presents as a perivascular fibrosis in

response to vascular hyperpermeability.[1, 2] Each of these responses are observed in the rat heart in response to pericardiotomy, insertion of silk ligature around the left coronary artery, with or without subsequent myocardial infarction (MI) following artery litigation, and are therefore reviewed herein as a model of the inflammation healing paradigm.

Pharmacological interventions, whether given intravenously or per os postinfarction, may influence any individual component of the inflammation healing response. Cardiologists therefore must be mindful of the potential effects, medications prescribed following infarction can have on healing tissue and whether they favor or hinder tissue repair. For example, it has been suggested that the incidence of myocardial rupture postinfarction is increased with thrombolytic therapy.[3] This remains to be fully confirmed. Clinically, it is known that following infarction, wall thinning and rupture are more likely to accompany the use of glucocorticoids and this has also been demonstrated experimentally.[4] Likewise, nonsteroidal anti-inflammatory agents lead to infarct expansion, a thinning and dilatation of the infarcted segment of myocardium in man as evidenced in an experimental model as well.[5] The efficacy and safety of angiotensin converting enzyme (ACE) inhibition postinfarction is presently under investigation in clinical trials conducted in the United States and abroad.[6–8] To date, the introduction of such an agent within the first week following infarction has proven

This work was supported in part by NIH Grant R01-HL-31701

effective in prolonging survival and reducing the subsequent appearance of ventricular dilatation and heart failure.[9] Administered on the day of infarction, on the other hand, the response to such an agent has been more variable and perhaps even detrimental.[10] Why might this be the case? Can answers be found in the inflammation healing paradigm? The perspective offered in this chapter seeks to address these questions based on lessons learned about inflammation and healing from snake venom, the subcutaneous injection of seaweed, and other experimental models.

Snake Venom and ACE Inhibitors

Bradykinin-Potentiating Factor

ACE inhibitors were introduced into clinical medicine as a result of research conducted by Ferreira, et al.[11] who examined the vasculotoxic consequences of snake bite. The venom of the Brazilian viper, *Bothrops jararaca*, induced systemic vasodilatation, together with an escape of intravascular fluid, and macromolecules into the extracellular space. Ferreira's, et al. search for the active component of the venom extract that served as the chemical mediator of this inflammatory-like response led to the discovery of bradykinin-potentiating factor and ultimately the isolation of bradykinin-potentiating peptides.[12] These peptides prevented the conversion of bradykinin (BK) into inactive metabolites and therefore they were inhibitors of kininase II (Fig. 1). They also would prevent the conversion of angiotensin I to Ang II and therefore were considered inhibitors of ACE (Fig. 1). Teprotide, a peptide isolated and purified from venom extract,[11] was studied extensively for its ability to augment the biological activities of BK and inhibit the formation of Ang II. Inhibition of ACE was subsequently found to also reduce the degradation of other substances, including substance P and enkephalins, each of which are mediators of inflammation.

ACE Inhibitors: Postinfarction and Heart Failure

In a clinical trial (SAVE), where an ACE inhibitor was given on days 3 to 16 following infarction to patients with impaired ejection fraction, despite the absence of symptomatic heart failure or myocardial ischemia, a reduction in all cause mortality and both fatal and nonfatal major cardiovascular events was observed.[9] This included a reduction in risk for the development of symptomatic heart failure and hospitalization for congestive heart failure in these patients, many of whom had also received thrombolytic therapy, aspirin, or beta-adrenergic receptor blockade. Long-term aspirin administration in association with ACE inhibitor treatment may, however, prove counterproductive.[13]

In the CONSENSUS II study, ACE inhibition introduced within 24 hours of the appearance of chest pain due to myocardial infarction did not prove efficacious. ACE inhibition was found not to alter survival at 1 or 6 months after infarction, compared to placebo, and this included death due to symptomatic heart failure.[10] Diverse outcomes have been reported with the early introduction of ACE inhibition following myocardial infarction.[6] Their role within 24 hours of infarction is therefore less certain.

In patients with left ventricular systolic dysfunction and advanced symptomatic failure, who were receiving diuretics and digitalis, a controlled multicenter trial (CONSENSUS I) demonstrated that interference with renin-angiotensin-aldosterone system (RAAS) activation by ACE inhibition, and reduction in plasma concentrations of Ang II and aldosterone, improved survival in comparison to conventional therapy plus placebo.[14, 15] Similar results were observed in the treatment trial of another controlled multicenter study (SOLVD) in patients with mild to moderate heart failure. Here mortality and morbidity due to symptomatic failure were reduced by ACE inhibition when combined with conventional therapy as compared to conventional therapy plus placebo.[16]

In the prevention trial of SOLVD, where an ACE inhibitor was given to previ-

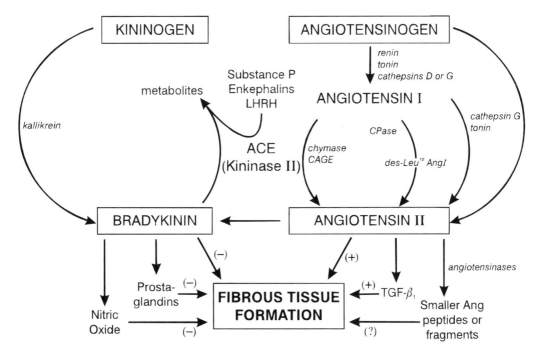

Figure 1. The generation of angiotensin II and bradykinin and their stimulatory (+) or inhibitory (−) influence on fibrous tissue formation. Bradykinin may also attenuate fibrosis through its influence on the production of prostaglandins and nitric oxide. Multiple pathways may be involved in the generation of angiotensin peptides. ACE is involved in the generation of angiotensin II and the hydrolysis of bradykinin, substance P, enkephalins, and luteinizing hormone releasing hormone (LHRH) (see text for details). CAGE = chymostatin sensitive angiotensin generating enzyme; CP = carboxypeptidase. Adapted from reference 158 with permission.

ously untreated, asymptomatic patients with evidence of left ventricular systolic dysfunction (i.e., ejection fraction ≤35%), a reduction in the incidence of heart failure and hospitalizations for symptomatic failure was observed.[17] A trend toward fewer deaths due to cardiovascular causes, albeit not statistically significant, was also reported.

In both the prevention and treatment trials of SOLVD, a significant reduction in the number of patients developing myocardial infarction or unstable angina was observed.[18] This provocative finding suggests that ACE inhibition may influence the atherosclerotic process[19] and/or the structural remodeling of coronary arteries[20]; it may also prevent cardiac myocyte necrosis associated with elevated plasma angiotensin II.[21-23] In patients with mild to moderately severe heart failure, receiving digoxin, diuretic, and ACE inhibitor, the rapid withdrawal of ACE inhibitor resulted in gradual worsening of heart failure.[24] Evidence of neurohormonal activation has been observed in many but not all patients with impaired ejection fraction following myocardial infarction.[25] Activation of the sterile normale saline and renin-angiotensin-aldosterone was most closely related to the clinical severity of left ventricular dysfunction (i.e., Killip class), ejection fraction, age, and diuretic usage during hospitalization.

Seaweed and Chemical Mediators of Inflammation

Patterns of Inflammation

Several different patterns of vascular hyperpermeability are known to accompany the early phase of inflammation. They involve different segments of the circulation and specific chemical mediators. An immediate transient response, involving venular capillaries, appears and disappears over the course of 1 hour. Vasoactive amines, such as histamine and serotonin, are released from mast cells to mediate this response. An immediate sustained response emerges over the course of 1 hour, while hyperpermeability of capillaries and smaller arterioles persists for up to 6 hours. This response involves the release of proteases and/or arachidonic acid metabolites. Chemical mediators include: Bradykinin; prostaglandins; anaphylatoxins of the complement system; components of the coagulation-fibrinolytic system; thromboxane; or leukotrienes. Endothelial cells represent an important source for many of these mediators. More recent evidence implicates a role for nitric oxide and Ang II in inflammatory reactions. A delayed and prolonged response does not occur for several hours but may persist for up to 6 hours. It follows overexposure to sunlight. Mediators of this response are less well understood.

Carrageenin Model of Inflammation

Various chemical agents have been used to address the release of chemical mediators of inflammation with a view toward the development of anti-inflammatory agents. Subcutaneous injection of egg white, dextran, or yeast have been associated with the immediate transient form of hyperpermeability and edema formation; each has been associated with the release of either histamine or serotonin.[26] The release of Bradykinin and Prostaglandins is associated with the immediate sustained response in vascular hyperpermeability and accompanies the injection of a polysaccharide derivative of seaweed, *Chondrus crispus*, also called (CARR) after the city in Ireland where it is distributed. Injected into the rat paw, carrageenin causes edema and the escape of plasma macromolecules over the course of 6 hours (Figure 2). Paw volume, measured in a plethysmograph, is used to assess the degree of edema formation. Urate crystals, uric acid, and kaolin are other

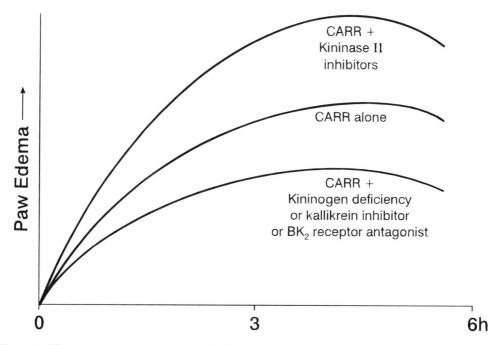

Figure 2. The subcutaneous injection of CARR into the rat paw is followed by interstitial edema and paw swelling over the course of 6 hours—an immediate, sustained pattern of inflammation. Edema formation is enhanced by pretreatment with a kininase II (ACE) inhibitor suggesting that bradykinin accumulation further augments vascular permeability. Edema is attenuated when the generation of bradykinin or binding to its B_2 receptor is disrupted.

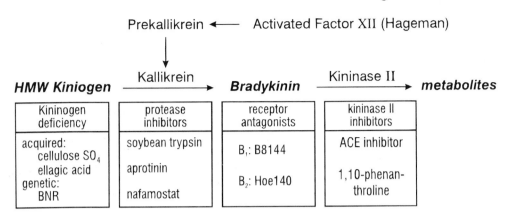

Figure 3. The generation of bradykinin (BK) and its degradation. Various pharmacological probes can be used to interfere with this cascade and to assess the role of BK in inflammation and healing. A substrain of the Brown Norway rat (BNR) has an inherited deficiency in kininogen. From Snakes Rev.

chemical agents that elicit this response. Because the seaweed (or carrageenin) model is also relevant to our consideration of inflammation and healing postmyocardial infarction (MI), it will be reviewed in some detail.

The rationale underlying studies that led to the identification of Bradykinin as a mediator of paw edema in the CARR model will be considered first (Fig. 3). Activated factor XII (Hageman factor), a component of the intrinsic coagulation cascade, together with prekallikrein (an inactive precursor of kallikrein formed in the liver, pancreas, and intestine) lead to the formation of kallikrein. Kallikrein, a serine protease found in plasma and tissue, converts high molecular weight kininogen to bradykinin. This cascade resembles the generation of Ang I, where aspartyl and/or serine proteases act on a larger molecular weight angiotensinogen precursor (Figure 1). Bradykinin, converted to inactive metabolites by kininase II (or ACE), has a very short half-life, however, it evokes a series of responses that elaborate other mediators of inflammation (Figure 1). Derived from endothelial cells or other mesenchymal cells (perhaps fibroblasts or fibroblast-like cells) via BK_2 receptor-ligand binding, these include: nitric oxide; and arachidonate metabolites, such as PGE_2.

The BK-generating pathway can be interrupted pharmacologically to create a kininogen deficiency or inhibition of kallikrein. A strain of Brown Norway rat having a genetic deficiency in kininogen provides a unique model. A recently developed stable BK_2 receptor antagonist (Hoe 140 or Icatibant) will interfere with receptor-ligand binding. Finally, an ACE inhibitor will attenuate kininase II activity and thereby increase local concentrations of BK and potentiate its effects.

Paw edema that normally appears over the course of 6 hours following CARR injection (Fig. 3) was attenuated in both the acquired (e.g., cellulose sulfate or ellagic acid) and genetic forms of kininogen deficiency[27, 28] by kallikrein inhibitors (e.g., soybean trypsin, aprotinin, and nafamostat),[28, 29] or with Hoe 140.[30] A BK_1 receptor antagonist (B8144) had no effect on edema formation following CARR injection. By retarding BK degradation, on the other hand, captopril increased CARR-induced paw edema; the same was true for the kininase II inhibitor phenanthroline.[28] Cobra venom factor, which depletes complement, did not alter paw edema following kaolin-induced paw swelling, indicating that the complement system is not participatory in this response.[31]

A role for prostaglandins in mediating hyperpermeability in the CARR model was examined from two different perspectives: the first was to use the cyclooxygenase inhibitor indomethacin; the second was to reduce membrane lipid precursors through long-term feeding with a diet deficient in essential fatty acids. In both cases, CARR-induced paw edema was reduced.[32]

Thus, chemical mediators associated with the immediate sustained form of hyperpermeability, accompany the early inflammatory response to CARR, is related to the release of Bradykinin and Prostaglandins. The source of these mediators is likely endothelial cells. Wiemer et al.[33] have shown that cultured endothelial cells produce and release Bradykinin. Provided Bradykinin degradation was prevented by ACE inhibition, the quantity of BK released by these cells produced a sustained stimulus of the autocoids Nitric Oxide and PGI_2. BK formation is therefore capable of eliciting a series of responses (Figure 1) by endothelial cells that could contribute to inflammation and healing. Given this diverse repertoire of endothelial cells, it is not surprising that inflammation and healing are fundamental properties of vascularized tissues.

Other Models of Inflammation

The presence of elevated serum ACE activity in patients with many chronic granulomatous diseases, such as sarcoidosis, leprosy, and Gaucher's disease,[34, 35] has drawn attention to the role of this hydrolase, angiotensin peptides, and substance P in inflammation. Granulomatous tissue is a chronic inflammatory condition, characterized by the accumulation and organization of activated macrophages and the formation of epithelioid cells. *Schistosoma mansoni* eggs have been injected into mice to create granulomatous disease of various organs. ACE activity was identified in such granulomas isolated from liver, colon, and lung and was greatest after the peak of the inflammatory cell response.[36] The maximum rise in serum ACE activity appeared to correlate with maximum granuloma size. Using immunofluorescent labeling, ACE has been detected in epithelioid cells and giant cells in granulomas found in sarcoidosis[37] and following *Schistosoma mansoni* infestation.[38] ACE activity is present in monocytes, macrophages, and epithelioid cells isolated from these granulomas.[39] In sarcoidosis, ACE binding and activity was inversely related to fibrous tissue at all

formation.[40, 41] This contrasts with ACE binding found in fibrous tissue that appears in the heart (vide infra).

The entire cascade involved in the generation of Angiotensin II peptides has been identified in macrophages.[38] Polymorphonuclear leukocytes and mast cells contain many of the proteases depicted in Figure 1 and which can generate Angiotensin peptides from two pathways[42–47]: conversion of Ang I from angiotensinogen, or direct conversion of Angiotensin II from this precursor. The generation of Angiotensin peptides by leukocytes is not inhibited by captopril, whereas enalapril and captopril each inhibit ACE activity and reduce Angiotensin II content in granulomas. Angiotensin II may be a direct or indirect (via its stimulation of Bradykinin, Prostaglandins, and/or Nitric Oxide) mediator of inflammation. It is now recognized that Nitric Oxide is generated by macrophages and polymorphonuclear leukocytes and that it contributes to inflammatory responses.[48] Evidence that Angiotensin II may be a direct mediator comes from multiple lines of investigation.[36, 39, 42, 43, 46, 49–51] For example, when generated by inflammatory cells, Angiotensin II alters macrophage migration and phagocytosis by receptor-ligand binding. Angiotensin II receptors have been identified by both radioligand assay and fluorescent labeling in macrophages and monocytes, but not eosinophils or lymphocytes.[50] T-lymphocytes contain high levels of membrane-bound ACE.[52] Angiotensin II binding activity has also been found in macrophage-enriched peritoneal exudate obtained from guinea pigs following administration of mineral oil.[53]

Substance P, a tachykinin involved in inflammatory responses, is also metabolized by ACE. This peptide modulates leukocyte activities and may regulate tissue repair by promoting fibroblast proliferation.[54] It has been identified in extracts of hepatic granulomas associated with *Schistosomiasis mansoni* infection in mice.[55] Little is known about the role of substance P in inflammatory and healing responses seen in the heart. However, recent evidence indicates that blockade of its receptor inhibited the formation of an inflammatory cytokine, tumor necrosis factor-α, within cardiac lesions associated with magnesium deficiency in rats.[56]

ACE inhibitors have been found to reduce granuloma size in the Schistosomiasis model, a nonreplicating antigenic moiety.[57] In the case of replicating pathogens (e.g., *Histolyticum capsulatum*), this intervention increased signs of infection and severity of disease.[58] Cell-mediated defenses may have been impaired by ACE inhibition and were rapidly restored with cessation of treatment.

Seaweed and Chemical Mediators of Healing

Fibrogenesis and Circulating Hormones

A role for circulating steroid hormones in fibrous tissue formation has been recognized for some time. In 1946, Selye[59] reported that chronic (>4 weeks) administration of the "stress hormone" deoxycorticosterone acetate (DOCA) led to a perivascular fibrosis of systemic and intramyocardial coronary arterioles. This reactive fibrous tissue response, or "perivascular granulomas" as he referred to them, was considered a disease of adaption. Chronic administration of aldosterone (ALDO) likewise is associated with a perivascular fibrosis of systemic organs and the heart.[60–62] This structural remodeling of the vasculature first appears at 4 weeks of treatment and continues, in a progressive manner, beyond this point.[62] It is found in patients with autopsy-proven adrenal adenoma as well.[63] The chronic deoxycorticosterone (DOC) excess state associated with androgen-induced 11α-hydroxylase inhibition is also associated with this fibrous tissue reaction in both rats[64, 65] and man.[66] Chronic androgen treatment is associated with increased collagen synthesis[67] detected as enhanced deposition of collagen in skin[68] and bone.[67] On the other hand, hypoaldosteronism, such as that which accompanies chronic heparin treatment, is associated with osteoporosis[69] and impaired wound healing.[70]

Selye's findings prompted others to address the role of steroid hormones in tissue repair.[71–74] In animals receiving a subcutaneous or intraperitoneal injection of various chemical agents (e.g., turpentine, CARR, or quartz) or following skin incision, it was found that cortisone inhibited collagen accumulation. Treatment with the mineralocorticoid DOCA, on the other hand, increased collagen synthesis in the granulomatous reaction and lead to larger granulomas. In adrenalectomized rats treated with DOCA the fibrous tissue response to subcutaneous CARR was enhanced beyond that seen with DOCA alone, suggesting the inhibitory role of cortisone had been withdrawn leaving unopposed effect of the mineralocorticoid on wound healing.

Mesenchymal cells contain the nuclear transcripts needed for the expression of type I and III collagens,[75] the major fibrillar collagens of most tissues save for bone where type II collagen predominates. Hormone-mediated regulation of fibrillar collagen transcription and translation requires receptor-ligand binding. In the case of Aldosterone or Deoxycotricosterone, mineralocorticoid receptors have been identified in fibroblasts of various tissues.[76–78] Because type I and II corticoid receptors have equal affinity for gluco- and mineralocorticoids, specificity to this promiscuous receptor needs to be conferred—a function achieved with the guardian enzyme 11α-hydroxysteroid dehydrogenase (11-HSD). This membrane-bound enzyme converts glucocorticoids into inactive 11-keto metabolites. In skin, lung, and cardiac fibroblasts, as well as osteoblasts, 11–HSD activity has been detected providing further evidence that these cells are targets for mineralocorticoid hormones. In serum-deprived cultured cardiac fibroblasts incubation with ALDO evokes a concentration-dependent increase in collagen synthesis which can be prevented by concomitant incubation with the type I corticoid receptor antagonist spironolactone. Chronic administration of Angiotensin II, associated with a rise in both plasma Angiotensin II and Aldosterone, is likewise associated with a perivascular fibrosis of systemic and coronary vessels.[62, 79] In this case, however, collagen synthesis rises early and fibrosis appears within 2 weeks of treatment and is progressive over the course of 6 weeks. A perivascular fibrosis is also seen with unilateral renal ischemia and activation of the Renin-angiotensin-aldosterone system.[61, 80, 81] Collagen mRNA expression and synthesis is increased in the heart following either suprarenal abdominal aorta constriction or unilateral renal ischemia.[82, 83]

To further address the role of Angiotensin II in promoting this reactive fibrosis, this peptide was administered to previously normal rats by implanted minipump.[84] The dose given did not elevate arterial pressure for several days. Macromolecular permeability was examined using an antibody to plasma fibronectin and the temporal appearance of myocardial fibrosis was examined using the picrosirius red stain, specific for fibrillar collagen.[1] On day 1 of the Angiotensin II infusion, intramyocardial coronary arterioles of both ventricles were morphologically intact and resembled untreated controls. On day 2, localized deposits of plasma fibronectin were evident within the media and adventitia of these vessels with protrusions into the adjacent interstitial space. Immunolabeling of large intramural arteries or veins was not detected. A cellular response was also now evident within the adventitia of these vessels and included fibroblasts and macrophages. On day 4, plasma fibronectin staining of the media and adventitia of arterioles was more extensive and widespread than that seen earlier, while its extension into the interstitial space was more advanced. On day 7 of Ang II, the walls of intramyocardial coronary arterioles had become thicker with diffuse fibronectin labeling evident in the media, adventitia and neighboring interstitial space. The increased cellularity of the adventitia was still evident in involved vessels on days 4 and 7. Although fibroblasts and macrophages were still apparent, polymorphonuclear leukocyte (PMNs) were no longer found on day 7.

By days 10 and 14 of the Ang II infusion, a widespread involvement of intramyocardial coronary arterioles was evident and plasma fibronectin labeling was present in the media and adventitia of these vessels. Again, larger intramural arteries and veins were not involved. The presence of an increased number of cells, presumably fibroblasts and macrophages, was still evident

while a perivascular fibrosis of arterioles, represented by an increased accumulation of fibrillar collagen, was evident on day 14.

By in situ hybridization, type I collagen mRNA-producing cells were found in the myocardium of both ventricles on days 4 and 7 of the Ang II infusion.[1] These cells were located in the adventitia and perivascular space of coronary arterioles. Within the interstitial space there were also mRNA synthesizing cells. Based on their morphological features, which included an elongated fusiform shape with elongated nuclei and prominent nucleoli, these cells appeared to be fibroblasts or a fibroblast-like phenotype. These cells were not seen in control animals. A perivascular fibrosis of intramural coronary vessels and endomyocardial scars were present in both the right and left ventricles by day 14. Each fibrous tissue response became more extensive over the course of 6-weeks Ang II treatment.[62] Mechanisms involved in promoting fibrogenesis require further investigation, but clearly implicate coronary vascular hyperpermeability.

Ang II receptors have likewise been identified in fibroblasts of various tissues.[85, 86] In serum-deprived cultured adult rat cardiac fibroblasts[87, 88] or mesangial cells,[89] Angiotensin II promotes an increase in collagen synthesis via AT_1 receptors.

Tissue Hormones

Various locally generated hormones appear to provide for a reciprocal regulation of cardiac fibroblast collagen turnover. This includes Angiotensin II, which not only augments collagen fibroblast synthesis but reduces its collagenolytic activity.[88] Each of these effects favor fibrous tissue formation. Similar responses have been observed in these cells for endothelin-1.[90] In other mesenchymal cells, including breast[91] and bone,[92] endothelin-1 likewise augments collagen synthesis. Inhibitors of collagen formation include BK and PG, each of which reduce cardiac fibroblast collagen synthesis, while augmenting collagenolytic activity.[93, 94] Local concentrations of Angiotensin II, Endothelin (ET), Bradykinin, and Prostaglandins are largely influenced by ACE. ACE therefore would appear to be central to the hormonal control of fibroblast collagen turnover and thereby fibrous tissue formation.

Components of an angiotensin II-generating system have been identified in granulocytes,[38] the heart,[95] and the vasculature.[96] This local hormonal system has been linked to homeostatic functions. Work from this laboratory would suggest an additional role, that includes the regulation of tissue structure under normal and pathological conditions. At sites where collagen turnover is normally high, such as heart valves and vascular adventitia, ACE binding is marked.[97] ACE binding and activity have been demonstrated in cultured valvular interstitial cells[98] and these cells contract in response to Angiotensin II.[99] For the first several weeks after birth, collagen production in the heart and vasculature is rapid. Treatment of 4-week-old rats with enalapril for 5 weeks, retarded normal collagen development in their right and left ventricles, aorta, and superior mesenteric artery.[100] High ACE binding activity is also found at sites of pathological fibrous tissue accumulation.[101, 102] Lisinopril attenuated the fibrous tissue response associated with the chronic administration of Angiotensin II[103] and following pericardiotomy.[104]

Cytokines or Growth Factors

Cytokines have a wide range of functions that contribute to the inflammatory phase of tissue repair in the heart. These include their role in mediating cell activation, cell proliferation and differentiation, chemotaxis, and phagocytosis. They further demonstrate functional redundancy between one another and have the capacity to interact with one another, in a synergistic or antagonistic manner. Cytokines, released locally at sites of cardiac myocyte necrosis, serve to contain the inflammatory response to the myocardium. Several are proinflammatory, such as platelet-derived growth factor and members of the interleukin series. Locally produced cytokines may also have systemic effects, such as the fever that accompanies acute myocardial infarction (AMI). The level and duration of cytokine expression will determine their contribution to the heart's response to injury, and

man's response to heart disease. The role of various cytokines in the inflammation-healing paradigm in the heart has not been fully explored and represents a fruitful area of research.

Within 48 hours following AMI, it has been found that the expression of transforming growth factor-α_1 (TGF-α_1) mRNA is increased in infarcted tissue.[105] Cells responsible for the expression of this cytokine and its contribution to the inflammation-healing response, postinfarction remain to be determined. TGF-α_1 is known to contribute to macrophage and fibroblast chemotaxis, fibroblast proliferation and their transformation to myofibroblasts, regulation of collagen turnover, and remodeling of scar tissue.[106–110] Factors regulating the expression of TGF-α_1 or other cytokines in the setting of myocardial infarction or other diseases of the heart have not been examined. Recent evidence indicates that in cultured neonatal rat cardiac fibroblasts, Angiotensin II will increase TGF-α_1 gene expression.[111]

Myocardial Infarction and Chemical Mediators of Inflammation

Inflammatory Response to Infarction

Mechanisms responsible for inflammatory and reparative phases of healing that follow myocardial infarction are not fully understood. The same is true for the relationship between infarct size and the extent of fibrosis that follows. A reparative fibrosis, or scarring, is essential to the heart and its structural integrity given that cardiac myocytes are thought to be terminally differentiated (i.e., they do not regenerate).

The rapidity with which infarcted myocardium is repaired, is dependent on the extent of cardiac myocyte necrosis and microvascular damage.[112] Within 24 hours of infarction, polymorphonuclear leukocytes are evident bordering on the site of necrotic myocytes and become most prominent by day 3. When the number of necrotic myocytes is small and the microvasculature spared, only macrophages are recruited into the reparative process.[112] The contribution of leukocytes to larger infarcts declines by day 4 and is replaced by macrophages, fibroblast-like cells (myofibroblasts), and the appearance of new blood vessels. Mediators of inflammatory cell and fibroblast chemotaxis in this setting are not well understood. They may include Bradykinin, Prostaglandins and Nitric Oxide, as well as components of the complement system,[113] platelet-derived growth factor, and the interleukins. Phenotypically transformed fibroblasts, called myofibroblasts, are characterized by the presence of α-smooth muscle actin. These cells are present on day 4 postinfarction and express mRNA for type I collagen,[114] a major component of subsequent scar tissue. These various responses involving inflammatory cells, fibroblasts and new blood vessels contribute to the formation of granulation tissue.

Bradykinin

Bradykinin has been implicated in a whole host of inflammatory conditions, including asthma, rheumatoid arthritis, and pancreatitis.[115] It also is considered a component of the early inflammatory response seen in the heart following myocardial infarction. The rapid degradation of circulating Bradykinin has made detection of this peptide difficult and its importance therefore has remained uncertain. Using an isolated, crystalloid perfused rat heart, Baumgarten et al.[116] have shown that BK is released from the heart and appears in coronary sinus effluent under basal conditions. Sinus BK concentration rises rapidly (severalfold) during myocardial ischemia. Administration of ramiprilat prior to the induction of ischemia served to increase the amount of BK appearing in the sinus effluent.

Some 20 years ago, Kimura et al.[117] reported that coronary sinus concentration of Bradykinin increased during the first 15 to 20 minutes following coronary ligation in the dog. Noda et al.[118] more recently have demonstrated a rise in BK concentration of the interventricular vein of the dog, following a 90-minute coronary artery occlusion and which is accentuated by captopril pretreatment. Nafamostat, a serine protease inhibitor, largely attenuated this response. In patients with myocardial infarction, Hashi-moto et al.[119] reported that an increase in plasma BK concentration could be detected during week 1 postinfarction. The interstitial edema of the myocardium associated with the release of BK following infarction was held responsible for the rapid rise in left ventricular filling pressure and fall in the first derivative of the rise in left ventricular systolic pressure, that appeared in dogs with coronary artery ligation and each response could be prevented by the protease inhibitor aprotinin.

The release of BK following infarction may be an integral feature of the natural inflammatory response of the myocardium. The associated coronary vascular hyperpermeability with interstitial edema, may have a detrimental effect on left ventricular diastolic and systolic function. Early potentiation of BK by ACE inhibition following myocardial infarction may further contribute to the decline in ventricular function and therefore could prove detrimental. Such an outcome would be similar to the augmented edema that accompanies subcutaneous administration of CARR in captopril-treated rats. It should be noted, however, that others[118, 120] have claimed that BK-mediated coronary vasodilatation serves to reduce the area at risk, following ischemia with reperfusion and hence the favorable effect seen with ramipril, was abrogated by the type 2 BK receptor antagonist Hoe 140. Future studies will be required to address these important issues.

Prostaglandins

Like BK, prostanoids are endogenous hormones. Their role as chemical mediators of inflammation is well recognized. PGI_2 and PGE_2 have each been detected in coronary sinus drainage. During myocardial ischemia and following infarction, PGE_2 release into sinus effluent rises several-fold.[121] Endothelial cells are able to elaborate various prostanoids and whether the early release of PGE_2 following infarction arises from the coronary vasculature and/or other cells is presently unknown. During the acute inflammatory phase that appears during the first several days after infarction, the release of PGE_2 is markedly increased by administration of BK suggesting, leukocytes may be involved.[121] Other mesenchymal cells are also able to synthesize prostanoids. These include squamous epithelial cells of visceral and parietal pericardium, pleura and peritoneum,[122–124] fibroblasts of various organs,[125–127] and cultured mesothelial cells of pericardium.[128] Whether these nonendothelial cells also release BK, a stimulus to PG synthesis[125] is yet uncertain. Both BK and PGE_2 alter cultured cardiac fibroblast collagen turnover.[93, 125, 129]

Nitric Oxide

The role of this reactive oxide of nitrogen in the inflammatory response that follows myocardial infarction is unknown. It is now appreciated that NO does contribute to inflammatory responses and that it is generated not only from endothelial cells, but polymorphonuclear leukocytes and macrophages.[48]

Angiotensin II

Noda et al.[118] have found Angiotensin II is released from the canine heart and appears in interventricular venous blood within 10–15 minutes, and remains elevated at 60 minutes, during a 90 minute occlusion of the canine left anterior descending coronary artery. This response was not blocked by captopril, but can be prevented by the serine protease inhibitor nafamostat and the cysteine protease inhibitor chymostatin. Plasma renin activity was unchanged in these dogs that underwent bilateral nephrectomy prior to the study. These important findings demonstrate that Angiotensin II generation in the heart is not dependent on renin, a serine protease. The cellular origin of Angiotensin II is uncertain. Potential candidates include macrophages, fibroblasts, and polymorphonuclear leukocytes. The mRNA expression of angiotensinogen is increased in the left ventricle on day 5 following infarction in the rat.[112, 130]

In using an AT_1 receptor antagonist administered at the time of left coronary ligation in rats, Smits et al.[131] demonstrated they could not prevent the proliferation of interstitial cells (likely fibroblast-like cells) at remote sites, involving the interventricular septum and right ventricle. The accumulation of collagen at these sites, however, was prevented by losartan as was the case for captopril, suggesting that the regulation of collagen turnover following infarction is separate from that regulating the mitogenic potential of mesenchymal cells.

Myocardial Infarction and Chemical Mediators of Healing

Healing Response to Infarction

Collagen degradation is an early component of tissue repair postinfarction. Within the necrotic segment of tissue is a marked reduction in collagen,[132] particularly within its neutral salt soluble fraction.[133] This implies proteolytic digestion of the structural protein assembly. Matrix metalloproteinases (MMPs) reside in the myocardium in latent form.[134, 135] When activated, MMP-1 (or interstitial collagenase) degrades fibrillar collagen into characteristic one- and three-quarter fragments; MMP-2 and MMP-9 are gelatinases that degrade these smaller fragments. A transient increase in collagenase activity appears in the infarcted rat left ventricle on day 2, peaks at day 7, and declines thereafter, together with a concomitant increase and contribution in collagenolytic activity of gelatinases.[136] An increase in collagenase (MMP-1) mRNA expression does not appear until day 7 and only in the infarcted ventricle, while changes in MMP-1 activity or mRNA expression are not observed at sites remote to the infarct. Tissue inhibitors of matrix MMPs neutralize collagenolytic activity. Transcription of TIMP mRNA occurs at 6 hours after coronary ligation in the infarcted rat ventricle, peaks on day 2, and slowly decreases thereafter. No change in TIMP mRNA expression is observed at remote sites. Fibroblast-like cells, not inflammatory or endothelial cells, are responsible for the transcription of MMP-1 and TIMP mRNAs.

The fibrogenic component of healing that follows the initial phase of collagen degradation is substitutive, replacing lost parenchymal cells. Collagen fibers are morphologically evident by day 7 postinfarction while an organized assembly of these fibers in the form of scar tissue becomes evident by day 14. Hydroxyproline concentration at the site of healing (or scarring) increases over 6 to 8 weeks.[137, 138] Scar tissue formation is accompanied by subsequent thinning and remodeling. Factors that regulate the fibrogenic phase of healing and subsequent remodeling of scar tissue are not well understood, but would appear to include components of a tissue hormonal system that includes Angiotensin II. This system could regulate collagen turnover and determine the tensile strength of scar tissue. A "weak" scar could lead to aneurysmal dilatation while the contraction of the scar, mediated by α-actin containing myofibroblasts and stimulated by Angiotensin II[139] could adversely influence ventricular chamber stiffness. The cellularity of scar tissue is transformed over time.[133] Myofibroblasts, an important component of early healing, are ultimately reduced in number, while smaller, mature fibroblasts, termed fibrocytes, remain. Collagen concentration at the site of infarction increases several-fold over several months[140] as does the degree of collagen crosslinking.[141] Ultimately, fibrous tissue undergoes retraction and/or resorption. Retraction is expressed as scar thinning and appears 6 weeks after myocardial infarction.[114,137] Irrespective of its etiologic basis, myocardial fibrosis is composed predominantly of type I collagen.[142,143]

Angiotensin II

The presence of Angiotensin II and its role in the fibrogenic phase of tissue repair requires that it be generated locally at functionally relevant concentrations, and that stereospecific Angiotensin II receptors be present in participatory cells that regulate collagen turnover. The association between ACE and tissue repair was examined using autoradiographic detection of ACE binding activity and morphological evidence of fibrosis that appeared in the heart under various conditions. Several different expressions of fibrosis, each having a diverse etiologic basis, were examined. These included: the scar that follows myocardial infarction; the endocardial fibrosis of the interventricu-

lar septum that appears postinfarction; the microscopic scarring and perivascular fibrosis found in the right ventricle remote to infarction; endomyocardial fibrosis following catecholamine-induced necrosis; pericardial fibrosis postpericardiotomy; perivascular fibrosis and microscopic scars associated with the chronic administration of AngII or ALDO; and the foreign body fibrosis associated with insertion of a silk ligature in the myocardium.

Our results confirm that marked ACE binding is coincident with fibrillar collagen accumulation. At the site of infarction, fibrillar collagen was first seen 1 week after coronary ligation. This is in keeping with the fibrogenic response following cardiac myocyte necrosis reported by others[137, 144–146] and expressed as a significant increase in hydroxyproline concentration and morphological appearance of a fibrillar collagen meshwork. As fibrous tissue, or formation, became more extensive over the course of 8 weeks, accompanied by thinning of the scar, ACE binding density increased correspondingly. The time-course to wound healing we observed in the infarcted rat left ventricle is similar to that seen in the dog postinfarction, where infarct contraction and thinning occur over 6 weeks together with ventricular dilatation.[137] Whether contraction of the scar is related to fibroblast-like cell contraction induced by Angiotensin II, as is the case for actin-containing valvular interstitial cells, remains to be defined.

We also observed that fibrous tissue, which appears remote to the infarction, is likewise a site of marked ACE binding. Previous studies in the human[147, 148] and rat[146] heart, indicate that collagen volume fraction is increased in both the right ventricle and interventricular septum following left ventricular infarction. Hirsch et al.[149] found biochemical evidence of increased ACE activity in tissue homogenates obtained from the right ventricle, and septum 12 weeks after left ventricular infarction. Their results further identified this to be a tissue-specific response with increased ACE mRNA expression confined to the right ventricle, not the pulmonary artery, aorta or kidney, while plasma renin concentration and serum ACE activity each remained no different from nonoperated controls. Our findings would suggest that this tissue-specific response in ACE transcription and activity is likely the result of fibrous tissue formation in the right ventricle and septum, expressed as a perivascular fibrosis of intramyocardial coronary arteries and as microscopic scars. The mechanism responsible for fibrogenesis at these remote sites, where vascular supply was presumably not compromised by left coronary artery ligation, remains to be elucidated. One possibility relates to the presence of "trophic" signals that arise at the site of infarction and which then traverse the interstitial space via its tissue fluid to distant sites (Figure 4). The interstitial space of the myocardium is continuous and involves the left ventricle, interventricular septum, and right ventricle. This is evidenced by the injection of Evans Blue into the left ventricle which is soon followed (15 to 30 minutes) by blue coloration of both ventricles. Tissue fluid is in dynamic equilibrium with cardiac lymph. Marked ACE binding was also observed within the endo-

myocardial fibrosis that appeared in the interventricular septum following left ventricular infarction. The mechanism for this response is uncertain.

In addition to the association between cardiac ACE and myocardial fibrosis, we found high density ACE binding in the pericardial fibrosis that followed pericardiotomy, and at the insertion of a silk ligature into the myocardium, irrespective of whether or not myocardial infarction followed.

Thus, and despite its diverse causality, fibrous tissue formation was anatomically coincident with high density ACE binding. The molecular characteristics and substrate utilization of cardiac ACE and its role in collagen turnover remain to be defined. This notwithstanding, Fabris et al.[150] have observed that ACE binding density in postinfarction scar tissue is reduced by quinapril. This suggests rat cardiac ACE is not a chymase.[151] Stauss et al.[152] reported that moexipril treatment, initiated 1 week prior to cor-

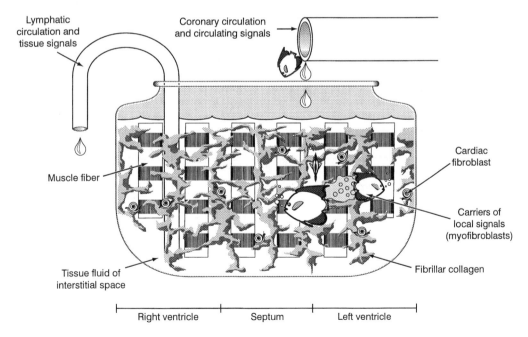

Figure 4. The cardiac interstitial space and its tissue fluid is a continuum that involves the right and left ventricular free wall and interventricular septum. Tissue fluid is in dynamic equilibrium with cardiac lymph. Signals that appear in tissue fluid are derived from the circulation or are activated locally. Following left ventricular infarction, such locally generated signals gain access to remote sites, such as the right ventricle, via their transport in tissue fluid or are carried to these sites by mobile cells, such as myofibroblasts. Reproduced from reference 159 with permission.

onary ligation in the rat, reduced infarct size as determined from the percentage of the left ventricular free-wall circumference occupied by transmural scar. These results could imply that this ACE inhibitor reduced cardiac myocyte necrosis. Alternatively, moexipril may also have retarded fibrous tissue formation postinfarction. In support of this latter premise, Michel et al.[153] found that perindopril treatment, begun 1 week after infarction, decreased the volume density of collagen found in the endomyocardium of the unscarred rat left ventricle. Van Krimpen et al.[146, 154] observed that captopril treatment, commenced in the rat at the time of left coronary artery ligation, prevented the expected proliferation of fibroblasts and subsequent accumulation of fibrillar collagen in the right ventricle and septum at 1 and 2 weeks postinfarction. In another model of myocardial fibrosis, Sun and co-worker,[103] reported that lisinopril attenuates fibrillar collagen formation within the perivascular space of intramural coronary arteries, and at sites of myocyte necrosis in the rat receiving angiotensin II. Thus, a compelling argument can be made to suggest that cardiac ACE is an integral component of a local hormonal system (Fig. 1) involved in tissue repair and that its inhibition reduces fibrillar collagen accumulation.

The cellular origin of cardiac ACE and its relationship to type I collagen-producing cells was identified by immunohistochemistry and in situ hybridization, respectively. At sites where fibrous tissue appeared in the heart, cells labeled with monoclonal ACE antibody were anatomically coincident with type I collagen mRNA-producing cells. Cells contributing type I fibrillar collagen in the heart normally include fibroblasts[75] and, following infarction, fibroblast-like cells.[155] We found that ACE-labeled fibroblasts in the vicinity of cell necrosis were large with prominent pale nuclei suggesting they were metabolically active. Fibroblasts removed from the leading edge of the healing response were smaller with dark nuclei and were ACE negative. Less metabolically active fibroblasts, such as those found in skeletal muscle tendon, do not demonstrate ACE binding.[97] Macrophages bordering the site of infarction were also labeled with monoclonal ACE anti-

body. Within existing new vessels that appeared at the site of tissue repair, endothelial cells demonstrated ACE labeling.

The presence of Angiotensin II receptor binding at each of the fibrous tissue sites, noted above for the rat infarct model, was examined by in vitro quantitative autoradiography.[104] The specific AngII receptor subtype involved was determined by displacement with an AT_1 (DuP 753, or losartan) and AT_2 (PD 123177) receptor antagonist. AT_1 receptor binding density was marked at the site of infarction, as well as remote sites involving the right ventricle, pericardium, and foreign body reaction. AT_2 receptors were not seen.

Bradykinin

The role of BK on scar tissue formation has not been systematically addressed. The ability of ACE inhibitors to reduce infarct or (scar) size may be related to their enhancing local concentrations of BK at the site of tissue repair. The elaboration of angiotensin peptides, BK or PGE_2 by myofibroblasts has not yet been determined. Nonetheless, receptor-ligand binding is a requisite if locally generated peptides are to influence fibrogenesis. Normally, high density AngII receptor binding in the heart is confined to its pacemaker and conduction tissue.[156] Depending on the experimental model examined, autoradiographic localization of type I Angiotensin II and Bradykinin receptor binding is anatomically coincident with sites of myocardial fibrosis and ACE binding.[97, 104]

The role of AngII and BK in regulating fibrogenesis can be inferred from in vivo studies wherein pharmacological agents that interfered with their elaboration or receptor binding were used. Six-week treatment with enalapril in 4-week-old rats retarded collagen formation in both the right and left ventricles, aorta, and superior mesenteric artery.[100] A small dose of quinapril, which did not prevent hypertension in 4–week-old spontaneously hypertensive rat (SHR), was found to inhibit aortic ACE activity by 60% without reducing plasma ACE activity. The expected rise in aortic collagen volume fraction, observed in untreated SHR at 30 weeks of age, was not seen in quinapril-treated animals.[79] As noted earlier, ACE inhibitors reduce fibrous tissue formation following infarction. The role of BK in this response remains to be elucidated.

Prostaglandins

Fibroblast-like cells, isolated from the site of infarction on day 7 postcoronary ligation, demonstrate increased cyclooxygenase activity and increased prostanoid production, including PGE_2.[157] At 30 days after infarction, BK-induced release of PGE_2 from the heart is increased.[121] Prostaglandin synthesis is increased in microsomes prepared from infarcted myocardium at 3 weeks and 3 months after coronary ligation. Thus, there is a persistence of PGE_2 production well beyond the inflammatory phase of tissue repair.

Summary

As in other organs, the heart is able to mount inflammatory and healing responses following parenchymal cell necrosis, tissue irritation, or invasion by foreign material or chemical toxin. A local hormonal system is involved in mediating each of these responses as is the case following snake bite or the subcutaneous injection of seaweed. Chemical mediators involved in each response appear to include AngII, BK, and PGE_2 and perhaps NO. Cells contributing to the healing response include α-smooth muscle actin containing myofibroblasts that express the mRNA for type I collagen, the major fibrillar collagen found in fibrous tissue formation. Pharmacological agents that interfere with either inflammatory or healing responses, may prove beneficial or detrimental in terms of their promoting or hindering the structural remodeling of the "injured" myocardium.

At present, a great deal needs to be learned about the specific nature of regulatory mechanisms involved in inflammation and tissue repair in the heart. This includes the identification and role played by specific peptide hormones, regulatory polypeptides (or cytokines), the extracellular matrix itself, and the interplay between these various factors.

References

1. Ratajska A, Campbell SE, Cleutjens JPM, Weber KT. Angiotensin II and structural remodeling of coronary vessels in rats. J Lab Clin Med 1994;124:408–415.
2. Laine GA, Allen SJ. Left ventricular myocardial edema: lymph flow, interstitial fibrosis and cardiac function. Circ Res 1991; 68:1713–1721.
3. Rovelli F, De Vita C, Feruglio GA, et al GISSI trial: early results and late follow-up. Gruppo Italiano per la Sperimentazione della Streptochinasi nell'Infarto Miocardico. J Am Coll Cardiol 1987;10(Suppl. B): 33B-39B.
4. Vivaldi MT, Eyre DR, Kloner RA, et al. Effects of methylprednisone on collagen biosynthesis in healing acute myocardial infarction. Am J Cardiol 1987;60:424–425.
5. Hammerman H, Schoen FJ, Braunwald E, et al. Drug-induced expansion of infarct: morphologic and functional correlations. Lab Invest 1984;69:611–617.
6. Weber KT, Brilla CG, Cleland JGF, et al. Cardioreparation and the concept of modulating cardiovascular structure and function. Blood Pressure 1993;2:6–21.
7. Hall AS, Tan L-B, Ball SG. Inhibition of ACE/kininase-II, acute myocardial infarction, and survival. Cardiovasc Res 1994;28: 190–198.
8. Ball SG, Hall A, Tan L-B. Inhibition of ACE/kininase-II after myocardial infarction—addendum. Cardiovasc Res 1994;28: 199–200.
9. Pfeffer MA, Braunwald E, Moyé LA, et al. Effect of captopril on mortality and morbidity in patients with left ventricular dysfunction after myocardial infarction. Results of the Survival and Ventricular Enlargement Trial. N Engl J Med 1992;327:669–677.
10. Swedberg K, Held P, Kjekshus J, Rasmussen K, et al. Effects of the early administration of enalapril on mortality in patients with acute myocardial infarction. Results of the Cooperative New Scandinavian Enalapril Survival Study II (CONSENSUS II). N Engl J Med 1992;327:678–684.
11. Ondetti MA, Cushman DW. Enzymes of the renin-angiotensin system and their inhibitors. Annu Rev Biochem 1982;51:283–308.
12. Ferreira LA, Henriques OB, Lebrun I, et al. Biologically active peptides from Bothrops jararacussu venom. Agents Actions Suppl 1992;36:209–214.
13. Hall D, Zeitler H, Rudolph W. Counteraction of the vasodilator effects of enalapril

by aspirin in severe heart failure. J Am Coll Cardiol 1992;20:1549–1555.

14. Swedberg K, Eneroth P, Kjekshus J, et al. Hormones regulating cardiovascular function in patients with severe congestive heart failure and their relation to mortality. CONSENSUS Trial Study Group. Circulation 1990;82:1730–1736.

15. Anon. Effects of enalapril on mortality in severe congestive heart failure. Results of the Cooperative North Scandinavian Enalapril Survival Study (CONSENSUS). The CONSENSUS Trial Study Group. N Engl J Med 1987;316:1429–1435.

16. Anon. Effect of enalapril on survival in patients with reduced left ventricular ejection fractions and congestive heart failure. The SOLVD Investigators. N Engl J Med 1991;325:293–302.

17. Anon. Effect of enalapril on mortality and the development of heart failure in asymptomatic patients with reduced left ventricular ejection fractions. The SOLVD Investigators. N Engl J Med 1992;327:685–691.

18. Yusuf S, Pepine CJ, Garces C, et al. Effect of enalapril on myocardial infarction and unstable angina in patients with low ejection fractions. Lancet 1992;340:1173–1178.

19. Chobanian AV. Pathophysiology of atherosclerosis. Am J Cardiol 1992;70:3G-7G.

20. Powell JS, Clozel JP, Muller RK, et al. Inhibitors of angiotensin-converting enzyme prevent myointimal proliferation after vascular injury. Science 1989;245:186–188.

21. Kremer D, Lindop G, Brown WCB, et al. Angiotensin-induced myocardial necrosis and renal failure in the rabbit: distribution of lesions and severity in relation to plasma angiotensin II concentration and arterial pressure. Cardiovasc Res 1981;15:43–46.

22. Tan LB, Jalil JE, Pick R, et al. Cardiac myocyte necrosis induced by angiotensin II. Circ Res 1991;69:1185–1195.

23. Ratajska A, Campbell SE, Sun Y, et al. Angiotenin II associated cardiac myocyte necrosis: role of adrenal catecholamines. Cardiovasc Res 1994;28:684–690.

24. Pflugfelder PW, Baird MG, Tonkon MJ, et al. Clinical consequences of angiotensin-converting enzyme inhibitor withdrawal in chronic heart failure: a double-blind, placebo-controlled study of quinapril. J Am Coll Cardiol 1993;22:1557–1563.

25. Rouleau JL, de Champlain J, Klein M, et al. Activation of neurohormonal systems in postinfarction left ventricular hypertrophy. J Am Coll Cardiol 1993;22:390–398.

26. Garcia Leme J, Hamamura L, Leite MP, et al. Pharmacological analysis of the acute inflammatory process induced in the rat's paw by local injection of carrageenin and by heating. Br J Pharmacol 1973;48:88–96.

27. Di Rosa M, Sorrentino L. Some pharmacodynamic properties of carrageenin in the rat. Br J Pharmacol 1970;38:214–220.

28. Damas J, Remacle-Volon G, Adam A. Inflammation in the rat paw due to urate crystals. Involvement of the kinin system. Naunyn Schmiedebergs Arch Pharmacol 1984;325:76–79.

29. Van Arman CG, Begany AJ, Miller LM, et al. Some details of the inflammation caused by yeast and carrageenin. J Pharmacol Exp Ther 1965;150:328–334.

30. Damas J, Remacle-Volon G. Influence of a long-acting bradykinin antagonist, Hoe 140, on some acute inflammatory reactions in the rat. Eur J Pharmacol 1992;211:81–86.

31. Noordhoek J, Nagy MR, Bonta IL. Involvement of complement and kinins in some non-immunogenic paw inflammations in rats. Agents Actions Suppl 1977;2:109–121.

32. Bonta IL, Bult H, Ven LL, et al. Essential fatty acid deficiency: a condition to discriminate prostaglandin and non-prostaglandin mediated components of inflammation. Agents Actions 1976;6:154–158.

33. Wiemer G, Scholkens BA, Becker RHA, et al. Ramiprilat enhances endothelial autocoid formation by inhibiting breakdown of endothelium-derived bradykinin. Hypertension 1991;18:558–563.

34. Lieberman J. Elevation of serum angiotensin-converting enzyme (ACE) level in sarcoidosis. Am J Med 1975;59:365–372.

35. Silverstein E, Friedland J. Elevated serum and spleen angiotensin converting enzyme and serum lysozyme in Gaucher's disease. Clin Chim Acta 1977;74:21–25.

36. Weinstock JV, Boros DL, Gee JB. Enhanced granuloma angiotensin I converting enzyme activity associated with modulation in murine schistosomiasis. Gastroenterology 1981;81:48–53.

37. Silverstein E, Pertschuk LP, Friedland J. Immunofluorescent localization of angiotensin converting enzyme in epitheloid and giant cells of sarcoidosis granulomas. Proc Natl Acad Sci USA 1979;76:6646–6648.

38. Weinstock JV, Blum AM. Synthesis of angiotensins by cultured granuloma macrophages in murine schistosomiasis mansoni. Cell Immunol 1987;107:273–280.

39. Weinstock JV. The significance of angiotensin I converting enzyme in granulomatous inflammation. Functions of ACE in granulomas. Sarcoidosis 1986;3:19–26.

40. Allen RKA, Chai SY, Dunbar MS, et al. In

vitro autoradiographic localization of angiotensin-converting enzyme in sarcoid lymph nodes. Chest 1986;90:315–320.

41. Pertschuk LP, Silverstein E, Friedland J. Immunohistologic diagnosis of sarcoidosis. Detection of angiotensin-converting enzyme in sarcoid granulomas. Am J Clin Pathol 1981;75:350–354.

42. Klickstein LB, Kaempfer CE, Wintroub BU. The granulocyte-angiotensin system. Angiotensin I-converting activity of cathepsin G. J Biol Chem 1982;257:15042–15046.

43. Wintroub BU, Klickstein LB, Dzau VJ, et al. Granulocyte-angiotensin system. Identification of angiotensinogen as the plasma protein substrate of leukocyte cathepsin G. Biochemistry 1984;23:227–232.

44. Hirayama K, Fukuyama K, Epstein WL. Angiotensin II-producing proteases from granulomatous tissue reaction in mice infected with *Schistosoma mansoni.* Comp Biochem Physiol 1990;96B:553–557.

45. Reilly CF, Tewksbury DA, Schechter NM, et al. Rapid conversion of angiotensin I to angiotensin II by neutrophil and mast cell proteinases. J Biol Chem 1982;15: 8619–8622.

46. Nozaki Y, Sato N, Iida T, et al. Prolyl endopeptidase purified from granulomatous inflammation in mice. J Biol Chem 1992;49: 296–303.

47. Schechter NM, Choi JK, Slavin DA, et al. Identification of a chymotrypsin-like proteinase in human mast cells. J Immunol 1986;137:962–970.

48. Nathan C. Nitric oxide as a secretory product of mammalian cells. FASEB J 1992;6: 3051–3064.

49. Weinstock JV, Blum AM. Isolated liver granulomas of murine *Schistosoma mansoni* contain components of the angiotensin system. J Immunol 1983;131:2529–2532.

50. Weinstock JV, Kassab JT. Functional angiotensin II receptors on macrophages from isolated liver granulomas of murine *Schistosoma mansoni.* J Immunol 1984;132: 2598–2602.

51. Ehlers MRW, Riordan JF. Angiotensin-converting enzyme: new concepts concerning its biological role. Biochemistry 1989;28: 5311–5318.

52. Costerousse O, Allegrini J, Lopez M, et al. Angiotensin I-converting enzyme in human circulating mononuclear cells: genetic polymorphism of expression in T-lymphocytes. Biochem J 1993;290:33–40.

53. Thomas DW, Hoffman MD. Identification of macrophage receptors for angiotensin: a potential role in antigen uptake for T lym-phocyte responses? J Immunol 1984;132: 2807–2812.

54. Payan DG. Neuropeptides and inflammation: the role of substance P. Annu Rev Med 1989;40:341–352.

55. Weinstock JV, Blum A, Walder J, et al. Eosinophils from granulomas in murine *Schistosomiasis mansoni* produce substance P. J Immunol 1988;141:961–966.

56. Weglicki WB, Mak IT, Phillips PM. Blockade of cardiac inflammation in Mg^{2+} deficiency by substance P receptor inhibition. Circ Res 1994;74:1009–1013.

57. Weinstock JV, Ehrinpreis MN, Boros DL, et al. Effect of SQ 14225, an inhibitor of angiotensin I-converting enzyme, on the granulomatous responses to *Schistosoma mansoni* eggs in mice. J Clin Invest 1981;67:931–936.

58. Deepe GS Jr, Taylor CL, Srivastava L, et al. Impairment of granulomatous inflammatory response to *Histoplasma capsulatum* by inhibitors of angiotensin-converting enzyme. Infect Immun 1985;48:395–401.

59. Selye H. The general adaptation syndrome and the diseases of adaptation. J Clin Endocrinol 1946;6:117–230.

60. Hall CE, Hall O. Hypertension and hypersalimentation. I. Aldosterone hypertension. Lab Invest 1965;14:285–294.

61. Brilla CG, Pick R, Tan LB, et al. Remodeling of the rat right and left ventricle in experimental hypertension. Circ Res 1990;67: 1355–1364.

62. Sun Y, Ratajska A, Zhou G, et al. Angiotensin converting enzyme and myocardial fibrosis in the rat receiving angiotensin II or aldosterone. J Lab Clin Med 1993;122: 395–403.

63. Campbell SE, Diaz-Arias AA, Weber KT. Fibrosis of the human heart and systemic organs in adrenal adenoma. Blood Pressure 1992;1:149–156.

64. Molteni A, Brownie AC, Skelton FR. Production of hypertensive vascular disease in the rat by methyltestosterone. Lab Invest 1969;21:129–137.

65. Skelton FR. The production of hypertension, nephrosclerosis and cardiac lesions by methylandrostenediol treatment in the rat. Endocrinology 1953;53:492–505.

66. Campbell SE, Farb A, Weber KT. Pathologic remodeling of the myocardium in a weightlifter taking anabolic steroids. Blood Pressure 1993;2:213–216.

67. Hassager C, Jensen LT, Podenphant J, et al. Collagen synthesis in postmenopausal women during therapy with anabolic steroid or female sex hormones. Metabolism 1990;39:1167–1169.

68. Brincat M, Moniz CJ, Studd JWW, et al. Long-term effects of the menopause and sex hormones on skin thickness. Br J Obstet Gynaecol 1985;92:256–259.
69. Wilson ID, Goetz FC. Selective hypoaldosteronism after prolonged heparin administration. Am J Med 1964;36:635–639.
70. Thompson RC Jr, Ludewig RM, Wangensteen SL, et al. Effects of heparin on wound healing. Surg Gynecol Obstet 1972;134:22–26.
71. Taubenhaus M, Amromin GD. Influence of steroid hormones on granulation tissue. Endocrinology 1949;44:359–367.
72. Robertson W van B, Sanborn EC. Hormonal effects on collagen formation in granulomas. Endocrinology 1958;63:250–252.
73. Schiller E. The influence of hormones on the development of silicotic nodules produced by intraperitoneal injection of quartz. Br J Indust Med 1953;10:1–8.
74. Pirani CL, Stepto RC, Sutherland K. Desoxycorticosterone acetate and wound healing. J Exp Med 1951;93:217–235.
75. Eghbali M, Blumenfeld OO, Seifter S, et al. Localization of types I, III, and IV collagen mRNAs in rat heart cells by in situ hybridization. J Mol Cell Cardiol 1989;21:103–113.
76. Slight S, Ganjam VK, Nonneman DJ, et al. Glucocorticoid metabolism in the cardiac interstitium: 11β-hydroxysteroid dehydrogenase activity in cardiac fibroblasts. J Lab Clin Med 1993;122:180–187.
77. Hammami MM, Siiteri PK. Regulation of 11β-hydroxysteroid dehydrogenase activity in human skin fibroblasts: enzymatic modulation of glucocorticoid action. J Clin Endocrinol Metab 1991;73:326–334.
78. Abramovitz M, Branchaud CL, Murphy BEP. Cortisol-cortisone interconversion in human fetal lung: contrasting results using explant and monolayer cultures suggest that 11β-hydroxysteroid dehydrogenase (EC 1.1.1.146) comprises two enzymes. J Clin Endocrinol Metab 1982;54:563–568.
79. Albaladejo P, Bouaziz H, Duriez M, et al. Angiotensin converting enzyme inhibition prevents the increase in aortic collagen in rats. Hypertension 1994;23:74–82.
80. Doering CW, Jalil JE, Janicki JS, et al. Collagen network remodeling and diastolic stiffness of the rat left ventricle with pressure overload hypertrophy. Cardiovasc Res 1988;22:686–695.
81. Jalil JE, Doering CW, Janicki JS, et al. Fibrillar collagen and myocardial stiffness in the intact hypertrophied rat left ventricle. Circ Res 1989;64:1041–1050.
82. Turto H, Lindy S. Digitoxin treatment and experimental cardiac hypertrophy in the rat. Cardiovasc Res 1973;7:482–489.
83. Chapman D, Weber KT, Eghbali M. Regulation of fibrillar collagen types I and III and basement membrane type IV collagen gene expression in pressure overloaded rat myocardium. Circ Res 1990;67:787–794.
84. Pearlman ES, Weber KT, Janicki JS, et al. Muscle fiber orientation and connective tissue content in the hypertrophied human heart. Lab Invest 1982;46:158–164.
85. Kimura B, Sumners C, Phillips MI. Changes in skin angiotensin II receptors in rats during wound healing. Biochem Biophys Res Commun 1992;187:1083–1090.
86. Katwa LC, Weber KT. Angiotensin type I and type II receptors in cultured adult rat cardiac fibroblasts. (Abstract) J Mol Cell Cardiol 1993;25(Suppl. III):S89.
87. Villarreal FJ, Kim NN, Ungab GD, et al. Identification of functional angiotensin II receptors on rat cardiac fibroblasts. Circulation 1993;88:2849–2861.
88. Brilla CG, Zhou G, Matsubara L, et al. Collagen metabolism in cultured adult rat cardiac fibroblasts: response to angiotensin II and aldosterone. J Mol Cell Cardiol 1994;26:809–820.
89. Wolf G, Neilson EG. Angiotensin II as a renal growth factor. J Am Soc Nephrol 1993;3:1531–1540.
90. Guarda E, Katwa LC, Myers PR, et al. Effects of endothelins on collagen turnover in cardiac fibroblasts. Cardiovasc Res 1993;27:2130–2134.
91. Schrey MP, Patel KV, Tezapsidis N. Bombesin and glucocorticoids stimulate human breast cancer cells to produce endothelin, a paracrine mitogen for breast stromal cells. Cancer Res 1992;52:1786–1790.
92. Tatrai A, Foster S, Lakatos P, et al. Endothelin-1 actions on resorption, collagen and noncollagen protein synthesis, and phosphatidylinositol turnover in bone organ cultures. Endocrinology 1992;131:603–607.
93. Zhou G, Tyagi SC, Weber KT. Bradykinin regulates collagen turnover in cardiac fibroblasts. (Abstract) Clin Res 1993;41:630A.
94. Dayer J-M, Roelke MS, Krane SM. Effects of prostaglandin E₂, indomethacin, trifluoperazine and drugs affecting the cytoskeleton on collagenase production by cultured adherent rheumatoid synovial cells. Biochem Pharmacol 1984;33:2893–2899.
95. Lindpaintner K, Jin M, Niedermaier N, et al. Cardiac angiotensin and its local activation in the isolated perfused beating heart. Circ Res 1990;67:564–573.
96. Dzau VJ. Circulating versus local renin-an-

giotensin system in cardiovascular homeostasis. Circulation 1988;77(Suppl. I):I-4-I-13.

97. Sun Y, Diaz-Arias AA, Weber KT. Angiotensin-converting enzyme, bradykinin and angiotensin II receptor binding in rat skin, tendon and heart valves: an in vitro quantitative autoradiographic study. J Lab Clin Med 1994;123:372–377.

98. Katwa LC, Ratajska A, Cleutjens JPM, et al. Angiotensin converting enzyme and kininase II-like activities in cultured valvular interstitial cells of the rat heart. Cardiovasc Res (In press).

99. Filip DA, Radu A, Simionescu M. Interstitial cells of the heart valves possess characteristics similar to smooth muscle cells. Circ Res 1986;59:310–320.

100. Keeley FW, Elmoselhi A, Leenan FHH. Enalapril suppresses normal accumulation of elastin and collagen in cardiovascular tissues of growing rats. Am J Physiol 1992; 262:H1013-H1021.

101. Yamada H, Fabris B, Allen AM, et al. Localization of angiotensin converting enzyme in rat heart. Circ Res 1991;68:141–149.

102. Johnston CI, Mooser V, Sun Y, et al. Changes in cardiac angiotensin converting enzyme after myocardial infarction and hypertrophy in rats. Clin Exp Pharmacol Physiol 1991;18:107–110.

103. Sun Y, Weber KT. Nonendothelial ACE and myocardial fibrosis in rats receiving angiotensin II: inhibition by lisinopril. (Abstract). Am J Hypertens 1993;6:4A.

104. Sun Y, Weber KT. Angiotensin II receptor binding following myocardial infarction in the rat. Cardiovasc Res 1994;28:1623–1628.

105. Thompson NL, Bazoberry F, Speir EH, et al. Transforming growth factor beta-1 in acute myocardial infarction in rats. Growth Factors 1988;1:91–99.

106. Lawrence WT, Diegelmann RF. Growth factors in wound healing. Clin Dermatol 1994; 12:157–169.

107. Reddy HK, Campbell SE, Tjahja IE, et al. Fibrillar collagen remodeling in infarcted human heart with progressive left ventricular dilatation and thinning. (Abstract) J Mol Cell Cardiol 1993;25(Suppl. III):S76.

108. Desmoulière A, Geinoz A, Gabbiani F, et al. Transforming growth factor-β1 induces α-smooth muscle actin expression in granulation tissue myofibroblasts and in quiescent and growing cultured fibroblasts. J Cell Biol 1993;122:103–111.

109. Ronnov-Jessen L, Petersen OW. Induction of α-smooth muscle actin by transforming growth factor-β1 in quiescent human breast gland fibroblasts. Implications for myofi-broblast generation in breast neoplasia. Lab Invest 1993;68:696–707.

110. Vyalov SL, Gabbiani G, Kapanci Y. Rat alveolar myofibroblasts acquire α-smooth muscle actin expression during bleomycin-induced pulmonary fibrosis. Am J Pathol 1993;143:1754–1765.

111. Sadoshima J, Izumo S. Molecular characterization of angiotensin II-induced hypertrophy of cardiac myocytes and hyperplasia of cardiac fibroblasts. Critical role of the AT$_1$ receptor subtype. Circ Res 1993;73:413–423.

112. Reimer KA, Jennings RB. Myocardial ischemia, hypoxia, and infarction. In: Fozzard HA, Haber E, Jennings RB, et al., eds. The Heart and Cardiovascular System. New York, NY: Raven Press, 1986: 1133–1201.

113. Kilgore KS, Friedrichs GS, Homeister JW, et al. The complement system in myocardial ischaemia/reperfusion injury. Cardiovasc Res 1994;28:437–444.

114. Sun Y, Cleutjens JPM, Diaz-Arias AA, et al. Cardiac angiotensin converting enzyme and myocardial fibrosis in the rat. Cardiovasc Res 1994;28:1423–1432.

115. Bhoola KD, Figueroa CD, Worthy K. Bioregulation of kinins: kallikreins, kininogens, and kininases. Pharmacol Rev 1992;44: 1–80.

116. Baumgarten CR, Linz W, Kunkel G, et al. Ramaprilat increases bradykinin outflow from isolated hearts of rat. Br J Pharmacol 1993;108:293–295.

117. Kimura E, Hashimoto K, Furukawa S, et al. Changes in bradykinin level in coronary sinus blood after the experimental occlusion of a coronary artery. Am Heart J 1973; 85:635–647.

118. Noda K, Sasaguri M, Ideishi M, et al. Role of locally formed angiotensin II and bradykinin in the reduction of myocardial infarct size in dogs. Cardiovasc Res 1993;27: 334–340.

119. Hashimoto K, Hirose M, Furukawa K, et al. Changes in hemodynamics and bradykinin concentration in coronary sinus blood in experimental coronary artery occlusion. Jpn Heart J 1977;18:679–689.

120. Hartman JC, Wall TM, Hullinger TG, et al. Reduction of myocardial infarct size in rabbits by ramiprilat: reversal by the bradykinin antagonist HOE 140. J Cardiovasc Pharmacol 1993;21:996–1003.

121. Evers AS, Murphree S, Saffitz JE, et al. Effects of endogenously produced leukotrienes, thromboxane, and prostaglandins on coronary vascular resistance in rabbit

myocardial infarction. J Clin Invest 1985;75: 992–999.

122. Herman AG, Claeys M, Moncada S, et al. Biosynthesis of prostacyclin (PGI$_2$) and 12L-hydroxy-5,8,10,14–eicosatetraenoic acid (HETE) by pericardium, pleura, peritoneum and aorta of the rabbit. Prostaglandins 1979;18:439–452.

123. Dusting GJ, Nolan RD. Stimulation of prostacyclin release from the epicardium of anaesthetized dogs. Br J Pharmacol 1981;74: 553–562.

124. Nolan RD, Dusting GJ, Jakubowski J, et al. The pericardium as a source of prostacyclin in the dog, ox and rat. Prostaglandins 1982; 24:887–902.

125. Goldstein RH, Polgar P. The effect and interaction of bradykinin and prostaglandins on protein and collagen production by lung fibroblasts. J Biol Chem 1982;257: 8630–8633.

126. Bareis DL, Manganiello VC, Hirata F, et al. Bradykinin stimulates phospholipid methylation, calcium influx, prostaglandin formation, and cAMP accumulation in human fibroblasts. Biochemistry 1983;80:2514–2518.

127. Ahumada GG, Sobel BE, Needleman P. Synthesis of prostaglandins by cultured rat hearts myocytes and cardiac mesenchymal cells. J Mol Cell Cardiol 1980;12:685–700.

128. Satoh K, Prescott SM. Culture of mesothelial cells from bovine pericardium and characterization of the arachidonate metabolism. Biochim Biophys Acta 1980;930: 283–296.

129. Baum BJ, Moss J, Breul SD, et al. Association in normal human fibroblasts of elevated levels of adenosine 3′:5′-monophosphate with a selective decrease in collagen production. J Biol Chem 1978;253:3391–3394.

130. Lindpaintner K, Lu W, Niedermajer J, et al. Selective activation of cardiac angiotensinogen gene expression in post-infarction ventricular remodeling in the rat. J Mol Cell Cardiol 1993;25:133–143.

131. Smits JFM, van Krimpen C, Schoemaker RG, et al. Angiotensin II receptor blockade after myocardial infarction in rats: effects on hemodynamics, myocardial DNA synthesis, and interstitial collagen content. J Cardiovasc Pharmacol 1992;20:772–778.

132. Factor SM, Robinson TF, Dominitz R, et al. Alterations of the myocardial skeletal framework in acute myocardial infarction with and without ventricular rupture. Am J Cardiovasc Pathol 1986;1:91–97.

133. Sekita S, Katagiri T, Sasai Y, et al. Studies on collagen in the experimental myocardial infarction. Jpn Circ J 1985;49:171–178.

134. Tyagi SC, Matsubara L, Weber KT. Direct extraction and estimation of collagenase(s) activity by zymography in microquantities of rat myocardium and uterus. Clin Biochem 1993;26:191–198.

135. Tyagi SC, Ratajska A, Weber KT. Myocardial matrix metalloproteinase(s): localization and activation. Mol Cell Biochem 1993; 126:49–59.

136. Cleutjens JP, Guarda E, Weber KT. Transcriptional and post-transcriptional regulation of interstitial collagenase after myocardial infarction in the rat heart. (Abstract) Circulation 1993;88(Suppl. I):I-380.

137. Jugdutt BI, Amy RWM. Healing after myocardial infarction in the dog: changes in infarct hydroxyproline and topography. J Am Coll Cardiol 1986;7:91–102.

138. Jugdutt BI. Left ventricular rupture threshold during the healing phase after myocardial infarction in the dog. Can J Physiol Pharmacol 1987;65:307–316.

139. Gabbiani G, Hirschel BJ, Ryan GB, et al. Granulation tissue as a contractile organ. A study of structure and function. J Exp Med 1972;135:719–734.

140. Mallory GK, White PD, Salcedo-Salgar J. The speed of healing of myocardial infarction. A study of the pathologic anatomy in seventy-two cases. Am Heart J 1939;18: 647–671.

141. McCormick RJ, Musch TI, Bergman BC, et al. Regional differences in LV collagen accumulation and mature cross-linking after myocardial infarction in rats. Am J Physiol 1994;266:H354-H359.

142. Bishop J, Greenbaum J, Gibson D, et al. Enhanced deposition of predominantly type I collagen in myocardial disease. J Mol Cell Cardiol 1990;22:1157–1165.

143. Weber KT, Janicki JS, Shroff SG, et al. Collagen remodeling of the pressure-overloaded, hypertrophied nonhuman primate myocardium. Circ Res 1988;62:757–765.

144. Judd JT, Wexler BC. Prolyl hydroxylase and collagen metabolism after experimental myocardial infarction. Am J Physiol 1975; 228:212–216.

145. Pick R, Jalil JE, Janicki JS, et al. The fibrillar nature and structure of isoproterenol-induced myocardial fibrosis in the rat. Am J Pathol 1989;134:365–371.

146. van Krimpen C, Smits JFM, Cleutjens JPM, et al. DNA synthesis in the non-infarcted cardiac interstitium after left coronary artery ligation in the rat heart: effects of captopril. J Mol Cell Cardiol 1991;23:1245–1253.

147. Volders PGA, Willems IEMG, Cleutjens JPM, et al. Interstitial collagen is increased in the non-infarcted human myocardium after myocardial infarction. J Mol Cell Cardiol 1993;25:1317–1323.

148. Beltrami CA, Finato N, Rocco M, et al. Structural basis of end-stage failure in ischemic cardiomyopathy in humans. Circulation 1994;89:151–163.

149. Hirsch AT, Talsness CE, Schunkert H, et al. Tissue-specific activation of cardiac angiotensin converting enzyme in experimental heart failure. Circ Res 1991;69:475–482.

150. Fabris B, Yamada H, Cubela R, et al. Characterization of cardiac angiotensin converting enzyme (ACE) and *in vivo* inhibition following oral quinapril to rats. Br J Pharmacol 1990;100:651–655.

151. Kinoshita A, Urata H, Bumpus FM, et al. Measurement of angiotensin I converting enzyme inhibition in the heart. Circ Res 1993;73:51–60.

152. Stauss HM, Zhu YC, Redlich T, et al. Early and late treatment of infarction-induced heart failure with a converting enzyme inhibitor: bradykinin potentiation versus angiotensin II reduction. (Abstract) Hypertension 1993;22:429.

153. Michel JB, Lattion AL, Salzmann JL, et al. Hormonal and cardiac effects of converting enzyme inhibition in rat myocardial infarction. Circ Res 1988;62:641–650.

154. van Krimpen C, Schoemaker RG, Cleutjens JPM, et al. Angiotensin I converting enzyme inhibitors and cardiac remodeling. Basic Res Cardiol 1991;86(Suppl. 1):149–155.

155. Cleutjens JPM, Kandala JC, Guarda E, et al. Regulation of collagen degradation in the rat myocardium after infarction. J Mol Cell Cardiol 1995 (In press).

156. Allen AM, Yamada H, Mendelsohn FAO. In vitro autoradiographic localization of binding to angiotensin receptors in the rat heart. Int J Cardiol 1990;28:25–33.

157. Weber DR, Stroud ED, Prescott SM. Arachidonate metabolism in cultured fibroblasts derived from normal and infarcted canine heart. Circ Res 1989;65:671–683.

158. Weber KT, Sun Y, Katwa LC, et al. Connective tissue: a metabolic entity? J Mol Cell Cardiol 1995;27 (In press).

159. Weber KT, Villarreal D, Griffing GT. Heart Failure: Pathophysiology, Aldosterone, and Anti-Aldosterone Therapy. Wilton, Conn: Medical Education Programs, Ltd., 1993.

Chapter 2

The Wound Healing Response After Myocardial Infarction: *Structural and Pharmacological Aspects*

Mat J.A.P. Daemen, J.F.M. Smits

Introduction

A myocardial infarction changes not only cardiac function, but also the structure of both the infarcted and noninfarcted myocardium. The beneficial effect of pharmacological interventions seems to be mediated, at least in part, by intervention in the complex changes in ventricular architecture after myocardial infarction, also referred to as "ventricular remodeling," and suggests a relationship between the structural and functional effects of the intervention. Most data in this respect are available for the effects of angiotensin-converting-enzyme ACE inhibitors, which are now used extensively in the treatment of myocardial infarction. Large studies have shown beneficial effects on morbidity and mortality[1] and there is clear evidence that ACE inhibitors do affect the structure of the infarcted heart. One example is the observation that immediate treatment may evoke adverse functional effects, due to an inhibition of the normal adaptive remodeling after the infarct.

From a theoretical point of view, questions relating to the mechanisms that mediate the response, such as the nature of the angiotensin receptors involved, and their localization in the heart or the periphery, need to be answered to understand the effect. Such knowledge may also help to solve practical questions related to the treatment of infarct patients.

In the present chapter we will focus on ventricular remodeling after myocardial infarction and describe structural and functional aspects of accepted pharmacological interventions.

Cardiac Remodeling Following Myocardial Infarction

Remodeling of the Infarct

Cardiomyocyte swelling and necrosis are early characteristics of an infarct. Myocyte necrosis is followed by a wound healing response, which involves a local inflammatory reaction, excessive extracellular matrix deposition, angiogenesis, and the appearance of myofibroblasts that increase the tensile strength of the infarct.[2] In general, the wound healing response of the heart to myocyte necrosis resembles the normal response of a parenchymatous tissue to injury, but with some special features, that are due to the unique microenvironment of the heart. One of these special features is that the expression of contractile proteins in myofibroblasts, present in the border zone between infarct and vital myocardium, is not transient, as it is in for instance dermal wound healing, but is maintained. This continuous expression of contractile proteins was found in different

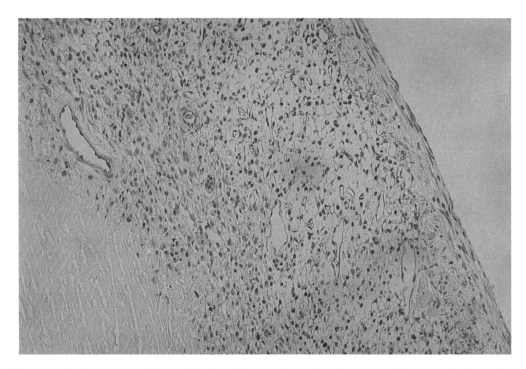

Figure 1. Photomicrograph (magnification 400 ×) of a section of a 4-day-old myocardial infarction in a rat stained with an antibody against ACE. Please note border zone of infarct and noninfarcted myocardium, where extensive ACE immunopositivity is found in endothelial cells lining capillaries as well as in myofibroblasts.

forms of cardiac injury in both animal and human studies,[2] and may give the scar contractile properties. In a recent study from our laboratory, smooth muscle actin, one of these contractile proteins, was found in human infarcts of more than 10 years of age.[3] The cyclic stretch and relaxation of the infarct is thought to induce and maintain the expression of contractile proteins in the myofibroblasts in the border zone. Recent in vitro and in vivo studies suggest that transforming growth factor beta, which is also expressed in the border zone of the infarct, modulates smooth muscle actin expression in the myofibroblast. Of interest in this respect is the recent observation that the mRNA and protein of angiotensin I converting enzyme (ACE) are also highly expressed in the border zone, suggesting a possible role of the renin-angiotensin-aldosterone system in the wound healing response of the infarcted myocardium (Figure 1, Passier, personal communication).

Dilatation and thinning, also called "in-farct expansion,"[1,4] are the most important architectural changes in the infarct region. Infarct expansion is not only caused by myocyte necrosis but also by myocyte slippage.[5,6] Infarct expansion is limited to the first weeks after myocardial infarction and can ultimately lead to a ventricular aneurysm. It correlates negatively with ventricular function and prognosis.

Remodeling of the NonInfarcted Ventricles

Ventricular Dilatation and Hypertrophy

Also the noninfarcted ventricle remodels to compensate for the loss of viable tissue and to maintain cardiac function. This remodeling involves ventricular dilatation which may initially be beneficial to maintain stroke volume. Ventricular dilatation, however, also increases ventricular wall stress, which may stimulate further ventricular enlargement.[1]

Hypertrophy of the noninfarcted ventricle is apparent within 1 week postinfarction. Hypertrophy involves all cellular compartments of the ventricle, including the myocyte, the vascular, and the extracellular matrix compartments. Hypertrophy early postmyocardial infarction is necessary to compensate for the loss of contractile tissue and to maintain cardiac function. In contrast, late hypertrophy may have adverse effects on cardiac function and may ultimately lead to heart failure.

The Myocyte Postmyocardial Infarction

In the noninfarcted myocardium, the volume and orientation of the myocytes changes.[7,8] Since the adult myocyte has lost the ability to undergo cell division, most authors believe that the number of cells does not increase. The myocyte can, however, still undergo nuclear division. Hypertrophy post MI is, indeed, associated with an increase in total DNA and DNA per myocyte. But the changes in myocyte mass, which are initiated by the increased wall stress do not fully compensate for the loss of viable tissue and for the loss of function. One of the possible explanations for this apparent paradox, i.e., more cardiac mass without an increased cardiac function, is that cardiac hypertrophy is associated with alterations in the quantity and quality of the expression of contractile, cytoskeletal, and neurohormonal genes.[9–11] This results in reexpression of the fetal phenotype i.e., the reexpression of proteins that were present in fetal life but had disappeared in adulthood. Extensive studies in this respect have been performed in (small) animals and similar changes have been documented in humans.[9] The expression of these fetal proteins is associated with a decreased contractility, but a lower energy demand of the cardiac muscle. For instance, the expression of the gene of the heavy chain of the contractile protein myosin changes from the α to the β chain, which contracts slower, but is less energy consuming.[12]

The Vascular Compartment

An increase in the number and length of capillaries has been documented in both animals and humans. It is found in the border zone between infarct and vital myocardium and in the noninfarcted hypertrophied myocardium. In the border zone, growth of new vessels is part of the normal wound healing response. The expression of ACE mRNA and protein is enhanced in these newly formed vessels, suggesting a relationship between vessel growth and the renin-angiotensin system (see below).

In the noninfarcted myocardium the increase in capillaries is insufficient to meet the increase in cardiomyocyte volume. The result is a decreased capillary to cardiomyocyte fiber ratio.[13] The increase in distance between capillaries and the decrease in density of capillary profiles during ventricular remodeling leads to a relative energy starvation[14] of the hypertrophied, noninfarcted myocardium. The expression of a less energy consuming phenotype (see above) may be regarded as an adaptation to the energy starvation of the hypertrophied cardiomyocyte, but is detrimental for contractility.

The Extracellular Matrix

Cardiac function is not only determined by the myocytes but also by the extracellular matrix, which connects the myocytes to each other and to surrounding capillaries. The fibrillar collagens, type I and type III, are the major components of the cardiac extracellular matrix. Changes in the amount and/or distribution of collagen can affect the function of the heart.[15] For instance an increased collagen fraction increases the stiffness of the heart, leading to a decreased compliance and diminished diastolic filling.[16] Increased intercellular and pericellular collagen fibers may limit myocyte motion and decrease the compliance of the ventricle. Also arrhythmias may result from increased collagen deposition. Fibrillar collagens accumulate in the cardiac interstitium during aging,[17] but also during cardiac hypertrophy induced by pressure overload.[18,19] The collagen amount increases also during ventricular remodeling after myocardial infarction in rats and humans.[20,21] In the rat model of myocardial infarction we found not only increases in collagen types I and III mRNA and protein, but also activation of collagen degradation[22,23] (See Chapter 19). Not only the absolute amounts but also the ratio between the amount of collagen type I and type III and the fraction of crosslinked collagen will affect cardiac function.[24] Inhibition of collagen synthesis or collagen crosslinking after induction of a myocardial infarction in the rat reduces cardiac function (Cleutjens, personal communication).

The amount of another extracellular matrix protein, fibronectin, which provides the scaffold for the deposition of collagen, also changes shortly after the induction of cardiac hypertrophy.[25,26] Also for this protein reexpression of the fetal phenotype occurs, although its consequence for function is not known.

In contrast to the changes in the myocyte compartment changes in the interstitium are associated with a change in DNA synthesis and cell number. In rats in which the left coronary artery was ligated to induce a myocardial infarction, DNA synthesis transiently increased within the first 2 weeks in both the noninfarcted left and right ventricles. DNA synthesis was maximal between days 7 and 14 and was found predominantly in fibroblasts and endothelial cells and only to a minor extent in cardiomyocytes.[27,28] In a rat model for cardiac hypertrophy induced by renovascular hypertension we observed such a response not only in the myocardium but also in cardiac valves.[29]

Pharmacology of the Response

Besides reopening of occluded coronary arteries with thrombolytic agents, there are nowadays at least three pharmacological strategies that are generally employed in the prevention of reinfarction and prevention and treatment of heart failure following infarction. These involve inhibition of platelet aggregation with aspirin, reduction of sympathetic input to the heart with beta-adrenoceptor blockers and reduction of mechanical load on the heart with vasodilating drugs. Especially ACE inhibitors have been proven successful in this respect.

These therapies may not only influence their primary targets but also the remodeling response of the heart. For aspirin, its antiinflammatory properties may be of importance in this respect. Here we will briefly discuss the evidence and implications for effects of antiinflammatory drugs on the remodeling response. ACE inhibitors will also be discussed in relation to their vasodilating effects. Effects of beta-blockers on cardiac remodeling following myocardial infarction have not been studied. One might, however, assume that part of the effect of these agents is related to their protective effect on catecholamine-induced cardiac myocyte necrosis and the ensuing microscarring of the myocardium.[30] Clearly, this subject deserves further study.

Antiinflammatory Drugs

The early healing response in the infarct area and the border zone involves inflammation and is associated with an enhanced expression of cell adhesion molecules. Recent studies with monoclonal antibodies against cell adhesion molecules indicate that prevention of leukocyte adhesion in the course of reperfusion profoundly limits the extent of the infarct.[31] This suggests that leukocyte invasion contributes substantially to the evolution of the necrotic area following ischemia. The data obtained in these studies are limited to the very short-term effects, i.e., infarct size in relation to the area at risk in the first hours after the infarct. Antiinflammatory drugs have been examined with respect to their long-term out come on myocardial infarction. Early administration of methylprednisolone was shown to decrease wall thickness in the infarct and induce ventricular dilatation in rats following coronary artery ligation.[32] Besides these topographic changes, which were related to cardiomyocyte slippage, these authors noted a reduction in collagen content in the infarct and border zone following 7-days methylprednisolone treatment. The effect of methylprednisolone on the collagen content may be multifactorial and might be related to the mineralocorticoid action of methylprednisolone; in later experiments, Weber and coworkers have shown that aldosterone, through its mineralocorticoid action, promotes collagen deposition in myocardial hypertrophy of a number of origins.[33-35] Inhibition of the inflammatory response, which may be related to the glucocorticoid effect does provide an alternative explanation. Thus, indomethacin[36] has also been shown to promote early thinning of the infarct. Similarly, some studies[37,38] indicate that ibuprofen also causes thinning of the infarct, whereas other studies failed to detect such a response.[39] Ibuprofen treatment does not seem to reduce myocardial collagen content following infarction,[38,39] although it does reduce pericardial collagen content.[40] The functional consequences of these effects of antiinflammatory agents are not clear; although there is some evidence for increased incidence of ventricular rupture,[38] there was no effect of ibuprofen on tensile strength in another study.[40] The fact that large scale studies with aspirin show clear improvement of patient survival suggests that, at least at low doses, there is no deleterious effect of this antiinflammatory agent. It remains, however, to be established whether these doses exert an antiinflammatory effect, besides their well established inhibition of platelet aggregation.

ACE Inhibitors: Involvement of the Renin-Angiotensin System in the Remodeling Response

The successful application of ACE inhibitors in the treatment of heart failure (CONSENSUS I) has prompted extensive research into the effects of these compounds following myocardial infarction.[41] Large clinical trials have yielded conflicting results. The SAVE trial with captopril indicated improved cardiac function associated with inhibition of ventricular remodeling.[42] In contrast, CONSENSUS-II was stopped because of an apparent lack of functional effect.[43] Several explanations for these discrepancies may be put forward. One is that CONSENSUS-II involved high-dose intravenous ACE inhibition, which may have resulted in hypotensive effects. Alternatively, the lack of selection of patients at risk may have contributed to the absence of a beneficial effect. Another explanation may be the

timing of the administration: in CONSENSUS-II, ACE inhibition was started within 24 hours after the occurrence of symptoms, whereas in the other (successful) studies treatment was delayed for several days. If the renin-angiotensin system is involved in the repair response of the heart to the loss of tissue, early ACE inhibition may have interfered in this process. We have addressed this possibility in a series of studies in rats following myocardial infarction after ligation of the coronary artery, in which we compared structural and functional effects of interventions in the renin-angiotensin system at different times following induction of the infarct. Our primary observations[44] were similar to those of Pfeffer et al.,[45] i.e., captopril treatment initiated 21 days after infarction almost causes normalization of cardiac function. They noted that the functional improvement was associated with inhibition of cardiac hypertrophy and dilatation, whereas cardiac stiffness did not increase.[45] In contrast to late treatment, when captopril treatment was started immediately after infarction, cardiac output was still depressed at 3 weeks after infarction[44]; furthermore, stroke volume was decreased at the expense of increased heart rate, suggesting further deterioration rather than improvement of cardiac function. In parallel studies we investigated structural effects of myocardial infarction as well as the response to ACE inhibition. Infarction resulted in necrosis and scarring of the infarcted area. The remnant myocardium exhibited a cellular response in both the myocyte and nonmyocyte compartment. In the latter, DNA synthesis was clearly increased.[27] Approximately 30% of the DNA-synthesizing cells in the interstitium could be identified as endothelial cells.[28] The fact that we observed collagen deposition, in parallel to DNA synthesis, suggests involvement of fibroblasts as well. This combination of effects, i.e., vascularization and collagen deposition may be considered as a wound healing response occurring outside the primarily injured area.

ACE inhibition with captopril during the phase of wound healing completely abolished DNA synthesis and collagen deposition following myocardial infarction.[27] This indicates that the endothelial as well as the fibroblast responses were inhibited. Interestingly, selective inhibition of the AT_1 receptors with losartan only partially mimicked the effects of captopril in spite of a similar blood pressure reduction: although collagen deposition was normalized, DNA synthesis was only partially inhibited.[46] Losartan did not affect cardiac function in any way. The discrepancy could be related to the fact that captopril not only interferes with angiotensin metabolism, but also with bradykinin metabolism. This is supported by the results of a study in the dog where the bradykinin antagonist HOE 140 blocked the effects of the ACE inhibitor ramiprilat on infarct size.[47] Detailed studies on the effects of bradykinin on cardiac remodeling processes after myocardial infarction are, however, not available. In a follow-up study the selective AT_2 antagonist PD123319 almost completely inhibited DNA synthesis.[48] Since AT_2 receptor blockade is not known to interfere with bradykinin metabolism it is unlikely that the bradykinin pathway is important in cardiac remodeling after myocardial infarction.

The renin angiotensin system is no longer considered an exclusive circulating hormone system. Evidence has accumulated that several tissues, including the heart, express all components to constitute local renin-angiotensin systems.[49] Expression of angiotensinogen, renin, and angiotensin I converting enzyme (ACE) have been demonstrated at the mRNA as well as the protein level in cardiac myocytes as well as cardiac fibroblasts. Of special interest are the observations that expression of angiotensinogen mRNA[50] and ACE mRNA[51] are increased in the remnant myocardium following myocardial infarction in rats. In fact, the increased wall stress in this situation correlated with angiotensinogen expression[52] and similarly, ACE expression correlated with the extent of myocardial infarction,[51] suggesting local regulation of the activity of the cardiac renin angiotensin system.

Angiotensin II may influence cardiac inotropy and chronotropy[53] although the inotropic response seems to be limited to atrial myocardium and could not be observed in human ventricular preparations.[54] The effects of angiotensin II on cardiac growth may be direct or indirect. The observation that the wound healing response after infarction is sensitive to ACE inhibition, but not limited to the left ventricle and also involves the right ventricle supports the idea that other factors may be involved. Possible indirect mechanisms are the vasoactive effects of angiotensin II, and the stimulatory effects of the peptide on the activity of the sympathetic nervous system. Alpha-adrenoceptor activation stimulates hypertrophy in neonatal rat cardiac myocytes[55] and DNA synthesis in vascular smooth muscle.[56] Moreover, at least part of the trophic effects of angiotensin II on vascular smooth muscle cells is mediated via the alpha-adrenoceptor.[57] Alternatively, angiotensin II could have direct effects on cardiac cells and the cardiac extracellular matrix. Angiotensin II is trophic for cardiomyocytes, and this effect is independent of its effect on blood pressure.[58] Because PD123319 did not affect blood pressure, combination of the effects of captopril, losartan, and PD123319 rules out mechanical load as a determinant of the cellular response, but not of the collagen deposition after myocardial infarction in the rat.

The trophic effect of angiotensin II on cardiomyocytes is mediated entirely through AT_1 angiotensin receptors.[58] The involvement of this pathway in cardiac hypertrophy following myocardial infarction in the rat was suggested by the total inhibition of hypertrophy we observed following infusion of the AT_1 antagonist losartan in infarcted rats.[46] Although cardiomyocytes represent the bulk of the mass of the heart, and changes in cardiac weight may be interpreted as changes in cardiac myocyte mass, cardiac fibroblasts and endothelial cells represent the bulk of the cell number. As mentioned above, these two cell types are indeed capable of replicating. Angiotensin II stimulates DNA synthesis and cell number in cultured cardiac fibroblasts.[59] Again, this response is mediated by AT_1 receptors. Angiotensin II also stimulates the synthesis of collagen types I and III and fibronectin in cultured fibroblasts.[60,61]

In this respect it is noteworthy that in a model for vascular neogenesis, the chick chorioallantoic membrane, angiotensin II induces a potent neovascularization response that is resistant to losartan and the nonpeptidergic AT_2 antagonist PD123319, but may be completely inhibited by the peptidic AT_2 antagonist CGP42112A.[62] This suggests involvement of a non-AT_1 receptor in this part of the response. These observations may provide an explanation for the paradoxical effects of captopril, losartan, and PD123319 on interstitial DNA synthesis and collagen deposition and suggest that collagen deposition is mediated by AT_1 receptors and endothelial cell proliferation by AT_2 receptors.

Conclusions

The heart exhibits an extensive remodeling response following myocardial infarction. Our knowledge about the response and the mechanisms underlying it are rapidly expanding; in parallel there is significant improvement of the therapeutic approach to patients suffering from myocardial infarction. Several important issues, such as dosing and timing of therapies, are, however, still a matter of debate. Further fundamental and clinical studies defining the role of the different regulatory mechanisms, as well as the functional consequences of selective intervention in parts of the remodeling response may aid in resolving these issues and may contribute to rationalization and consequent improvement of therapy of this vulnerable patient population.

References

1. Pfeffer MA, Braunwald E. Ventricular remodeling after myocardial infarction. Experimental observations and clinical implications. Circulation 1990;81:1161–1172.
2. Vracko R, Thorning D. Contractile cells in rat myocardial scar tissue. Lab Invest 1991;65:221–227.
3. Willems EMG, Havenith MH, De Mey JGR, et al. Alpha smooth muscle actin positive cells in healing human myocardial scars. Am J Pathol 1994, 145,060–075.
4. Hutchins GM, Bulkey BH. Infarct expansion versus extension: two different complications of acute myocardial infarction. Am J Cardiol 1978;41:1127–1132.
5. Cooper G 4th, Mercer WE, Hoober JK, et al. Load regulation of the properties of adult feline cardiocytes. The role of substrate adhesion. Circ Res 1986;58:692–705.
6. Tsutsui H, Urabe Y, Mann DL, et al. Effects of chronic mitral regurgitation on diastolic function in isolated cardiocytes. Circ Res 1993;72:1110–1123.
7. Anversa P, Beghi C, Kikkawa Y, et al. Myocardial response to infarction in the ratmorphometric measurement of infarct size and myocyte cellular hypertrophy. Am J Pathol 1985;118:484–492.
8. Capasso JM, Bruno S, Cheng W, et al. Ventricular loading is coupled with DNA synthesis in adult cardiac myocytes after acute and chronic myocardial infarction in rats. Circ Res 1992;71:1379–1389.
9. Lompre AM, Mercadier JJ, Schwartz K. Changes in gene expression in cardiac growth. Intern Rev Cytol 1991;124:137–186.
10. Boheler KR, Schwartz K. Gene expression in cardiac hypertrophy. Trends Cardiovasc Med 1992;2:176–182.
11. Chien KR, Knowlton KU, Zhu H, et al. Regulation of cardiac gene expression during myocardial growth and hypertrophy. Molecular studies of an adaptive physiological response. FASEB J 1991;5:3037–3046.
12. Schwartz K, Boheler KR, De La Bastie D, et al. Switches in cardiac muscle gene expression as a result of pressure and volume overload. Am J Physiol 1992;262:R364-R369.
13. Olivetti G, Anversa P. Long term pressure induced cardiac hypertrophy: capillary and mast cell production. Am J Physiol 1989;257:H1766-H1772.
14. Katz A. Cardiomyopathy of overload. N Engl J Med 1990;322:100–110.
15. Caulfield JB, Norton P, Weaver RD. Cardiac dilatation associated with collagen alterations. Mol Cell Biochem 1992;118:171–179.
16. Brilla CG, Janicki JS, Weber KT. Impaired diastolic function and coronary reserve in genetic hypertension. Circ Res 1991;69:107–115.
17. Chapman D, Weber KT, Eghbali M. Regulation of fibrillar collagen types I and II and basement type IV collagen gene expression in pressure overloaded rat myocardium. Circ Res 1990;67:787–794.
18. Weber KT, Brilla CG. Pathological hypertrophy and cardiac interstitium. Circulation 1991;83:1849–1865.
19. Weber KT, Anversa P, Armstrong PW, et al. Remodeling and reparation of the cardiovascular system. J Am Coll Cardiol 1992;20:3–16.
20. Michel J, Lattion A, Salzmann J, et al. Hormonal and cardiac effects of converting en-

zyme inhibition in rat myocardial infarction. Circ Res 1988;62:641–650.

21. Volders PGA, Willems IEMG, Cleutjens JPM, et al. Interstitial collagen is increased in the non-infarcted myocardium after myocardial infarction. J Mol Cell Cardiol 1993;25: 317–323.

22. Collagen remodeling after myocardial infarction in the rat heart Cleutjens JPM, Verluylen MJA Smits JFM, Daemen MJAP. Am J Pathol 1995 in press.

23. Regulation of collagen degradation in the rat myocardium after infarction. Cleutjens JPM, Kandala JC, Guarda E, Guntaka RV Weber KT. JMOL Cell Cardiol 1995 in press.

24. Limoto D, Covell J, Harper E. Increase in cross-linking of type I and type III collagens associated with volume-overload hypertrophy. Circ Res 1988;63:399–405.

25. Shekhonin BV, Guriev SB, Irgashev SB, et al. Immunofluorescence identification of fibronectin and fibrinogen/fibrin in experimental myocardial infarction. J Mol Cell Cardiol 1990;22:533–541.

26. Samuel JL, Barrieux A, Dufour S, et al. Accumulation of fetal fibronectin mRNAs during the development of rat cardiac hypertrophy induced by pressure overload. J Clin Invest 1991;88:1737–1746.

27. van Krimpen C, Smits JFM, Cleutjens JPM, et al. DNA synthesis in the non-infarcted cardiac interstitium is increased after left coronary artery ligation in the rat. Effects of captopril. J Mol Cell Cardiol 1991;23:1245–1253.

28. Kuizinga MC, Cleutjens JPM, Smits JFM, et al. Griffonia simplicifolia I (GSI): a suitable rat cardiac microvascular marker on paraffin embedded tissue.(Abstract) J Mol Cell Cardiol 1992;24(Suppl. V):S57.

29. Willems EMG, Havenith MH, Smits JFM, et al. Structural alterations in heart valves during left ventricular overload in the rat. Lab Invest 1994;71:127–133.

30. Pick R, Jalil J, Janicki J, et al. The fibrillar nature and structure of isoproterenol-induced myocardial fibrosis in the rat. Am J Pathol 1989;134:365–371.

31. Byrne JG, Smith WJ, Murphy MP, et al. Complete prevention of myocardial stunning, contracture, low reflow and edema after heart transplantation by blocking neutrophil adhesion molecules during reperfusion. J Thorac Cardiovasc Surg 1992σ04:1589–1596.

32. Mannisi JA, Weisman HF, Bush DE, et al. Steroid administration after myocardial infarction promotes early infarct expansion. J Clin Invest 1987;79:1431–1439.

33. Brilla CG, Weber KT. Mineralocorticoid ex-

cess, dietary sodium, and myocardial fibrosis. J Lab Clin Med 1992;120:893–901.

34. Kocher O, Skalli O, Bloom W, et al. Cytoskeleton of rat aortic smooth muscle cells. Lab Invest 1980;50:645–652.

35. Brilla C, Janicki JS, Weber KT. Cardioreparative effects of lisinopril in rats with genetic hypertension and left ventricular hypertrophy. Circulation 1991;83:1771–1779.

36. Hammerman H, Kloner RA, Schoen FJ, et al. Indomethacin-induced scar thinning following experimental myocardial infarction. Circulation 1983;67:1290–1295.

37. Judgutt BI. Delayed effects of early infarct-limiting therapies on healing after myocardial infarction. Circulation 1985;72:907–914.

38. Judgutt BI. Effect of nitroglycerin and ibuprofen on left ventricular topography and rupture threshold during healing after myocardial infarction in the dog. Can J Physiol Pharmacol 1988;66:385–395.

39. Cannon RO, Rodriguez ER, Speir E, et al. Effect of ibuprofen on the healing phase of experimental myocardial infarction in the rat. Am J Cardiol 1985;55:1609–1613.

40. Przylenk K. Effect of chronic ibuprofen therapy on early healing of experimentally induced acute myocardial infarction. Am J Cardiol 1989;63:1146–1148.

41. Swedberg K, Kjekshus J. Effects of enalapril on mortality in severe heart failure: results of the Cooperative North Scandinavian Enalapril Survival study. Am J Cardiol 1988;62: 60A-66A.

42. Pfeffer MA, and the SAVE investigators. Effect of captopril on mortality and morbidity in patients with left ventricular dysfunction after myocardial infarction. N Engl J Med 1992;327:669–677.

43. Swedberg K, Held P, Kjekdhus J, et al. Effects of the early administration of enalapril on mortality in patients with acute myocardial infarction-results of the cooperative New Scandinavian Enalapril Survival study (CONSENSUS II). N Engl J Med 1992;327: 678–684.

44. Schoemaker RG, Debets JJM, Struyker-Boudier HAJ, et al. Delayed but not immediate captopril therapy improves cardiac function in conscious rats, following myocardial infarction. J Mol Cell Cardiol 1991;23:187–197.

45. Pfeffer JM, Pfeffer MA, Braunwald E. Influence of chronic captopril therapy on the infarcted left ventricle of the rat. Circ Res 1985; 57:84–95.

46. Smits JF, van Krimpen C, Schoemaker RG, et al. Angiotensin II receptor blockade after myocardial infarction in rats: effects on hemodynamics, myocardial DNA synthesis,

and interstitial collagen content. J Cardiovasc Pharmacol 1992;20:772–778.

47. Martorana P, Kettenbach B, Breipohl G, et al. Reduction of infarct size by local angiotensin converting enzyme inhibition is abolished by a bradykinin antagonist. Eur J Pharmacol 1990;182:395–396.

48. Daemen MJAP, Smits JFM. Inhibition of myocardial DNA synthesis after coronary artery ligation in the rat heart by the angiotensin subtype 2 receptor antagonist PD123319. (Abstract) Eur Heart J 1993;76: A2351.

49. Lee YA, Lindpaintner K. The cardiac renin angiotensin system; from basic research to clinical relevance. Drug Res 1993;43:201–206.

50. Lindpaintner K, Lu W, Neidermajer N, et al. Selective activation of cardiac angiotensinogen gene expression in post-infarction ventricular remodeling in the rat. J Mol Cell Cardiol 1993;25:133–143.

51. Hirsch AT, Talsness CE, Schunkert H, et al. Tissue-specific activation of cardiac angiotensin converting enzyme in experimental heart failure. Circ Res 1991;69:475–482.

52. Beutler B, Cerami A. Cachectin: more than a tumor necrosis factor. N Engl J Med 1987;16: 379–385.

53. Dzau VJ. Tissue renin-angiotensin system in myocardial hypertrophy and failure. Arch Intern Med 1993;153:937–942.

54. Du XY, Schoemaker R, Saxena PR. Different responses in human atrial and ventricular tissue.(Abstract) Pharmacol World Sci 1993; 15(Suppl. I):15.

55. Simpson P. Stimulation of hypertrophy of cultured neonatal rat heart cells through an alpha 1-adrenergic receptor and induction of beating through an alpha 1- and beta 1-adrenergic receptor interaction. Evidence for independent regulation of growth and beating. Circ Res 1985;56:884–894.

56. Yamori Y, Massayuki M, Nara Y, et al. Catecholamine-induced polyploidization in vascular muscle cells.(Abstract) Circulation 1987;75(Suppl. I):I92.

57. Van Kleef EM, Smits JF, De Mey JG, et al. Alpha 1 adrenoreceptor blockade reduces the angiotensin II induced vascular smooth muscle cell DNA synthesis in the rat thoracic aorta and carotid artery. Circ Res 1992;70: 1122–1127.

58. Dostal DE, Baker KM. Angiotensin II stimulation of left ventricular hypertrophy in adult rat heart. Mediation by the AT1 receptor. Am J Hypertens 1992;5:276–280.

59. Schorb W, Booz GW, Dostal DE, et al. Angiotensin II is mitogenic in neonatal cardiac fibroblasts. Circ Res 1993;72:1245–1254.

60. Sadoshima JI, Izumo S. Molecular characterization of angiotensin II induced hypertrophy of cardiac myocytes and hyperplasia of cardiac fibroblasts. Critical role of AT1 receptor subtype. Circ Res 1993;73:413–423.

61. Crawford DC, Chobanian AV, Brecher P. Angiotensin II induces fibronectin expression associated with cardiac fibrosis in the rat. Circ Res 1994;74:727–728.

62. Le Noble FA, Schreurs NH, van Straaten HW, et al. Evidence for a novel angiotensin II receptor involved in angiogenesis in chick embryo chorioallantoic membrane. Am J Physiol 1993;264:R460-R465.

Chapter 3

Wound Healing After Myocardial Infarction

Peter Whittaker, Ph.D.

" . . . the infarcted area gradually acquires a gelatinous, ground-glass, gray appearance, eventually converting into a shrunken, thin, firm scar, which whitens and firms progressively with time."[1]

Most studies of myocardial infarction have focussed on the acute effects, such as the determinants of myocyte necrosis and therapies to prevent or minimize muscle injury. More recently attention has also been devoted to examination of the remodeling process that occurs after myocardial infarction, particularly the possibility of limiting the progressive ventricular dilation that occurs in the months to years after infarction. In contrast, very little attention has been paid to the healing process. The above quotation is typical of the amount of attention and even interest given to scar healing after myocardial infarction. Certainly the image of a gray, gelatinous mass does not suggest a topic worthy of interest. However, in this chapter, I would like to demonstrate that the healing process is dynamic and important.

The time-course of the early cellular events in healing after myocardial infarction such as infiltration of the infarct by polymorphonuclear leukocytes and other inflammatory cells has been extensively reviewed in many papers and textbooks (for example see Mallory et al.[2] or Pasternak et al.[1]), and so will not be covered here. Instead I will concentrate on the production and organization of the scar's major structural protein, collagen. We will examine the time-course of collagen production, how much and what type of collagen is present, the degree and nature of collagen cross-links, and how the collagen fibers are organized in the scar. All of these factors are important in determining the properties of the scar. We will then consider how the healing process might be affected or modified by various external factors, how the progression of healing might be monitored in vivo, and finally how the presence of a scar might affect the rest of the heart.

Collagen in the Scar

Time-Course of Collagen Accumulation

The healing process starts very quickly. Expression of messenger RNA (mRNA) for types I and III collagen was found to be elevated on the second day after infarction in rabbits.[3] Collagen mRNA expression was preceded, 24 hours earlier, by expression of mRNA for fibronectin,[3] which is thought to play an important role in the subsequent organization of collagen in the scar.[4] New collagen fibers produced by fibroblasts can be seen at the edge of the scar in rats by the third or fourth day after infarction, which corresponds to the time at which increased levels of tissue hydroxyproline are found.[5] Many studies have shown that the amount of collagen in the scar increases with time after injury. For example, Jugdutt and Amy[6] found a progressive increase in scar hydroxyproline (a biochemical marker for col-

From Weber KT, MD *Wound Healing in Cardiovascular Disease*, Armonk, NY, Futura Publishing Company Inc., © 1995.

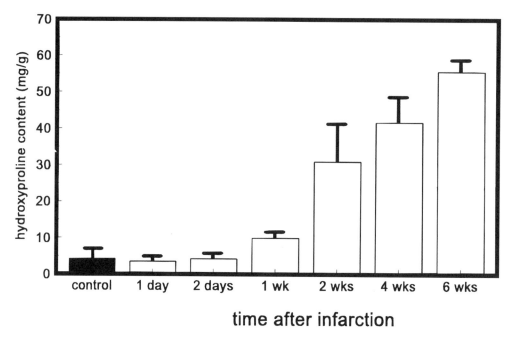

time after infarction

Figure 1. Temporal changes in myocardial hydroxyproline content in the center of the infarct. Hydroxyproline content was increased significantly above control levels at 7 days after myocardial infarction. Figure adapted with permission from Jugdutt and Amy,[6] J Am Coll Cardiol, 1986;7: 91–102.

lagen) over the first 6 weeks after permanent coronary artery occlusion in dogs (Fig. 1). The increase in hydroxyproline at the center of the infarct was significantly increased over that in noninfarcted myocardium 7 days after infarction. At 6 weeks after infarction collagen content had increased by a factor of five over the 1 week level. Although they did not examine changes at later times, the increase in collagen content appeared to reach a plateau at 6 weeks. Regional differences in hydroxyproline content indicated that the process was more than a simple uniform deposition of collagen. At 1 week after infarction, the relative distribution of collagen across the wall was similar to that seen in noninfarcted hearts, while at 6 weeks after infarction, there appeared to be a relative decrease in the amount of hydroxyproline in the subendocardial layer. Also at 6 weeks after infarction there appeared to be a greater concentration of collagen at the center of the infarct than at the edge[7]; however, the reasons for such regional variation are unknown. These investigators also found that there was a

correlation between the size of the infarct and the amount of hydroxyproline present at each time point examined—the larger the infarct the greater the amount of collagen required.[6]

The appearance of collagen in the infarcted tissue is a significant event because the mechanical properties of collagen are very different than those of muscle. The tensile strength of collagen approaches that of steel (50 to 100 MPa versus approximately 500 MPa). In addition, the stiffness of collagen, depending on its source, would appear to be 4 to 5 orders of magnitude greater than that of cardiac muscle (calculated from data published by Brady[8]). That the amount of collagen in the heart will significantly determine its passive mechanical properties has been demonstrated by Przyklenk et al.,[9] who found that the tensile strength of tissue taken from the infarct in dog hearts 24 hours after coronary artery occlusion correlated significantly with the collagen content of the tissue—the more collagen present, the stronger the tissue. Similarly, Lerman et al.[5] found a correlation between the passive stiffness of rabbit hearts examined 1 to 8 days after myocardial infarction and their hydroxyproline content. Thus, the increase in collagen content of the scar will lead to a progressive increase in tensile strength and stiffness.

Collagen Type Composition

The type of collagen in a tissue is also an important determinant of the tissue's mechanical properties. For example, type I collagen is the principal component of tissues that require stiffness and high tensile strength such as tendon. In contrast, tissues that require greater compliance, such as skin, have a higher proportion of type III collagen. The normal ratio of type I to type III collagen in myocardium is approximately 7:1,[10] but the early stages of wound repair are associated with an increase in the amount of type III collagen. Vivaldi et al.[11] found that the relative content of scars formed 4 weeks after permanent coronary artery occlusion in rats, estimated by densitometry of electrophoretic gels, was 40% type I, 35% type III, and 25% type V. The relatively large amount of type V collagen is in sharp contrast to values of under 3% found in subcutaneous granulation tissue 3 weeks after injury.[12] Although the large amount of type V collagen found in the scar is surprising, it could be explained in that its presence has been associated with angiogenesis, may be involved in cellular migration, and is found in hypertrophic scars (reviewed in Hering et al.[12]). The two former situations would certainly be found in myocardial scars, while the third may be supported by our observation of "whorls" or "nodules" of collagen fibers in myocardial scars.[13] Such structures are often found in hypertrophic dermal scars.[14] The presence of type V collagen has also been noted in other myocardial scars. After ventriculotomy, in which a longitudinal myocardial incision was sutured closed, Kawahara et al.,[15] using immunohistochemical methods, observed fibroblasts which stained positive for type V collagen in the first few days after surgery, and extracellular type V collagen 3 to 4 weeks later. Although they also observed collagen types IV and VI, the bulk of the scar was composed of types I and III.

Further work is needed to fully investigate the amounts and time-course of collagen type changes in the scar and their functional significance.

Scar Collagen Crosslinks

The degree and nature of collagen crosslinks can significantly alter mechanical properties. For example, abnormalities in collagen crosslinking are associated with human diseases indicating reduced structural integrity such as congenital dislocation of the hip (reviewed by Last et al.[16]). Several studies have examined changes in collagen crosslinking after infarction. Connelly et al.[17] examined scar collagen crosslinks 3 weeks after infarction by measuring the concentration of aldol and hydroxynorleucine in rabbit hearts that were permanently occluded and in those where the artery was reperfused 3 hours after occlusion. The concentration of aldol crosslinks was significantly lower in the reperfused hearts. Furthermore, there was a statistically significant correlation between aldol crosslink concentration, expressed per microgram of hydroxyproline, and the tensile strength of the scar. Although there was also a reduction in hydroxynorleucine concentration in the reperfused hearts, the difference was not significant. Vivaldi et al.[11] found that the increase in collagen content in the scars from rats examined 2 and 4 weeks after permanent coronary artery occlusion was accompanied by a 2 to 3-fold increase in the concentration of hydroxypyridinium crosslinks. Scar collagen examined 13 weeks after myocardial infarction contained a substantial increase in the concentration of hydroxylysylpyridinoline crosslinks when compared with noninfarcted control tissue.[18] These crosslink changes reflect, in the former study, increasing maturity of the scar and in the latter study, a potential increase in the tensile strength of the collagen. Although there appear to be considerable changes in collagen crosslinks in the scar during the first months after myocardial infarction, the precise functional significance of these changes is not known.

Collagen Fiber Organization

The role of collagen organization in the mechanical properties of tissue can be illus-

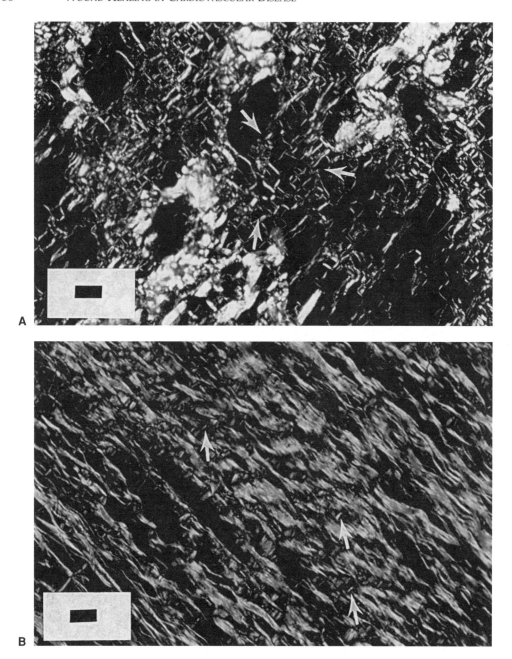

Figure 2. Micrographs of collagen fibers in canine myocardial scars 6 weeks after infarction. The tissue sections were stained with picrosirius red and viewed with polarized light [bar = 20 μm]. Panel A: A region where cellular debris was still present (represented by the black spaces between the bright collagen fibers). Thin collagen fibers are organized in a lattice (the arrows indicate such a region). Some thick collagen fibers can be seen in the lower left and upper right of the figure. Panel B: A region with more complete healing than shown in Panel A. Thick collagen fibers running from upper left to lower right appear to be woven through the thin fiber lattice. The arrows indicate thin collagen fibers in the lattice that are aligned perpendicular to the orientation of the thick fibers.

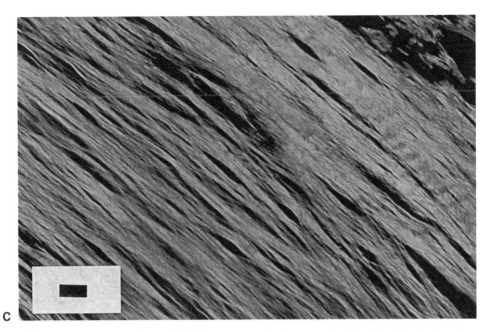

C

Figure 2. *(continued).* Panel C: A region in the center of the scar. The thin fiber lattice is no longer present. Figure reprinted with permission from the original color figure in Whittaker et al.,[13] Am J Pathol 1989;134:879–893.

trated by comparing tendon and skin. The unidirectional organization of collagen fibers in tendon confers strength and stiffness parallel to the tendon's long axis, while the relatively complex three-dimensional weave of fibers found in skin provides multiaxial compliance.

The organization of collagen fibers in myocardial scars changes at different stages of development.[13] In regions where debris from necrotic myocytes was still present, we observed that the collagen fibers were arranged into a lattice-like organization (Figure 2A). The fibers in this lattice structure appeared green when stained with picrosirius red and viewed with polarized light. Under these conditions the color of the collagen fibers depends on their thickness; with increasing fiber thickness the color changes from green to yellow to orange.[19] Therefore the lattice fibers are thin. Although the picrosirius red/polarized light method cannot definitively distinguish type I from type III collagen,[20] it is known that type III collagen fibers are usually thinner than type I fibers.[21] As we have also seen that type III collagen is found in relatively

high concentration during the early phases of wound healing, it is tempting to speculate that the lattice represents type III collagen. However, the possibility that the green fibers represent thin type I fibers cannot be discounted. In regions where the myocyte debris has been removed and the bulk of the area was occupied by collagen, the green fiber lattice was still present, but now thicker yellow and orange fibers could also be seen which appeared to be "woven" through the lattice (Figure 2B). In regions still further removed from areas of myocyte debris, the lattice was no longer present (Figure 2C). Instead we found parallel arrays of collagen fibers. We have also seen the presence of the lattice organization in developing scars in the hearts of hamsters with hereditary cardiomyopathy, and its absence in scars that appear to be fully healed (Davison et al., unpublished data). It is possible that the lattice plays the role of scaffolding in organizing the collagen fibers in the scar; its presence may be required in the "building" stage, but once construction is completed the scaffolding would no longer be required. Further work needs to be done to fully understand this component of the healing process.

In addition to the changes reported above, there were also differences in collagen organization across the thickness of the scar. We measured the three-dimensional organization of collagen in transmural scars from dog hearts 6 weeks after permanent coronary artery occlusion using a Universal stage, which permits rotation of the tissue sections around three orthogonal axes.[13] The collagen was organized into three separate layers, which appeared to correspond to the three layers of muscle that had occupied the space before infarction. The collagen in the midmyocardium was aligned circumferentially, while the subepi- and subendocardial collagen was aligned obliquely to the midmyocardial tissue. Collagen fibers in wounds tend to be aligned parallel to directions of stress,[22] and so it may be that the wall stress produced by the remaining muscle may be responsible for the alignment of fibers in the scar. A similar trilayered structure has been observed in human hearts after infarction.[23] Whether this structure is altered in situations where healing is abnormal is not known, but given the influence of organization on mechanical properties, the potential exists for considerable variation in scar stiffness.

Modification of the Healing Process

The above discussion has illustrated that healing of the infarct is a dynamic process and so it would be reasonable to expect that the process can be influenced by external intervention. In this section, I will consider the effect on scar healing of several procedures, interventions, or circumstances that may be encountered in patients. I will first consider the effect of reperfusion on healing, then the influence of various pharmacological therapies, and finally the influence of existing conditions such as diabetes and aging.

Reperfusion

Early reperfusion of an occluded artery is known to limit the amount of myocyte necrosis. Moreover, there appears to be some benefit to patients if the artery is reperfused at a time when it is no longer possible to salvage any muscle. Could this effect be because of enhanced scar healing? Miura and colleagues[24] assessed the degree of infarct organization, a term they used to indicate the area of the infarct occupied by granulation tissue and fibrosis, measured 7 days after infarction in rabbits with and without reperfusion. In rabbits with permanent occlusions, there was an inverse relationship between organization and infarct size; that is, the larger the infarct the less the degree of organization (Figure 3A). This appears reasonable because the larger the infarct, the further the fibroblasts will have to travel to reach all parts of the infarct. Reperfusion 30 minutes after occlusion did prevent some myocyte death and so the infarcts were not as large. However, the relationship between infarct size and organization was shifted upwards, so that for any given infarct size there was a greater degree of organization. A similar upward shift was found when reperfusion occurred 60 minutes after occlusion, a time at which there was no reduction in infarct size. In a similar study, Morita et al.[25] examined the effect of late reperfusion on healing in rats examined 7 days after infarction. They found that the amount of unresorbed necrotic myocardium was reduced by both early and late reperfusion (Figure 3B). Infiltration of neutrophils and macrophages into the infarct was increased by reperfusion; events consistent with enhanced removal of necrotic tissue. Despite the observed enhancement of healing, late reperfusion provided no protection against expansion of the infarct. On the other hand, some studies have found no enhancement of collagen content in reperfused versus nonreperfused hearts in either rabbits, examined 3 weeks after infarction,[17] or in dogs 2 weeks after infarction.[26] Whether reperfusion influences the organization of collagen fibers in the scar is unknown.

There has been speculation that very late reperfusion may be detrimental. Honan et al.[27] used meta-analysis to examine data from four trials using intravenous streptokinase and found a correlation between the incidence of myocardial rupture and the

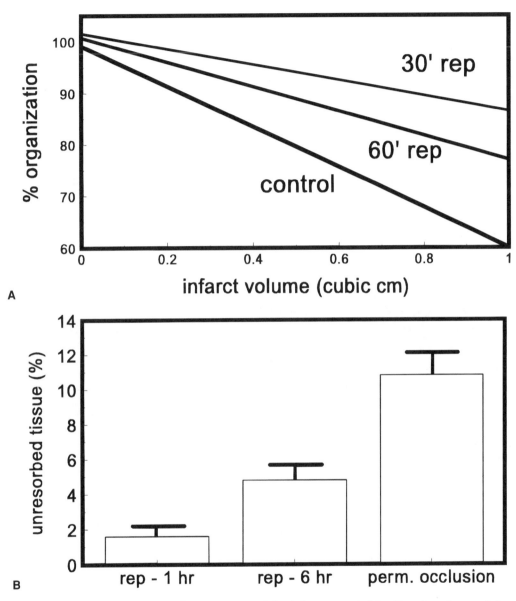

Figure 3. Panel A: Graph shows the percentage of the infarct occupied by fibrosis and granulation tissue (organization) as a function of infarct volume in rabbit hearts examined 7 days after infarction. Regression lines are shown for data obtained after permanent occlusion (control), and after reperfusion (30 or 60 minutes after occlusion). Figure adapted with permission from Miura et al.,[24] Can J Cardiol 1991;7:146–154. Panel B: Graph shows the amount of unresorbed necrotic tissue present in rat infarcts 7 days after myocardial infarction. The amount of unresorbed necrotic tissue was significantly reduced by either early (1 hour) or late (6 hours) reperfusion of the occluded artery versus that found after permanent occlusion. Figure adapted with permission from Morita et al.,[25] Am J Pathol 1993;143:419–430.

time between the onset of chest pain and the start of thrombolytic therapy. The risk of rupture appeared to be greater for patients receiving streptokinase if the treatment was started more than 11 hours after the onset of symptoms. Several studies have shown that damage to the heart's original collagen matrix increases with time after occlusion,[28,29] and there is also evidence that some aspect of reperfusion may instigate collagen damage.[30,31] Thus, it may be possible that there is a time beyond which any reperfusion-mediated enhancement of healing is counteracted by enhanced collagen degradation.

Pharmacological Therapy

Most of the attention on pharmacological influences has focussed on the apparent disruption of the normal healing process by antiinflammatory agents. Such agents are often used to treat pericarditis, inflammation of the pericardium, which is relatively common in the first few days after myocardial infarction. However, many antiinflammatory agents have been found to cause scar thinning.[32,33] The mechanism of such adverse healing is unclear; collagen content in the scar was not reduced several weeks after infarction[33] and in fact was found to increase in ibuprofen-treated rats.[34] Nor was tensile strength and collagen content decreased 30 hours after infarction.[35] Mannisi et al.[36] speculated that methylprednisolone exacerbated scar thinning before any new collagen was produced by reducing the amount of edema in the infarct. Aspirin, which is also an antiinflammatory agent, did not cause scar thinning after infarction,[32] and so provides a potentially safer alternative treatment for pericarditis. Nevertheless, the potential deleterious effects of antiinflammatory agents on the healing process should certainly be considered.

Many other drugs are commonly given to patients after a heart attack, usually to limit the progressive dilatation of the left ventricular after myocardial infarction. The angiotensin-converting-enzyme (ACE) inhibitor captopril has been shown to be effective in reducing mortality after infarction,[37] presumably in part because of its limitation of ventricular remodeling. It is possible that captopril could exert an effect on the scar, but this possibility has not been examined. In contrast, we found that another ACE inhibitor, quinapril, given immediately after infarction in spontaneously hypertensive rats, produced scars that contained thinner collagen fibers than those found in nontreated hearts examined 9 weeks later.[38] Further work must be done to examine the potential effect of ACE inhibitor therapy on scar healing. In addition, because we do not know when the healing process is completed, it is possible that healing could be affected even when drugs are given months after infarction.

We have seen that reperfusion of an occluded artery may enhance the healing process, but are there any pharmacological interventions that can promote healing? This is not a new idea. Almost 30 years ago Dr. Richard Bing's group demonstrated enhanced protein synthesis in the scar by administration of bovine growth hormone.[39] More recently, it was suggested that growth hormone treatment could decrease the incidence of ventricular aneurysm formation after myocardial infarction in rats.[40] Unfortunately, there were significant differences in infarct size between the treated and untreated groups in this study, which may well confound the results. We performed a similar study and found that growth hormone treatment started before or after coronary artery occlusion in rats produced an increase in collagen content of the scar examined one week after occlusion; however, there was no reduction in the degree of infarct expansion.[41] It may prove difficult to enhance healing in animal models such as the rat because they naturally heal quite rapidly. In this regard, it should be noted that attempts to enhance wound healing in other tissues (most notably the skin where immediate access to the bulk of the tissue is readily attained by topical application of the wound enhancing agent) have been most successful in situations where the normal healing process has been compromised. For example, Beck et al.[42] found that transforming growth factor-β1 was able to increase the breaking strength of skin wounds in both old rats and rats treated with methylprednisolone. Without the growth factor, the breaking strength of wounds from both of these groups was lower than in non-treated mature animals. Dermal wound healing has also been enhanced in diabetic mice using platelet-derived growth factor and basic fibroblast growth factor[43]; however, the use of such agents to enhance myocardial repair in subjects with compromised healing has not been investigated.

Existing Conditions

Finally in this section, I will briefly mention two special circumstances that might adversely affect healing after myocardial infarction; diabetes and aging. Kranz et al.[44] found that infarcts in alloxan-diabetic rats were associated with the presence of myocardial abscesses surrounded by loose connective tissue. It is well-known that diabetic patients have a worse outcome after myocardial infarction even when their usually higher incidence of risk factors is taken into account.[45] The precise reasons for the increased mortality with diabetes are unknown; however, it is possible that impairment of the normal healing process may be involved. Similarly, the reasons for the association of age with poor outcome after infarction are unclear. It is known that healing is impaired with increasing age,[42] but there has been limited examination of myocardial scar healing in old subjects. Kranz et al.[46] noted few changes except for a decrease in the number of fibroblasts synthesizing collagen precursors in old rats; however, they did not assess collagen content, type, crosslinks, or organization.

Detection of Collagen Changes In Vivo

The above discussions have examined many methods to assess changes in the scar in vitro, which although useful in enhancing our understanding of the healing process, are not practical for in vivo assessment. The three most promising noninvasive methods to assess scar tissue characteristics in vivo are nuclear magnetic resonance, acoustic analysis, and biochemical analysis of blood samples.

Magnetic Resonance

Changes in myocardial collagen content have been associated with changes in atomic nuclei relaxation times obtained using nuclear magnetic resonance. Specifically, T2 (spin-spin) relaxation times in the hearts of spontaneously hypertensive rats correlated with myocardial hydroxyproline content.[47] Additionally, Wisenberg et al.[48] found that T2 relaxation times remained elevated in nonreperfused dogs examined 3 weeks after myocardial infarction when compared to those measured in dogs reperfused 2 hours after coronary artery occlusion (Figure 4A). Because the water content of the scars, a significant determinant of relaxation times, was the same in reperfused and nonreperfused groups, they speculated that the observed difference in relaxation times might be due to differences in the collagen content or ultrastructure. Although these observed differences do not yet provide sufficient information for clinical decision making, the use of high resolution magnetic resonance techniques such as those used to examine skin[49] may allow more detailed structural information to be obtained.

Acoustic Analysis

Two-dimensional echocardiography is perhaps the most useful method to image the heart in vivo. Correlations have been found between the amount of myocardial collagen and echocardiographic assessment of regional echo amplitude in both fibrotic[50] and nonfibrotic hearts.[51] Furthermore, two-dimensional echocardiography has, on the basis of increases in pixel brightness in images of the heart, been shown to be capable of distinguishing between "recent" (within 48 hours) and "healed" (later than 4 weeks) infarcts.[52] More detailed examination of acoustic properties of the heart such as attenuation and backscatter of ultrasonic signals have revealed additional information. Mimbs et al.[53] found that collagen content in myocardial infarcts in dog hearts examined at 2, 4, and 6 weeks after infarction correlated with an in vitro assessment of ultrasonic attenuation. Moreover, this corre la-

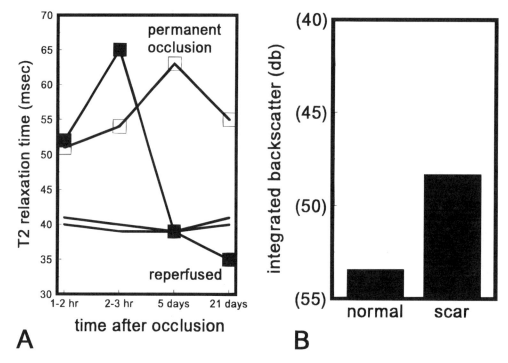

Figure 4. Examples of nuclear magnetic resonance and acoustic differences found in myocardial scar tissue. Panel A: Temporal changes in T2 relaxation times, obtained using nuclear magnetic resonance, in the infarcts of dogs after permanent coronary artery occlusion (open boxes) and in dogs reperfused 2 hours after occlusion (closed boxes). T2 relaxation times in control, noninfarcted tissue did not change (lines without symbols). Figure adapted with permission from data presented in Wisenberg et al.,[48] Am Heart J 1988;115:510–518. Panel B: Greater angle averaged ultrasonic backscatter (parentheses indicate negative numbers) was found in scar versus normal tissue. Figure adapted with permission from Wickline et al.,[23] Circulation 1992;85:259–268, copyright 1992 American Heart Association.

tion improved with time after infarction. They also found that after perfusing rabbit hearts with collagenase, neither the hydroxyproline content nor the ultrasonic attenuation changed. In contrast, ultrasonic backscatter decreased significantly in collagenase perfused hearts. These findings illustrate the importance of the physical configuration of the collagen on acoustic properties. This point was emphasized in a study by Wickline et al.,[23] who found transmural differences in ultrasonic backscatter in formalin fixed myocardial scars from patients who underwent cardiac allograft transplantation for end-stage ischemic heart disease (Figure 4B). They attributed the changes in backscatter to changes in collagen fiber orientation across the scar. Specifically, the results were consistent with a trilayered struc-

ture, which in turn is consistent with the three collagen layers found in our morphological study of scars in canine hearts.[13] Although the two studies assessing backscatter of acoustic signals were performed *in vitro*, the methods are approaching the point where they might be used *in vivo* to enhance the currently available echocardiographic methods.

Biochemical Analysis

It may be possible to use biochemical analysis to follow changes in the healing process. Jensen et al.[54] measured the blood serum content of a procollagen type III amino-terminal peptide (PIIINP) after myocardial infarction. This extension peptide of type III procollagen is cleaved off during conversion to type III collagen, and then passes into the extracellular fluid. Elevated serum levels of the peptide would reflect either increased synthesis or degradation of type III collagen. They compared serum levels of the peptide in 16 patients with acute myocardial infarction and 15 control patients. Significantly elevated levels of PIIINP were found on the second day after infarction. Although the levels peaked anytime from days 2 through 7, they remained elevated for at least 4 months, suggesting that infarct healing is a protracted process. The levels had returned to normal values 22 to 24 months after infarction. The peak serum PIIINP level correlated with infarct size estimated by both lactate dehydrogenase and creatine kinase isoenzyme MB, a finding consistent with the correlation of infarct size and tissue hydroxyproline content shown by Jugdutt and Amy.[6] Another clinical biochemical analysis of blood after transmural myocardial infarction followed the serum levels of the collagen-associated amino acids hydroxyproline and hydroxylysine.[55] Serum levels of both amino acids were significantly lower 24 hours after infarction than control values, but then increased. The levels were still elevated between 3 and 4 weeks later, consistent with the previous study. Whether such analysis would be a practical method to diagnose abnormal healing remains to be seen. However, Jensen et al.[54] observed higher than expected levels of PIIINP 2 days after infarction in a patient who subsequently developed a septal aneurysm. This patient's PIIINP levels started to increase again 7 days after infarction, in contrast to the other patients who did not develop aneurysms. Although a single case, it does suggest that biochemical analysis may be useful to identify abnormal healing.

Effects of Healing on NonInfarcted Myocardium

It would be naive to think that the healing process occurs in isolation from the rest of the heart. There is growing evidence that the structural changes that occur in the scar have a profound effect on the rest of the heart. Although this is a topic that will be covered by some of the other chapters in this book, there are some aspects of these changes that are worth emphasizing.

Collagen Changes in Noninfarcted Myocardium

In addition to the increase in collagen content in the scar, several groups have reported an increase in the collagen content of noninfarcted tissue. Volders et al.[56] used morphometric methods to compare collagen content in patients who died between 6 weeks and 13 years after myocardial infarction (mean 5.6 years), with age and gender matched control hearts without cardiovascular disease. They found an approximate 2.5-fold increase in collagen in the noninfarcted intraventricular septum (in the mid-septal region the increase was from 4% to 10%). Hypertrophied hearts from hypertensive patients (defined as systolic blood pressure >140 mmHg and diastolic pressure >90 mmHg) contained a similar increase in collagen while hypertrophied hearts in the absence of hypertension showed no collagen increase. These findings suggested that the hypertrophy associated with myocardial infarction was not necessarily responsible for the increase in collagen content, and the authors speculated that another factor, perhaps increased levels of angiotensin II or catecholamines may play a role. In contrast, Jugdutt and Amy[6] found no increase in the collagen content of noninfarcted canine tissue, but the analysis was performed only 6 weeks after infarction.

There is also evidence for changes in collagen type composition and collagen crosslinking. Bishop et al.[57] found that there was a significant reduction in the proportion of type III collagen present in nonscarred regions of patients with a history of transmural myocardial infarction who were undergoing orthotopic heart transplantation (35% ± 2% versus 42% ± 1% in control hearts). This decrease in the proportion of type III collagen occurred despite a slight increase in the actual amount of type III collagen; there was a substantial increase in the amount of type I collagen. In noninfarcted tissue examined 13 weeks after permanent coronary artery occlusion in rats, McCormick et al.[18] not only found an increase in collagen content in both the viable freewall and interventricular septum, but also noted an increase in the concentration of hydroxylysylpyridinoline crosslinks.

Myocyte Disorganization in Noninfarcted Myocardium

It is not only the collagen in the noninfarcted tissue that is affected by the presence of myocardial infarction. In the mid-myocardium of normal hearts, the myocytes are highly organized and are aligned virtually parallel to each other. In contrast, we found that viable muscle in the regions adjacent to the scar tissue in dogs loses this organization[13] (Figure 5A). We found evidence of disarray as early as 4 to 5 days after infarction and the degree of muscle disorganization increased with time (Figure 5B). In fact, we found no region of muscle adjacent to the scar 6 weeks after infarction that had a normal organization. Such disorganization was found as far as 1.2 cm from the edge of the scar, which if present on both sides of the scar would represent a substantial percentage of the circumference of the remaining viable muscle.

Functional Consequences of Structural Changes in Noninfarcted Myocardium

It is likely that the structural changes to both collagen and muscle will have functional consequences. Increased collagen content, crosslinking, and a greater proportion of type I collagen will probably increase myocardial stiffness and hence could reduce contractility. Muscle disarray is also likely to reduce contractility, a concept supported by studies that found infarct size was overestimated by two-dimensional echocardiography (muscle disarray results in dyskinesis or even akinesis adjacent to the scar and so the noncontracting area will include both scar and viable muscle). In addition, the structural changes could produce conduction abnormalities in the heart. Electrical signals will not propagate in the normal way if the muscle is disorganized (conduction parallel to the long axis of a myocyte is twice as fast as perpendicular conduction), and increased collagen concentration will reduce or block intercellular connections between myocytes. Bélichard et al.[58] demonstrated that rats with moderate or large transmural infarcts were far more susceptible to ventricular tachycardia or fibrillation by programmed electrical stimulation 5 weeks after myocardial infarction than noninfarcted hearts. Captopril treatment which resulted in less ventricular dilation, less hypertrophy, and reduced collagen content in the noninfarcted tissue, significantly reduced the susceptibility to arrhythmias. A similar reduction in susceptibility was found in rats treated with the beta-blocker, propranolol. Despite a reduction in hypertrophy, propranolol did not reduce ventricular dilation and increased the collagen content of noninfarcted tissue. Although it is possible that the reduction in hypertrophy was the key factor (the authors did not examine muscle organization), it is unclear how such different effects on remodeling of the heart after infarction could produce similar results. In addition, Vracko et al.[59] found evidence of nerve growth after infarction from areas of viable muscle into and along the edge of the scar with nerve densities greater than normally seen. Such changes in noninfarcted tissue could also play a role in the development of lethal arrhythmias after myocardial infarction.

These last studies illustrate the complexity of the process initiated by myocardial infarction. We are only just beginning to appreciate that the infarcted and noninfarcted region cannot be considered as separate entities. The mechanism of how these two regions are interconnected will be a promising area for future research.

Summary

Wound healing is an underappreciated component of myocardial infarction. The healing phase is, in fact, dynamic and multifaceted. Healing begins soon after the onset of ischemia with the infiltration of inflammatory cells into the infarct. A mixture of types I and III collagen, possibly with other types as well, is produced in accumulating amounts starting a few days after infarction. The collagen molecules undergo increasing

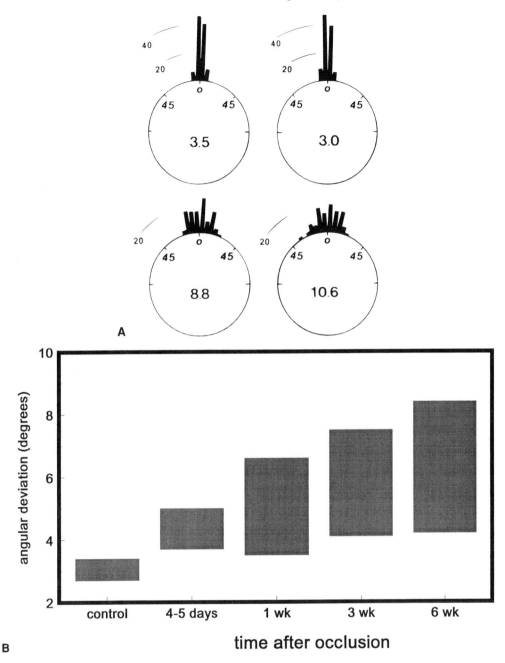

Figure 5. Illustration of the loss of the normal highly organized arrangement of myocytes in regions adjacent to scar tissue. Panel A: Circular histograms showing myocyte orientation in noninfarcted hearts (upper histograms) and in areas adjacent to scar tissue 6 weeks after myocardial infarction (lower histograms). Each orientation distribution is divided into 5° intervals. The mean orientation of each distribution coincides with 0°, while the angular deviation (a measure of the spread of the data) is indicated in the center of the circles. The scale indicates the percentage of cells with a particular orientation. Figure reprinted with permission from Whittaker et al.,[13] Am J Pathol 1989; 134:879–893. Panel B: Graph showing progressive disorganization of muscle adjacent to scar tissue. The angular deviation of individual orientation distributions is plotted as a function of time after permanent coronary artery occlusion. The shading represents the range of angular deviations obtained at each time period.

crosslinking, while the collagen fibers are arranged in an organized fashion. These changes result in increased stiffness and tensile strength. This process can be modified by external factors such as reperfusion of the occluded artery, treatment with various drugs or growth factors, or by preexisting disease or age. In addition, it is unwise to consider healing of the infarct as an isolated event, because profound changes occur in the noninfarcted regions too. Although the starting point of the healing process is well-defined, we do not yet know when (or if) this process is ultimately completed. Thus, in contrast to the gray, gelatinous object alluded to in the opening quotation, the scar formed after myocardial infarction is an important and dynamic entity that exerts considerable influence on both the structure and function of the heart.

References

1. Pasternak RC, Braunwald E, Sobel BE. Acute myocardial infarction. In: Braunwald E, ed. Heart Disease: A Textbook of Cardiovascular Medicine. 4th ed. Philadelphia, Pa: WB Saunders, 1992:1202.
2. Mallory GK, White PD, Salcedo-Salgar J. The speed of healing of myocardial infarction. A study of the pathologic anatomy in seventy-two cases. Am Heart J 1939;18:647–671.
3. Knowlton AA, Connelly CM, Romo GM, et al. Rapid expression of fibronectin in the rabbit heart after myocardial infarction with and without reperfusion. J Clin Invest 1992;89:1060–1068.
4. Casscells W, Kimura H, Sanchez JA, et al. Immunohistochemical study of fibronectin in experimental myocardial infarction. Am J Pathol 1990;137:801–810.
5. Lerman RH, Apstein CS, Kagan HM, et al. Myocardial healing and repair after experimental infarction in the rabbit. Circ Res 1983;53:378–388.
6. Jugdutt BI, Amy RWM. Healing after myocardial infarction in the dog: changes in infarct hydroxyproline and topography. J Am Coll Cardiol 1986;7:91–102.
7. Jugdutt BI, Khan MI. Impact of increased infarct transmurality on remodeling and function during healing after anterior myocardial infarction in the dog. Can J Physiol Pharmacol 1992;70:949–958.
8. Brady AJ. Passive elastic properties of cardiac myocytes relative to intact cardiac tissue. In: Robinson TF, Kinne RKH, eds. Cardiac Myocyte-Connective Tissue Interactions in Health and Disease. Basel, Switzerland: S Karger AG, 1990:37.
9. Przyklenk K, Connelly CM, McLaughlin RJ, et al. Effect of myocyte necrosis on strength, strain, and stiffness of isolated myocardial strips. Am Heart J 1987;114:1349–1359.
10. Medugorac I. Collagen type distribution in the mammalian left ventricle during growth and aging. Res Exp Med (Berl) 1982;180:255–262.
11. Vivaldi MT, Eyre DR, Kloner RA, et al. Effects of methylprednisolone on collagen biosynthesis in healing acute myocardial infarction. Am J Cardiol 1987;60:424–425.
12. Hering TM, Marchant RE, Anderson JM. Type V collagen during granulation tissue development. Exp Mol Pathol 1983;39:219–229.
13. Whittaker P, Boughner DR, Kloner RA. Analysis of healing after myocardial infarction using polarized light microscopy. Am J Pathol 1989;134:879–893.
14. Kischer CW, Brody GS. Structure of the collagen nodule from hypertrophic scars and keloids. Scan Electr Microsc 1981;III:371–376.
15. Kawahara E, Mukai A, Oda Y, et al. Left ventriculotomy of the heart: tissue repair and localization of collagen types I, II, III, IV, V, VI and fibronectin. Virchows Archiv A 1990;417:229–236.
16. Last JA, Armstrong LG, Reiser KM. Biosynthesis of collagen cross-links. Int J Biochem 1990;22:559–564.
17. Connelly CM, Vogel WM, Wiegner AW, et al. Effects of reperfusion after coronary artery occlusion on postinfarction scar tissue. Circ Res 1985;57:562–577.
18. McCormick RJ, Musch TI, Bergman BC, et al. Regional differences in LV collagen accumulation and mature crosslinking after myocardial infarction in rats. Am J Physiol 1994;266:H354-H359.
19. Junqueira LCU, Montes GS, Sanchez EM. The influence of tissue section thickness on the study of collagen by the picrosirius-polarization method. Histochemistry 1982;74:153–156.
20. Piérard GE. Sirius red polarization method is useful to visualize the organization of connective tissues but not the molecular composition of their fibrous polymers. Matrix 1989;9:68–71.
21. Carrasco FH, Montes GS, Krisztan RM, et al. Comparative morphologic and histochemical studies on the collagen of vertebrate arteries. Blood Vessels 1981;18:296–302.
22. Forrester JC, Zederfeldt BH, Hayes TL, et al.

Wolff's law in relation to the healing skin wound. J Trauma 1970;10:770–779.

23. Wickline SA, Verdonk ED, Wong AK, et al. Structural remodeling of human myocardial tissue after infarction. Quantification with ultrasonic backscatter. Circulation 1992;85: 259–268.

24. Miura T, Shizukuda Y, Ogawa S, et al. Effects of early and later reperfusion on healing speed of experimental myocardial infarct. Can J Cardiol 1991;7:146–154.

25. Morita M, Kawashima S, Ueno M, et al. Effects of late reperfusion on infarct expansion and infarct healing in conscious rats. Am J Pathol 1993;143:419–430.

26. Roberts CS, Schoen FJ, Kloner RA. Effect of coronary reperfusion on myocardial hemorrhage and infarct healing. Am J Cardiol 1983; 52:610–614.

27. Honan MB, Harrell FE Jr, Reimer KA, et al. Cardiac rupture, mortality and the timing of thrombolytic therapy: a meta-analysis. J Am Coll Cardiol 1990;16:359–367.

28. Whittaker P, Boughner DR, Kloner RA. Role of collagen in acute myocardial infarct expansion. Circulation 1991;84:2123–2134.

29. Takahashi S, Barry AC, Factor SM. Collagen degradation in ischaemic rat hearts. Biochem J 1990;265:233–241.

30. Zhao M, Zhang H, Robinson TF, et al. Profound structural alterations of the extracellular collagen matrix in postischemic dysfunctional ("stunned") but viable myocardium. J Am Coll Cardiol 1987;10:1322–1334.

31. Whittaker P, Boughner DR, Kloner RA, et al. Stunned myocardium and myocardial collagen damage: differential effects of single and repeated occlusions. Am Heart J 1991;121: 434–441.

32. Brown EJ Jr, Kloner RA, Schoen FJ, et al. Scar thinning due to ibuprofen administration after experimental myocardial infarction. Am J Cardiol 1983;51:877–883.

33. Hammerman H, Kloner RA, Schoen FJ, et al. Indomethacin-induced scar thinning after experimental myocardial infarction. Circulation 1983;67:1290–1295.

34. Cannon RO III, Rodriguez ER, Speir E, et al. Effect of ibuprofen on the healing phase of experimental myocardial infarction in the rat. Am J Cardiol 1985;55:1609–1613.

35. Przyklenk K. Effect of chronic ibuprofen therapy on early healing of experimentally induced myocardial infarction in dogs. Am J Cardiol 1989;63:1146–1148.

36. Mannisi JA, Weisman HF, Bush DE, et al. Steroid administration after myocardial infarction promotes early infarct expansion. J Clin Invest 1987;79:1431–1439.

37. Pfeffer MA, Braunwald E, Moyé LA, et al. Effect of captopril on mortality and morbidity in patients with left ventricular dysfunction after myocardial infarction. Results of the survival and ventricular enlargement trial. N Engl J Med 1992;327:669–677.

38. Zdrojewski T, Gaudron P, Whittaker P, et al. Divergent effects of ACE-inhibition on hemodynamics and scar healing after myocardial infarction in spontaneously hypertensive rats. (Abstract) J Am Coll Cardiol 1994; 23:412A.

39. Gudbjarnason S, Fenton JC, Wolf PL, et al. Stimulation of reparative processes following experimental myocardial infarction. Arch Intern Med 1966;118:33–40.

40. Castagnino HE, Toranzos FA, Milei J, et al. Preservation of myocardial collagen framework by human growth hormone in experimental infarctions and reduction in the incidence of ventricular aneurysms. Int J Cardiol 1992;35:101–114.

41. Whittaker P, Kloner RA. Growth hormone treatment accelerates collagen deposition in myocardial scars. (Abstract) Circulation 1990;82(Suppl.III):289.

42. Beck LS, DeGuzman L, Lee WP, et al. One systemic administration of transforming growth factor-β1 reverses age-or glucocorticoid-impaired wound healing. J Clin Invest 1993;92:2841–2849.

43. Greenhalgh DG, Sprugel KH, Murray MJ, et al. PDGF and FGF stimulate wound healing in the genetically diabetic mouse. Am J Pathol 1990;136:1235–1246.

44. Kranz D, Hecht A, Fuhrmann I, et al. The influence of diabetes mellitus and hypercorticism on the wound healing of experimental myocardial infarction in rats. Exp Pathol Bd 1977;14:1–8.

45. Stone PH, Muller JE, Hartwell T, et al. The effect of diabetes mellitus on prognosis and serial left ventricular function after acute myocardial infarction: contribution of both coronary disease and diastolic left ventricular dysfunction to the adverse prognosis. J Am Coll Cardiol 1989;14:49–57.

46. Kranz D, Hecht A, Fuhrmann I. The influence of age on the wound healing of experimental myocardial infarction. Exp Pathol Bd 1975;11:107–114.

47. Grover-McKay M, Scholz TD, Burns TL, et al. Myocardial collagen concentration and nuclear magnetic resonance relaxation times in the spontaneously hypertensive rat. Invest Radiol 1991;26:227–232.

48. Wisenberg G, Prato FS, Carroll SE, et al. Serial nuclear magnetic resonance imaging of acute myocardial infarction with and with-

out reperfusion. Am Heart J 1988;115: 510–518.

49. Richard S, Querleux B, Bittoun J, et al. In vivo proton relaxation times analysis of the skin layers by magnetic resonance imaging. J Invest Dermatol 1991;97:120–125.

50. Shaw TRD, Logan-Sinclair RB, Surin C, et al. Relation between regional echo intensity and myocardial connective tissue in chronic left ventricular disease. Br Heart J 1984;51:46–53.

51. Lythall DA, Bishop J, Grenbaum RA, et al. Relationship between myocardial collagen and echo amplitude in non-fibrotic hearts. Eur Heart J 1993;14:344–350.

52. Chandraratna PAN, Ulene R, Nimalasuriya A, et al. Differentiation between acute and healed myocardial infarction by signal averaging and color encoding two-dimensional echocardiography. Am J Cardiol 1985;56: 381–384.

53. Mimbs JW, O'Donnell M, Bauwens D, et al. The dependence of ultrasonic attenuation and backscatter on collagen content in dog and rabbit hearts. Circ Res 1980;47:49–58.

54. Jensen LT, Horslev-Petersen K, Toft P, et al. Serum aminoterminal type III procollagen peptide reflects repair after acute myocardial infarction. Circulation 1990;81:52–57.

55. Kucharz E, Drozdz M, Cerazy B, et al. Collagen metabolism in patients with myocardial infarction. Cor Vasa 1982;24:339–344.

56. Volders PGA, Willems IEMG, Cleutjens JPM, et al. Interstitial collagen is increased in the non-infarcted human myocardium after myocardial infarction. J Mol Cell Cardiol 1993;25:1317–1323.

57. Bishop JE, Greenbaum R, Gibson DG, et al. Enhanced deposition of predominantly type I collagen in myocardial disease. J Molec Cell Cardiol 1990;22:1157–1165.

58. Bélichard P, Savard P, Cardinal R, et al. Markedly different effects of ventricular remodeling result in a decrease in inducibility of ventricular arrhythmias. J Am Coll Cardiol 1994;23:505–513.

59. Vracko R, Thorning D, Frederickson RG. Nerve fibers in human myocardial scars. Hum Pathol 1991;22:138–146.

Chapter 4

Myocardial Rupture Postinfarction

Scott E. Campbell, Ph.D., Alberto A. Diaz-Arias, M.D.,
Karl T. Weber, M.D.

Introduction

Hospital survival in patients presenting with acute myocardial infarction (AMI) and either ventricular dysfunction or arrhythmias has improved over the past decade, a circumstance attributed to more aggressive management, including pharmacological and mechanical reperfusion techniques applied early after presenting symptoms and signs of AMI. At the same time, and despite interventional therapy for acute coronary occlusion, the incidence of myocardial rupture worldwide has increased.[1-3] Myocardial rupture is reported to be the second or third most common cause of death following AMI.[4,5] Literature reports indicate that 3% to 45% of patients with AMI experience cardiac rupture.[4-7] Particularly troublesome is the fact that patients presenting with rupture are more likely to have experienced their first transmural infarction which is not complicated by ventricular dysfunction or arrhythmias[2,5] and who should, therefore, otherwise survive their infarction.

Clinical Data

Age/Sex

Myocardial rupture occurs most often in the elderly patient population, primarily individuals 70 years or older. Data from the GISSI-2 trial[8] indicated the frequency of rupture in patients with their first myocardial infarction increased from 19% in patients <60 years of age to 86% among patients >70 years of age. In patients who rupture, there may be a predilection for male gender prior to the age of 60.[5,9] However, Dellborg et al.[4] found the highest incidence of rupture in patients <70 years of age in females.

The majority of clinical investigations have found that an equal number of men and women experience rupture following AMI.[5,7,10,11] However, epidemiologic data indicates that myocardial infarction occurs more frequently in men than women.[5] Accordingly, the general perception is that women, particularly elderly women, are more prone than men to rupture following AMI.

Previous Myocardial Infarction

The overwhelming majority of clinical studies have indicated that patients with previous myocardial infarction are less likely to rupture than those experiencing their first infarction.[2,5,10,11] It has been suggested that scars and/or interstitial fibrosis provide increased tensile strength to the myocardium,[12-14] thereby conferring an increased resistance to ventricular wall rupture. The predominant absence of scars secondary to previous infarction would suggest that coronary disease, e.g., atherosclerosis, would be less extensive in patients who rupture. Batts et al.[5] found

This work was supported in part by NHLBI grant R01-31701.

From Weber KT, MD *Wound Healing in Cardiovascular Disease,* Armonk, NY, Futura Publishing Company Inc.,
© 1995.

critical (grade 4) multivessel coronary disease in 81% of patients who ruptured, while Mann and Roberts[11] reported an incidence of 63%. However, Mann and Roberts[11] also found total or near occlusion and narrowing of coronary arteries to be significantly less in patients who experienced septal or free wall ruptures following AMI compared to those who did not rupture.

Infarct Expansion

Infarct expansion is defined as a fixed, permanent, disproportionate regional thinning and dilatation of the infarct zone.[15] It occurs in approximately 35% to 42% of anterior transmural infarcts, is overrepresented in patients who die within 30 days of myocardial infarction, and rarely occurs in nontransmural infarcts.[15] Although infarct expansion usually develops in large infarcts, it is the extent of the transmural necrosis, not the absolute infarct size, that predicts its occurrence. Schuster and Bulkley[16] found that 43% of patients with infarct expansion ruptured, while only 2% of patients without expansion ruptured. They determined that 96% of patients who ruptured in their study had infarct expansion.

The development of infarct expansion is relatively rapid. Rat studies have reported that 80% of experimentally infarcted animals develop expansion within 24 hours.[17] The severity of expansion increases from days 1 to 5 and its prevalence plateaus at 1 week. The anterior and anteroapical ventricular wall appear to be more prone to infarct expansion and rupture or late aneurysm than other sites.[18] Both cell stretch and myocyte slippage have been proposed as mechanisms to explain the occurrence of expansion. The anteroapical wall is thinner than other ventricular regions and may be more susceptible to myocyte slippage under abnormal loading conditions.[15] Infarcts in the anterior and anteroapical regions tend to be larger and perhaps are affected more by differences in ventricular load than other regions.

Experimental and clinical data have established a putative relationship between treatment with antiinflammatory agents and infarct expansion. In experimental studies, corticosteroid treatment has been shown to cause late aneurysm formation in association with infarct expansion.[19] Nonsteroidal antiinflammatory agents have also been shown to cause late scar thinning and regional dilatation. Hammerman et al.[20,21] reported greater infarct expansion and thinner scars following coronary occlusion in dogs when treated with indomethacin. Ibuprofen has also been shown to increase infarct thinning in dogs[22] and increase the incidence of septal rupture in humans following acute anterior myocardial infarction.[23]

Location of Rupture Site

Published reports categorize patients with myocardial rupture into three classifications based on site of rupture: papillary muscle; interventricular septum; and free wall. Rupture of the papillary muscle is relatively rare, occurring in 1.5% of in-hospital deaths and 8% of all ruptures,[4] and can lead to acute mitral incompetency with >90% mortality.[24]

Rupture of the interventricular septum is more common, reportedly comprising 10% to 20% of all ruptures.[4,25] Mann and Roberts[26] found less severe coronary artery narrowing in patients with AMI and septal rupture compared to patients with AMI who did not rupture. Septal rupture appears to be more frequently associated with posterior wall AMI,[26] although a relationship between anteroseptal apical infarcts and ventricular septal rupture has also been reported.[27] The time course from onset of AMI to septal rupture is relatively long, with 3 to 10 days most often reported.[4,26,27] Accordingly, with early diagnosis, surgical repair can be successful and the prognosis for recovery good.[28]

Rupture of the ventricular free wall is most common, comprising 50% to 75% of all ruptures.[4,5] Various preferential locations for the site of rupture in the ventricular free wall have been reported. Both anterior wall[10,11] and lateral wall[5] have been proposed as primary sites for rupture postinfarction. Although Mann and Roberts[11] found anterior wall locations for myocardial infarction and rupture to predominate, they did find that a significantly higher incidence of lateral wall infarctions occurred in ruptured compared to nonruptured myocardium. Free wall ruptures are almost always fatal, with the majority of deaths after onset of symptoms occurring within the first week.[5,7,11] However, as many as 22% of free wall ruptures,[10] and 30% of ruptures in general,[4] occur within the first 24 hours of AMI.

Thrombolytic Therapy

Lewis et al.[10] reported 92% of infarcted areas in ruptured patients were hemorrhagic. Prior to the advent of therapies designed to produce reperfusion postinfarction, hemorrhagic infarcts were reportedly fewer in number.[29,30] It has been suggested that hemorrhage can increase the extent of necrosis and delay healing.[31,32] The results of the ISIS-2 study indicated that the frequency of myocardial rupture was apparently higher in patients treated with streptokinase 24 hours after onset of chest pain compared to those receiving placebo.[33] However, several other studies could not find any difference in frequency of rupture between patients who received thrombolytic therapy and control groups.[30,34,35] Honan et al.[36] performed a meta-analysis of several thrombolytic treatment trials postinfarction. They concluded that early thrombolytic therapy postinfarction improves survival and decreases the risk of cardiac rupture, while late administration of thrombolytics also improves survival but may increase the risk of cardiac rupture.

Histopathology

Identification of the histologic substrate for myocardial rupture is a necessary step for the identification of its pathophysiological basis. A better understanding of the predisposing factors to this unsuccessful wound healing process may allow for the development of preventative measures. The issues of myocyte necrosis, inflammatory cell response, role of fibrillar collagen, and the impact of its breakdown must be addressed.

Myocyte Necrosis

Most ruptures occur in the latter half of the first week following infarction. This time course has lead many investigators to hypothesize that rupture occurs in infarcted myocardium when myocyte necrosis is extensive and the tissue is at its weakest point.[9,10,27] However, morphological data has indicated that myocyte necrosis need not necessarily be present for rupture to occur. Up to 30% of ruptures can occur in the first 24 hours of infarction,[4] preceding appreciable neutrophilic infiltration and coagulation necrosis. In studies of infarcted and normal myocardial strips from dogs 24 hours after occlusion of the left anterior descending coronary artery, Przyklenk et al.[37] found no difference in material properties, i.e., tensile strength, strain and stiffness, between normal and infarcted tissue. This lead them to conclude that myocyte necrosis, per se, did not appreciably affect tensile strength of the myocardium and implicated a weakness in the collagenous framework as more contributory to ventricular rupture. Lerman et al.,[38] examining normal and infarcted rabbit left ventricle 1 to 8 days after coronary occlusion, also found no decrease in the rupture threshold in infarcted hearts compared to normal. Following transmural infarction in the rabbit and either no reperfusion or late (i.e., 3 hours postinfarction) reperfusion, Connelly et al.[39] tested the tensile strength of infarcted tissue strips, the force required to initiate a tear in the central infarcted region, and the intracavitary pressure required to rupture the infarcted ventricle. They determined that within 24 hours, reperfused strips had less tensile strength than those with permanent occlusion, but tear threshold and response to increased left ventricular pressure was not influenced by reperfusion. At 3 days postinfarction, reperfused strips had equal tensile strength, greater resistance to tearing and were able to withstand greater left ventricular distending pressures that nonreperfused tissue. By 7 days postinfarction, all parameters tested were equal between nonreperfused and late reperfused myocardial tissue. This lead the authors to conclude that late reperfusion can accelerate myocardial healing postinfarction and may be beneficial in preventing rupture. These apparent beneficial effects of reperfusion may be related to the fact that fewer neutrophils are found in reperfused infarcts compared with permanently ischemic infarcts.[40] The importance of these inflammatory cells in myocardial rupture will be subsequently discussed.

Inflammatory Cells

The wound healing response to myocardial infarction involves migration and proliferation of inflammatory cells. Their contribution to myocardial rupture is still uncertain. Appreciable infiltration of neutrophils following AMI in man occurs within 24 hours,[29] reaching its peak on days 3 to 4. By 5 to 7 days, degradation of neutrophils is evident.[29] Eosinophils and macrophages are found between days 4 to 6, with macrophages persisting 2 to 3 weeks postinfarction.[29] A significant increase in infarct mass has been reported the first few days following infarction related to edema and inflammatory cell infiltration.[41] It has been proposed that this interstitial edema and cell infiltration may impede myocyte slippage early after infarction, thereby leading to less infarct expansion and possibility of rupture.[15,42] Antiinflammatory agents may promote rupture by reducing tissue edema and cellular infiltration, causing greater infarct expansion and predisposing to rupture. Inflammatory cells, particularly neutrophils, possess proteases including collagenase that may breakdown collagen and increase the possibility of rupture at later time points post-infarction. However, reduction of the inflammatory cell response following AMI in rats can lead to a reduction in collagen degradation within 24-hour-old infarcts.[43] The potential importance of collagenase and collagen degradation will be discussed in more detail below.

Fibrillar Collagen

A preliminary report in five postmortem human hearts drew attention to an additional important component of rupture that had previously been neglected, namely an absence of fibrillar collagen at the site of the rupture that appeared 3 to 10 days after AMI.[44] The collagen network of the myocardium has been morphologically defined using scanning electron microscopy[45,46] and shown to consist of predominantly type I and III fibrillar collagen.[47,48] This structural protein network is responsible for the alignment of myocytes to one another, as well as to their surrounding blood and lymph containing vasculature[13]; it thereby serves as a major determinant of myocardial architecture and geometry. Type I collagen, the major fibrillar collagen found in the myocardium,[47,48] is thought to have a tensile strength that approximates steel,[49] while type III collagen provides a resilience to the tissue.[50] A structural or biochemical defect of these fibrillar collagens is thought to predispose cardiovascular tissue to abnormal thinning and dilatation[51] and/or rupture.[13,44,52] For example, the loss of collagen strands between groups of myocytes was found in reperfused and stunned canine myocardium with segmental wall motion abnormality[53] and in the dilated, thin walled human heart with primary myocardial disease.[51] Cardiovascular aneurysm and rupture have been reported in several species, including man, associated with a copper deficient diet.[52] This was attributed to an impairment in collagen crosslinking associated with the copper-dependent enzyme lysyl oxidase.[54]

We wished to test the hypothesis that a loss of fibrillar collagen significantly contributed to the structural alterations resulting in ruptured myocardium. To determine whether such a loss of fibrillar collagen represented an integral component of the ruptured human myocardium seen after AMI and to compare the histopathologic profile amongst ruptured myocardium that presented clinically at variable intervals of time after AMI, we undertook a retrospective morphologic study of postmortem tissue available at this medical center over the past 20 years. To test this hypothesis we utilized the collagen specific stain, Sirius Red F3BA, together with polarization microscopy, to identify the structural integrity of fibrillar collagen in postmortem human tissue in which myocardial rupture following infarction was documented at autopsy. We also wished to address the element of time, i.e., the clinical presentation of rupture, as it pertained to the integrity of this collagen network (Table 1). The results of our study indicate that irrespective of time, a virtual absence of fibrillar collagen was found in the myocardium bordering the rupture tract following AMI (Figs. 1 and 2). The area of myocardium exhibiting this loss of collagen and the extent of myocyte necrosis was,

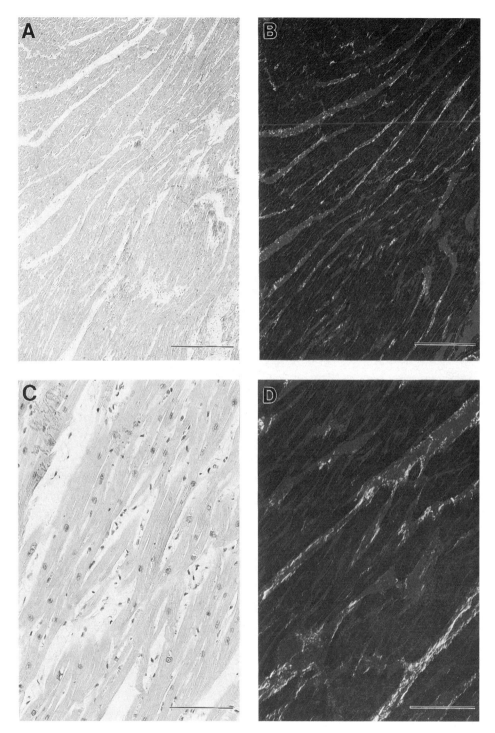

Figure 1. Light photomicrographs of normal myocardial tissue remote from the site of ventricular rupture. Panels A (H&E) and B (PSR; polarized light and first order filter): Equivalent tissue sections at low power. Note extent of interstitial collagen (bright areas between dark staining myocytes) in Panel B. Magnification bar = 0.5 mm. Panels C (H&E) and D (PSR; polarized light and first order filter): Equivalent tissue sections at high power. Note normal striated appearance of cardiac myocytes in both panels. Normally distributed interstitial and perivascular (solid arrowhead) collagen fibrils appear bright in Panel D. Magnification bar = 100 μm.

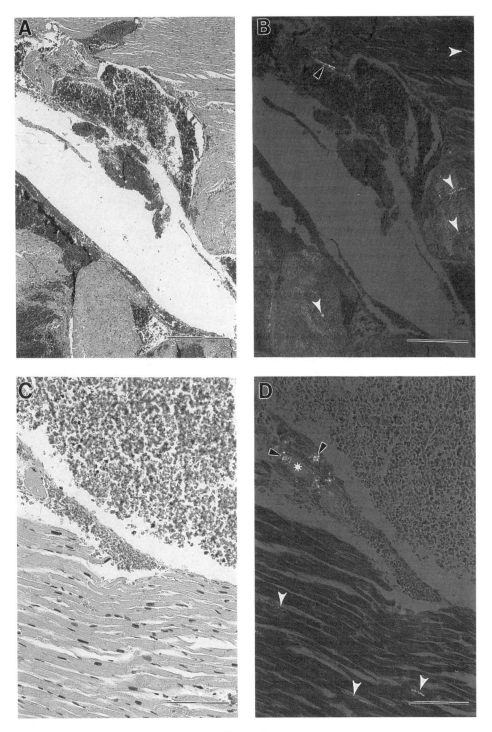

Figure 2.

—legend on facing page—

Table 1

Patients with Myocardial Rupture Following Acute Myocardial Infarction

Time to Rupture (days)	Age (years)	Sex	Heart Weight (g)	Rupture Site
1–2	70 ± 2	2M/3F	436 ± 38	3 anterior; 2 posterior
3–5	65 ± 3	4M/3F	511 ± 53	1 anterior; 5 posterior; 1 posterior septal/apical
6–10	67 ± 5	8M	563 ± 43	3 anterior lateral; 2 posterior; 1 posterior lateral; 1 lateral; 1 inferior septal

Values mean ± SEM; M = male; F = female

however, greater the longer the interval between infarction and appearance of rupture.

Our data indicate that a significant amount of collagen has disappeared within the site of rupture as early as 24 hours following AMI (Fig. 2). Even more rapid alterations in the connective tissue matrix have been reported. Sato et al.[55] found fibrillar collagen damage within 40 minutes of ischemia produced by occlusion of the left anterior descending coronary artery in porcine myocardium. Similar early collagen damage has been found in a canine model of coronary reperfusion.[53,56] Additionally, glycoproteins and glycosaminoglycans bound to collagen fibers may be equally important in maintaining the integrity of the collagen network. Sato et al.[55] documented disappearance of this material early after the onset of myocardial ischemia, leading to the suggestion that the earliest manifestation of damage to the connective tissue network was a loss of ground substance.[57] Whittaker et al.[58] reported evidence using a left coronary artery occlusion model in the rat to support this contention. They found a significant correlation between the reduction in collagen birefringence, assessed using silver-stained sections and polarized light, and the time after occlusion. This loss of birefringence was thought related to degradation of ground substance attached to collagen.

Collagenase

The rapid loss of fibrillar collagen following AMI is not likely to be solely a result of mechanical factors. In order to physically disrupt collagen fibers in the arrested rat myocardium, Factor et al.[59] had to introduce intraventricular pressures in excess of 100 mm Hg. However, Whittaker et al.[58] were unable to find collagen strut damage using the same distending pressure. More likely, proteolytic digestion provides for the rapid disappearance of fibrillar collagen from the infarcted myocardium. Immunohistochemical techniques have demonstrated that the myocardium contains collagenase.[60,61] Moreover, inflammatory cells that invade infarcted myocardium contain

Figure 2. Light photomicrographs of ventricular myocardium from hearts that ruptured within 48 hours postinfarction. Panels A (H&E) and B (PSR; polarized light and first order filter): Equivalent tissue sections from rupture site at low power. RBCs and PMNs can be seen in the rupture tract and bordering myocardium. In Panel B, solid white arrowheads indicate short strands of fibrillar collagen and solid black arrowheads denote perivascular collagen in bordering myocardium. Magnification bar = 0.5 mm. Panels C (H&E) and D (PSR; polarized light and first order filter): Equivalent tissue sections from rupture site at high power. Normally striated myocytes predominate in the myocardium bordering the rupture tract. In Panel D, solid white arrowheads indicate strands of fibrillar collagen and solid black arrowheads perivascular collagen. The white asterisk appears in the lumen of a coronary vessel; normally striated and necrotic myocytes are present surrounding the vessel. Magnification bar = 100 μm.

various proteases that could contribute to fibrillar collagen degradation.[62,63] Charney et al.[64] have reported collagen loss in stunned canine myocardium following 3 hours of repeated occlusion-reperfusion and a subsequent 90-minute reperfusion period. This was attributed to activation of latent collagenase or procollagenase in the myocardium, with polymorphonuclear contribution unlikely. Finally, oxygen metabolites that may be generated during infarction, with or without coronary reperfusion, are known to stimulate such proteolytic enzyme systems.[65]

Conclusions and Future Directions

Prediction of Myocardial Rupture

Considering the severity of the consequences of myocardial rupture, it is of great importance to be able to identify patients who may be susceptible to rupture postinfarction. Beyond the aforementioned patient profile, i.e., patient (more female than male) >70 years of age with a first time infarct, several studies have sought to further identify clinical signs that may predict rupture. In addition to a low occurrence or absence of previous myocardial infarction, Herlitz et al.[6] concluded that patients who rupture have a lower incidence of angina pectoris and their pain course during the acute phase of the infarction is more severe than patients with myocardial infarction who do not rupture. In a recent study by Oliva et al.,[66] patients who ruptured postinfarction were found to have a significantly greater incidence of pericarditis, repetitive emesis, and restlessness and agitation compared to patients without rupture. In addition, one or more episodes of abrupt, transient hypotension and bradycardia were common and unexpected alterations in T waves on the electrocardiogram (ECG) were often found. Failure of the T wave to invert, or reversal of polarity of inverted T waves, during the first 24 to 72 hours after transmural infarction were thought due to subepicardial ischemia progressing to necrosis or a slow, outward advancement of intramyocardial hemorrhage preceding rupture.[66]

Considering the importance of fibrillar collagen in maintaining structural integrity postinfarction and the deleterious effects of its degradation, it is tempting to speculate that the monitoring of collagen degradation following AMI might serve to identify patients at risk for developing myocardial rupture. Collagen breakdown has been monitored by serum samples following streptokinase therapy.[67] Experimental[68] and clinical[69] studies have shown that plasma hydroxyproline is increased within the first week following acute myocardial necrosis. Whether patients who develop rupture would have a greater than expected rise in collagen degradation products in their plasma remains to be examined.

Putative Therapeutic Regimens

A reduction in the incidence of myocardial rupture may be accomplished by proper pharmacological strategies. Stimulation of processes which aid the initial wound healing and diminish detrimental long-term consequences, e.g., progressive myocardial fibrosis, may improve survival in this patient population.

The potential benefit of thrombolyic therapy in preventing rupture has already been discussed. While earlier studies indicated a potential increase in the frequency of rupture with early thrombolytic intervention, i.e., the ISIS-2 trial, the majority of studies to date indicate a potential benefit of thrombolytic intervention.[36,70] It is generally believed that the decrease in amount of necrotic tissue, prevention of transmural infarction, and stimulation of an earlier healing process will lessen the chances of rupture postinfarction.

The systemic renin-angiotensin system is activated following AMI. Furthermore, unloading of the ventricle is considered important in preventing infarct expansion and late ventricular dilatation, events known to predispose to rupture. Treatment with angiotensin converting enzyme ACE inhibitors postinfarction can block these events and may also prove beneficial in prevention of myocardial rupture. Several experimental and clinical trials have shown that ACE inhibitors can modulate ventricular remodeling postinfarction. The apparent benefit and optimal timing for initiation of ACE inhibition postinfarction remain undetermined.

Clinical trials designed to determine the benefit of early intervention with ACE inhibitors are inconclusive. The CONSENSUS-II study randomized patients with AMI to receive early treatment (within 24 hours) with either placebo or enalaprilat/enalapril.[71] The study was stopped by the Safety Monitoring Committee before completion because it was felt that continuation of the study would fail to separate drug from placebo. At closure, the number of patients who died by the 6-month follow-up was greater in the ACE inhibitor group than those receiving placebo, although the difference was not statistically significant. A post-hoc analysis of patients 70 years of age or older indicated a trend towards "harm." In contrast, the SMILE (Survival of Myocardial Infarction Long-Term Evaluation) study found beneficial effects of early ACE inhibitor treatment postinfarction.[72] Patients were randomized to receive either oral zofenopril or placebo with 24 hours of acute anterior myocardial infarction. By 6 weeks, mortality was reduced and the frequency of refractory congestive heart failure was significantly less than placebo controls. Differences in these studies were thought to relate to selection of patients, route of administration of drug, or characteristics of each ACE inhibitor.[73] Further early ACE inhibitor treatment trials are ongoing. The ISIS-4 trial is comparing placebo to captopril treatment, and the GISSI-3 trial placebo to lisinopril, within 24 hours of myocardial infarction. Considering the importance of fibrillar collagen to structural integrity of the ventricular wall postinfarction and that effector hormones of the renin-angiotensin system can stimulate collagen synthesis, ACE inhibitors might interfere with the normal wound healing process early on and prevent necessary collagen deposition. This possibility remains to be investigated.

Delayed ACE inhibitor treatment following myocardial infarction has also been investigated. The SAVE (Survival and Left Ventricular Enlargement) trial administered captopril to patients within 3 to 16 days of infarction.[74] This study showed a 19% reduction in total cumulative mortality in the captopril treated group compared to placebo control, but no clear survival benefit was apparent until 1 year of treatment. The incidence of both fatal and nonfatal cardiovascular events was also reduced in the captopril group. The results of other delayed treatment trials postinfarction, i.e., the TRACE study administering trandolapril and the AIRE study treating with ramipril, have yet to be reported. Whether delayed treatment has a beneficial effect on late myocardial rupture has not been determined.

Finally, more experimental treatment regimens may be initiated. Modulation of lipid chemoattractant factors that govern the inflammatory cell response postinfarction might provide a possible interventional measure to prevent fibrillar collagen degradation.[75] It may be necessary to consider pharmacological strategies that could inhibit collagenase activation. Regulation of specific cytokines may help modulate the wound healing process postinfarction. Tranforming growth factor (TGF)-β has been proposed to play an important role in the response to myocardial infarction.[76] This cytokine is known to facilitate other types of wound healing[77] and can stimulate collagen synthesis and inhibit collagenase activity.[78] The possibility of exogenous TGF-β delivery to the site of cardiac injury in order to accelerate tissue repair should be considered.

Summary

Myocardial rupture is an important cause of death following AMI. Patients 70 years or older, predominantly female, and experiencing their first infarction are more prone to rupture. Infarct expansion is commonly associated with rupture and may result from myocyte slippage. Antiinflammatory agents can exacerbate infarct expansion and predispose to rupture. Ventricular free wall rupture is the most common, with anterior and lateral walls most frequently involved. Transmural infarcts are a prerequisite for rupture; however, myocyte necrosis, per se, does not seem to play an important role. Inflammatory cells can contribute to myocardial rupture, perhaps by releasing collagenase which degrades fibrillar collagen. Serum monitoring of patients postinfarction may predict those susceptible to rupture. Thrombolytic therapy appears to be beneficial in preventing rupture, although timing of treatment is an important consideration. ACE inhibitors may also prove useful in preventing rupture, but definitive conclusions from clinical trials remain to be reported. Pharmacological agents that can modify collagen turnover and/or specific cytokines known to promote wound healing need to be considered as therapeutic strategies in prevention of myocardial rupture.

References

1. ISIS-1 (First International Study of Infarct Survival) Collaborative Group. Mechanisms for the early mortality reduction produced by beta-blockade started early in acute myocardial infarction: ISIS-1. Lancet 1988;1: 921–923.
2. Reddy SG, Roberts WC. Frequency of rupture of the left ventricular free wall or ventricular septum among necropsy cases of fatal acute myocardial infarction since introduction of coronary care units. Am J Cardiol 1989;63:906–911.
3. Rovelli F, De Vita C, Feruglio GA, et al. GISSI trial: early results and late follow-up. J Am Coll Cardiol 1987;10:33B-39B.
4. Dellborg M, Held P, Swedberg K, et al. Rupture of the myocardium. Occurrence and risk factors. Br Heart J 1985;54:11–16.
5. Batts KP, Ackermann DM, Edwards WD. Postinfarction rupture of the left ventricular free wall: clinicopathologic correlates in 100 consecutive autopsy cases. Hum Pathol 1990; 21:530–535.
6. Herlitz J, Samuelsson SO, Richter A, et al. Prediction of rupture in acute myocardial infarction. Clin Cardiol 1988;11:63–69.
7. Solberg S, Nordrum I, Fausa D, et al. Cardiac ruptures in northern Norway. Acta Med Scand 1988;224:303–310.
8. Maggioni AP, Maseri A, Fresco C, et al. Age-related increase in mortality among patients with first myocardial infarctions treated with thrombolysis. N Engl J Med 1993;329: 1442–1448.
9. Shapira I, Isakov A, Burke M, et al. Cardiac rupture in patients with acute myocardial infarction. Chest 1987;219:219–223.
10. Lewis AJ, Burchell HB, Titus JL. Clinical and pathologic features of postinfarction cardiac rupture. Am J Cardiol 1969;23:43–53.
11. Mann JM, Roberts WC. Rupture of the left ventricular free wall during acute myocardial infarction: analysis of 138 necropsy patients and comparison with 50 necropsy patients with acute myocardial infarction without rupture. Am J Cardiol 1988;62:847–859.
12. Lerman RH, Apstein CS, Kagan HM, et al. Myocardial healing and repair after experimental infarction in the rabbit. Circ Res 1983; 53:378–388.
13. Weber KT. Cardiac interstitium in health and disease: the fibrillar collagen network. J Am Coll Cardiol 1989;13:1637–1652.
14. Weber KT, Janicki JS, Shroff SG et al. Collagen compartment remodeling in the pressure overloaded left ventricle. J Appl Cardiol 1988;3:37–46.
15. Weisman HF, Healy B. Myocardial infarct expansion, infarct extension, and reinfarction: pathophysiologic concepts. Prog Cardiovasc Dis 1987;30:73–110.
16. Schuster EH, Bulkley BH. Expansion of transmural myocardial infarction: a pathophysiologic factor in cardiac rupture. Circulation 1979;60:1532–1538.
17. Hochman JS, Bulkley BH. Expansion of acute myocardial infarction: an experimental study. Circulation 1982;65:1446–1450.
18. Bulkley BH. Site and sequelae of myocardial infarction. N Engl J Med 1981;305:337–338.
19. Mannisi JA, Weisman HF, Bush DE, et al. Steroid administration after myocardial infarction promotes early infarct expansion: a study in the rat model. J Clin Invest 1987;79: 1431–1439.
20. Hammerman H, Kloner RA, Schoen FJ, et al. Indomethacin-induced scar thinning after experimental myocardial infarction. Circulation 1983;67:1290–1295.
21. Hammerman H, Schoen FJ, Braunwald E, et al. Drug-induced expansion of infarct: morphologic and functional correlations. Circulation 1984;69:611–617.
22. Brown EJ, Kloner RA, Schoen FJ, et al. Scar thinning due to ibuprofen administration after experimental myocardial infarction. Am J Cardiol 1983;51:877–883.
23. Boden WE, Sadaniantz A. Ventricular septal rupture during therapy for pericarditis after acute myocardial infarction. Am J Cardiol 1985;55:1631–1632.
24. Sanders RJ, Neubuerger KT, Ravin A. Rupture of papillary muscles: occurrence of rupture of the posterior muscle in posterior myocardial infarction. Chest 1957;31: 316–323.
25. Christensen DJ, Ford M, Reading J, et al. Effect of hypertension on myocardial rupture

after acute myocardial infarction. Chest 1977;72:618–622.

26. Mann JM, Roberts WC. Acquired ventricular septal defect during acute myocardial infarction: analysis of 38 unoperated necropsy patients and comparison with 50 unoperated necropsy patients without rupture. Am J Cardiol 1988;62:8–19.

27. Hackel DB, Wagner GS. Acute myocardial infarction with ventricular septal rupture. Clin Cardiol 1993;16:143–146.

28. Daggett WM, Guyton RA, Mundth ED, et al. Surgery for post-myocardial infarct ventricular septal defect. Ann Surg 1977;186:260–271.

29. Lautsch EV, Lanks KW. Pathogenesis of cardiac rupture. Arch Pathol 1967;84:264–271.

30. Gertz SD, Kalan JM, Kragel AH, et al. Cardiac morphologic findings in patients with acute myocardial infarction treated with recombinant tissue plasminogen activator. Am J Cardiol 1990;65:953–961.

31. Bresnahan GF, Roberts R, Shell WE, et al. Deleterious effects due to hemorrhage after myocardial reperfusion. Am J Cardiol 1974;33:82–86.

32. Twidale N, Morphett A, Henry L, et al. Hemorrhagic myocardial infarction complicated by free wall rupture: a case associated with unusual clinical features following intravenous thrombolytic therapy. Aust NZ J Med 1989;19:138–140.

33. ISIS-2 Collaborative Group. Randomised trial of intravenous streptokinase, oral aspirin, both, or neither among 17,187 cases of suspected acute myocardial infarction ISIS-2. Lancet 1988;2:349–360.

34. Yusuf S, Collins R, Peto R, et al. Intravenous and intracoronary fibrinolytic therapy in acute myocardial infarction: overview of results on mortality, reinfarction and side-effects from 33 randomized controlled trials. Eur Heart J 1985;6:556–585.

35. The ISAM Study Group. A prospective trial of intravenous streptokinase in acute myocardial infarction (ISAM): mortality, morbidity, and infarct size at 21 days. N Engl J Med 1986;314:1465–1471.

36. Honan MB, Harrell FE Jr, Reimer KA, et al. Cardiac rupture, mortality and the timing of thrombolytic therapy. A meta-analysis. J Am Coll Cardiol 1990;16:359–367.

37. Przyklenk K, Connelly CM, McLaughlin RJ, et al. Effect of myocyte necrosis on strength, strain, and stiffness of isolated myocardial strips. Am Heart J 1987;114:1349–1359.

38. Lerman RH, Apstein CS, Kagan HM, et al. Myocardial healing and repair after experi-

mental infarction in the rabbit. Circ Res 1983;53:378–388.

39. Connelly CM, Ngoy S, Schoen F, et al. Biomechanical properties of reperfused transmural myocardial infarcts in rabbits during the first week after infarction. Implications for left ventricular rupture. Circ Res 1992;71:401–413.

40. Roberts CS, Schoen FJ, Kloner RA. Effect of coronary reperfusion on myocardial hemorrhage and infarct healing. Am J Cardiol 1983;52:610–614.

41. Reimer KA, Jennings RB. The changing anatomic reference base of evolving myocardial infarction. Underestimation of myocardial collateral blood flow and overestimation of experimental anatomic infarct size due to tissue edema, hemorrhage and acute inflammation. Circulation 1979;60:866–876.

42. Jugdutt BI, Basualdo CA. Myocardial infarct expansion during indomethacin and ibuprofen therapy for symptomatic post-infarction pericarditis. Influence of other pharmacologic agents during early remodeling. Can J Cardiol 1989;5:211–221.

43. Cannon RO III, Butany JW, McManus BM, et al. Early degradation of collagen after myocardial infarction in the rat. Am J Cardiol 1983;52:390–395.

44. Factor SM, Robinson TF, Dominitz R, et al. Alterations of the myocardial skeletal framework in acute myocardial infarction with and without ventricular rupture. A preliminary report. Am J Cardiovasc Path 1986;1:91–97.

45. Borg TK, Caulfield JB. The collagen matrix of the heart. Fed Proc 1981;40:2037–2041.

46. Borg TK, Sullivan T, Ivy J. Functional arrangement of connective tissue in striated muscle with emphasis on cardiac muscle. Scan Electron Microsc 1982;4:1775–1784.

47. Medugorac I, Jacob R. Characterisation of left ventricular collagen in the rat. Cardiovasc Res 1983;17:15–21.

48. Weber KT, Janicki JS, Shroff SG, et al. Collagen remodeling of the pressure overloaded, hypertrophied nonhuman primate myocardium. Circ Res 1988;67:757–765.

49. Burton AC. Relation of structure to function of the tissues of the wall of blood vessels. Physiol Rev 1954;34:619–642.

50. Parry DAD, Craig AS. Collagen fibrils during development and maturation and their contribution to the mechanical attributes of connective tissue. In: Nimni ME, ed. Collagen. vol. 2, Biochemistry and Biomechanics. Boca Raton, Fla: CRC Press, 1988:1–23.

51. Weber KT, Pick R, Janicki JS, et al. Inade-

quate collagen tethers in dilated cardiopathy. Am Heart J 1988;116:1641–1646.

52. Shields GS, Coulson WF, Kimball DA, et al. Studies on copper metabolism. XXXII. Cardiovascular lesions in copper-deficient swine. Am J Pathol 1962;41:603–621.

53. Zhao M, Zhang H, Robinson TF, et al. Profound structural alterations of the extracellular collagen matrix in postischemic dysfunctional ("stunned") but viable myocardium. J Am Coll Cardiol 1987;10:1322–1334.

54. Dawson R, Milne G, Williams RB. Changes in the collagen of rat heart in copper-deficiency-induced cardiac hypertrophy. Cardiovasc Res 1982;16:559–565.

55. Sato S, Ashraf M, Millard RW, et al. Connective tissue changes in early ischemia of porcine myocardium: an ultrastructural study. J Mol Cell Cardiol 1983;15:261–275.

56. Whittaker P, Boughner DR, Kloner RA, et al. Stunned myocardium and myocardial collagen: differential effects of single and repeated occlusions. Am Heart J 1991;121:434–441.

57. Whittaker P. Role of collagen in myocardial ischemia, infarction, and healing. Heart Failure 1990;6:151–157.

58. Whittaker P, Boughner DR, Kloner RA. Role of collagen in acute myocardial infarct expansion. Circulation 1991;84:2123–2134.

59. Factor SM, Flomenbaum M, Zhao M-J, et al. The effects of acutely increased ventricular cavity pressure on intrinsic myocardial connective tissue. J Am Coll Cardiol 1988;12:1582–1589.

60. Chakraborty A, Eghbali M. Collagenase activity in the normal rat myocardium. Histochemistry 1989;92:391–396.

61. Tyagi SC, Ratajska A, Weber KT. Myocardial matrix metalloproteinases: localization and activation. Mol Cell Biochem 1993;126:49–59.

62. Cochrane CG. Immunologic tissue injury mediated by neutrophilic leukocytes. Adv Immunol 1968;9:97–162.

63. Harris ED, Krane SM. Collagenases. N Engl J Med 1974;291:557–563, 605–609, 652–661.

64. Charney RH, Takahashi S, Zhao M, et al. Collagen loss in the stunned myocardium. Circulation 1992;85:1483–1490.

65. Lucchesi BR. Myocardial ischemia, reperfusion and free radical injury. Am J Cardiol 1990;65:14I-23I.

66. Oliva PB, Hammill SC, Edwards WD. Cardiac rupture, a clinically predictable compli-

cation of acute myocardial infarction: report of 70 cases with clinicopathologic correlations. J Am Coll Cardiol 1993;22:720–726.

67. Peuhkurinen KJ, Risteli L, Melkko JT, et al. Thrombolytic therapy with streptokinase stimulates collagen breakdown. Circulation 1991;83:1969–1975.

68. Takahashi S. A study on myocardial fibrosis in myocardial infarction and in idiopathic cardiomyopathy: a measurement of hydroxyproline level in plasma and in myocardium. Jpn Circ J 1979;43:913–921.

69. Kucharz E, Drozdz M, Cerazy B, et al. Collagen metabolism in patients with myocardial infarction. Cor Vasa 1982;24:345–353.

70. Gertz SD, Kragel AH, Kalan JM, et al. Comparison of coronary and myocardial morphologic findings in patients with and without thrombolytic therapy during fatal first acute myocardial infarction. Am J Cardiol 1990;66:904–909.

71. Swedberg K, Held P, Kjekshus J, et al. Effects of the early administration of enalapril on mortality in patients with acute myocardial infarction. N Engl J Med 1992;327:678–684.

72. Ambrosioni E, Borghi C, Magnani B, et al. Early treatment of acute myocardial infarction with angiotensin-converting enzyme inhibition: safety considerations. Am J Cardiol 1991;68:101D-110D.

73. Hall AS, Tan L-B, Ball SG. Inhibition of ACE/kininase-II, acute myocardial infarction, and survival. Cardiovasc Res 1994;28:190–198.

74. Pfeffer MA, Braunwald E, Moye LA, et al. Effect of captopril on mortality and morbidity in patients with left ventricular dysfunction after myocardial infarction. N Engl J Med 1992;327:669–677.

75. Schreiner GF, Rovin B, Lefkowith JB. The antiinflammatory effects of essential fatty acid deficiency in experimental glomerulonephritis. J Immunol 1989;143:3192–3199.

76. Thompson NL, Bazoberry F, Speir EH, et al. Transforming growth factor beta-1 in acute myocardial infarction in rats. Growth Factors 1988;1:91–99.

77. Sporn MB, Roberts AB. Peptide growth factors and inflammation, tissue repair and cancer. J Clin Invest 1986;78:329–332.

78. Roberts AB, Sporn MB. The transforming growth factor-βs. In: Sporn MB, Roberts AB, eds. Peptide Growth Factors and Their Receptors, Vol. I. Berlin: Springer-Verlag, 1993:419–472.

Chapter 5

Chronic Ischemic Heart Disease

A. Martin Gerdes, Ph.D.

Introduction

Chronic ischemic heart disease (IHD) is a common disorder often leading to heart failure. The term ischemic cardiomyopathy (ICM) is used when there is significant impairment of left ventricular function caused by atherosclerotic coronary artery disease.[1] The failing heart is characterized by ventricular dilation, with diffuse areas of myocardial damage consisting of replacement fibrosis, interstitial fibrosis, and myocyte hypertrophy.[2] The response of cardiac myocytes to chronic ischemia is of particular importance due to the mechanical role of these cells in pump function. This chapter will focus largely on myocyte remodeling to determine the contribution of these cells to the progression to failure as a result of chronic IHD.

In recent years, reliable methods have been developed and used to document changes in cardiac myocyte shape.[3] These techniques have allowed accurate characterization of changes in cell shape during postnatal growth, aging, hypertrophy, and failure.[4] Cumulatively, these data have provided important insight into the adaptive growth of cardiac myocytes. Isolated cell data from patients with heart failure due to chronic IHD suggest that maladaptive changes in cardiac myocyte shape underlie the adverse changes in ventricular geometry characteristic of this disease.[5] Since this earlier report, we have collected additional isolated cell data from patients with congestive failure due to ICM and nonfailing controls. All available isolated cell data collected from ICM patients in our laboratory will be analyzed and discussed in detail in this chapter.

Methods

Isolated myocytes of high quality (e.g., >70% rod-shaped cells) were collected from 11 patients with failure due to IHD (cardiomyopathy) and 5 nonfailing controls. The cell isolation procedure has been outlined in detail previously.[5] Briefly, freshly explanted tissue was placed into ice-cold cardioplegic solution for transportation to the lab. An epicardial vessel (usually a vein) was cannulated for perfusion of media followed by media plus collagenase. Distal epicardial branches were ligated to allow better perfusion of penetrating vessels. Digested tissue was minced and agitated to disperse myocytes. Cells were fixed immediately in glutaraldehyde for subsequent analysis of myocyte dimensions.

Myocyte dimensions were determined in the following manner: cell length was measured using a microscope; cell volume was measured using a Coulter Channelyzer; and myocyte cross-sectional area was calculated from cell volume and length (cross-sectional area = volume/length). Myocyte diameter was also calculated from cross-sectional area using the formula for a circle (area = πr^2; diameter = 2r). A detailed description of these methods and extensive documentation of their reliability have been reported.[3]

Results

Hearts from patients with ICM had significant coronary artery disease and diffuse

From Weber KT, MD *Wound Healing in Cardiovascular Disease*, Armonk, NY, Futura Publishing Company Inc., © 1995.

Table 1

ICM (Ischemic Cardiomyopathy), and C (Unsuitable Donors With Patent Coronary Arteries and Non-Failing, Non-Dilated Ventricles)

Patient Number	Age	Sex	BW (Kg)	HW (Gm)	LVEF (%)
ICM					
2344	57	M	76	465	19
2471	57	M	97	485	15
2516	49	M	82	575	22
2520	41	M	64	415	24
2522	62	M	96	685	16
2538	53	M	92	440	31
2569	47	M	78	480	16
2577	55	M	74	431	26
2605	41	M	77	344	12
2624	60	M	66	603	12
2635	53	M	83	616	15
Mean	52		80	503	19
C					
2523	46	F	53	NA	62
2524	49	F	57	380	58
2617	41	F	46	NA	70
2787	58	F	54	NA	70
2840	21	M	77	NA	NA
Mean	43		57		65

Body weight, BW; Heart weight, HW; LVEF, left ventricular ejection fraction; NA, not available. Data from Tables 1 and 2 were modified from Gerdes et al. (5) with permission from the American Heart Association.

and localized areas of myocardial fibrosis. Left ventricular ejection fraction averaged 19% for patients with ICM and 65% for non-failing controls (Table 1). Four patients with ICM had a prior history of hypertension (patient numbers 2522, 2569, 2605, 2624). Unsuitable donor hearts with widely patent coronary arteries, normal ejection fractions, and normal chamber volumes, served as nonfailing controls. Two of these patients were "true" controls with no prior history of heart disease (patient numbers 2617 and 2840). Hearts from these patients became electrically unstable and were not transplanted. Three unsuitable donors had hypertension but were used as controls since their hearts were nondilated and nonfailing (patient numbers 2523, 2524, and 2787).

Changes in left ventricular myocyte dimensions are shown in Table 2. A representative example of an isolated myocyte from a normal and failing heart is shown in (Figure 1). Myocyte volume was 25% greater in hearts from patients with ICM but the change did not reach statistical significance. Cell length was increased 42%. Cross-sectional area, cell width, and sarcomere length were unchanged. Cell length/width ratio was increased 55%. Thus, cardiac myocyte shape was significantly altered primarily due to a dramatic increase in cell length.

Discussion

Patients with congestive heart failure due to ICM typically have an increase in chamber diameter of approximately 40%.[6] Data from our patients indicated a similar increase in cardiac myocyte length (42%) suggesting that cell lengthening alone may account for all of the chamber dilation in these failing hearts. This should not be surprising since recent isolated myocyte data from hypertrophied hearts with volume and pressure overload have clearly demonstrated that changes in myocyte length and width parallel known alterations in chamber diameter and wall thickness, respectively.[4,7] Data from other laboratories, however, have suggested that slippage of myocytes past one another also contributes to the chamber dilation.[2] While isolated cell data alone cannot resolve this issue, it is clear that remodeling of myocyte shape is a major contributor to the characteristic alterations in ventricular geometry.

Recent data from experimental animals and humans have shown that myocyte shape, or more specifically length/width ratio, is tightly regulated within a narrow range (approximately 7 to 9). This ratio is maintained during normal physiological growth associated with postnatal development and during developing and compensated hypertrophy due to various types of overloading conditions.[4] Myocyte length/width ratio is a very useful parameter for comparison of individual data since it represents a normalized value and is the cellular analog to chamber diameter/wall thickness ratio which typically increases in failing hearts. In fact, an increase in this

Table 2

Isolated Myocyte Data

Patient Number	Cell Volume (μm^3)	Cell Length (μm)	C.S. Area (μm^2)	Cell Width (μm)	Cell L/W Ratio	Sarcomere Length (μm)
ICM						
2344	47,313	176	269	18.5	9.5	1.99
2471	50,300	216	233	17.2	12.6	2.05
2516	33,963	180	189	15.5	11.6	2.03
2520	43,039	187	230	17.1	10.9	2.12
2522	86,090	221	390	22.3	9.9	2.07
2538	42,167	204	207	16.2	12.6	2.06
2569	63,766	187	341	20.8	9.0	2.09
2577	27,627	183	151	13.9	13.2	2.05
2605	89,333	215	416	23.0	9.3	2.04
2624	66,573	201	331	20.5	9.8	2.05
2635	18,651	183	102	11.4	16.1	2.05
Mean	51,711(25)	196(42)*	260(13)	17.9(7)	11.3(55)*	2.05(2)
±S.E.	6,849	5	30	1.1	0.7	0.01
C						
2523	53,039	159	334	20.6	7.7	1.97
2524	45,002	131	344	20.9	6.3	2.01
2617	25,178	132	191	15.6	8.5	2.05
2787	55,509	133	417	23.0	5.8	1.95
2840	28,205	133	212	16.4	8.1	2.01
Mean	41,387	138	300	19.3	7.3	2.00
±S.E.	6,281	5	43	1.4	0.5	0.02

L/W, length/width; ( ), % difference from C; *, $P < 0.01$.

parameter appears to be specific for chronic remodeling associated with a dilated, relatively thin-walled ventricle.

It is clear that the appropriate myocyte adaptation to elevated afterload (e.g., pressure) is an increase in cross-sectional area.[4,7] Elevations in preload (e.g., volume) induce a proportional increase in cell length and diameter.[4,7] It appears that these adaptive growth reactions help return wall stress toward normal. The mechanism by which mechanical signals are transduced into parallel (e.g., increased diameter) and series (e.g., increased cell length) addition of new contractile units is very poorly understood. The unique architecture of myocyte cytoskeletal elements and myocyte-myocyte interconnections via collagen struts offers an enticing explanation. Cardiac myocytes are connected laterally by collagen struts which insert into the sarcolemma near the Z lines.[8] Within myocytes, radially oriented cyto-

skeletal elements associated with the Z lines of myofibrils connect the sarcolemma to the nucleus.[9] It is likely that the myocyte nucleus can instantaneously sense changes in wall stress via this mechanism. Although the mechanisms by which such signals may be converted into new series and parallel contractile units is unknown, increased pressure on the myocyte nucleus is known to stimulate mRNA synthesis.[10] It is possible that a disruption in this mechanical linkage could lead to a reduced signal for cross-sectional growth and produce the maladaptive change in cardiac myocyte shape characteristic of heart failure. Indeed, Weber et al.[11] have noted a reduction in intermyocyte collagen struts in failing human hearts. Schaper et al.[12] have also observed changes in the appearance and distribution of desmin within cardiac myocytes from failing human hearts. Obviously, this is an area of research that merits further investigation.

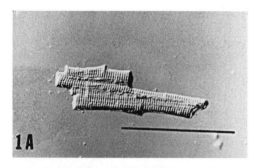

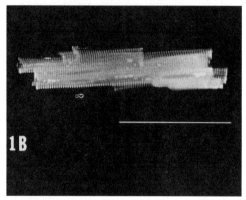

Figure 1. Panel A: Representative isolated myocyte from nonfailing human left ventricle. Nomarski optics: bar = 100 μm. Panel B: Representative isolated myocyte from the left ventricle of a patient with ischemic cardiomyopathy. Cell is labeled with rhodamine-phalloidin to show actin (same magnification as Panel A). Reprinted from Gerdes et al.[5] with permission from the American Heart Association.

Without exception, individual cell size data from the patients involved in this study demonstrated a perfect correlation between cell shape and ventricular architecture related to specific cardiovascular history. This is also the case with cells collected from other patients with idiopathic DCM.[13] Data from the two controls with no prior history of heart disease (e.g., "true" controls) are virtually indistinguishable from control data collected from other mammalian species (e.g., rats, cats, guinea pigs, and hamsters.)[14,15] Three other patients with hypertension were included in the "control" group because they had nonfailing, nondilated ventricles. As would be predicted, cell length was normal but myocyte cross-sectional area was elevated in these individu-

als. It is also interesting to note cellular dimensions of the four patients in the ICM group with prior hypertension. These patients had increased myocyte cross-sectional area values similar to the hypertensive, nonfailing group (means of 370 and 365 μm², respectively). They also had the highest values for myocyte length. Consequently, myocyte length/width ratio was increased to a comparable extent as in the other ICM patients without a prior history of hypertension. Myocyte cross-sectional area for the two "true" controls and the seven ICM patients without a previous history of hypertension were also the same (means of 202 and 197 μm², respectively). Cumulatively, these data suggest that progression to failure due to IHD is related to a selective and maladaptive increase in cell length without a concomitant change in cross-sectional area. This appears to be true irrespective of preexisting disease upon which ICM is superimposed (e.g., hypertension). It is also worth noting that identical changes in cell shape were observed in hearts from patients with similar gross anatomical remodeling due to idiopathic DCM.[13] Since those patients had no significant coronary artery disease, it is more difficult to conclude that chronic ischemia and/or hypoxia is directly responsible for the abnormal myocyte remodeling in these diseases. The fact that similar maladaptive changes in cardiac myocyte shape occur in both (ICM) and idiopathic DCM, however, suggests that a common final pathway may be involved.

Wall stress is directly proportional to ventricular pressure and chamber radius and inversely proportional to wall thickness.[7] Patients with failure due to ICM usually have elevated end-diastolic pressure, normal systolic pressure, increased chamber radius, and normal or reduced wall thickness. Although systolic and diastolic wall stress are increased, there does not appear to be an appropriate increase in myocyte cross-sectional area. The underlying reason for this maladaptation is not clear at this time. It is possible that transverse growth of myocytes is limited by inadequate microvascular blood flow in ICM. This problem would be exacerbated if diffusion distance were increased due to capillary spreading from increased myocyte cross-sectional growth. Alternatively, the series addition of contractile units (e.g., increased cell length) may not adversely affect diffusion distance if such a change were associated with a parallel increase in capillary length. An increase in cell length without an accompanying increase in myocyte diameter, however, would lead to further chamber dilation and increased diastolic wall stress (which is believed to be the stimulus for series addition of sarcomeres). It is generally believed that cardiac myocytes in adults have lost their ability to divide. Animal data from our lab have repeatedly shown that myocyte volume and heart mass increase proportionally in cardiomegaly suggesting that cell number remains constant.[4] Some investigators, however, have suggested that myocyte hyperplasia may be part of the adaptive response.[16-18] Typically, ICM produces an increase in heart mass of approximately 80%–90%.[2] Compared to the two "true" controls, cell volume was 94% greater in our pool of ICM patients. This suggests that hypertrophy alone may have been responsible for the heart enlargement. It is worth noting, however, that several patients with severe cardiomegaly had myocytes that were normal or below normal in size (e.g., patient numbers 2577, 2516, and 2635). On the other extreme, patient number 2605 had the smallest heart in the ICM group and the greatest extent of myocyte enlargement. Clearly, it is very difficult to reach a conclusion regarding possible changes in myocyte number based on morphometric measurements collected from a population with such great heterogeneity. It is easier to assess possible changes in myocyte number in controlled animal experiments where genetic variability can be minimized.[4] In the unlikely case that myocyte hyperplasia occurred in any of the human hearts in our study, it seemed to be of little value in attenuating or preventing heart failure.

Data from experimental animals indicate that cardiac myocytes are capable of at least doubling in size.[19] Some of the patients with ICM in this study had cardiac myocytes with volumes within the normal range. Therefore, it appears that myocytes from failing hearts have not necessarily exhausted their potential for adaptive growth. Altered cell shape, not cell size, appears to be the problem.

Summary

Myocyte length and length/width ratio were increased in patients with ICM. These changes reflect the gross anatomical alterations in wall thickness and chamber volume that are typical of ICM. Future research into the mechanism by which cardiac myocytes regulate cell shape may lead to improved therapies which attenuate or prevent this maladaptive change.

The cell sizing methods used here could be of diagnostic value in differentiating between acute versus chronic remodeling in patients with various types of heart disease. Unfortunately, a good method for isolating myocytes from biopsy samples is currently unavailable.

Acknowledgments: The author is grateful to Lawrence Miller, Lee Langley, Trish Carroll, and Tom Nolte from Lifelink of Florida (Tampa, FL) for their valuable assistance in obtaining cardiac tissue. I would also like to acknowledge the assistance of Jo Ann Moore, Linda Clark, and Dr. Douglas D. Schocken. This protocol was approved by the University of South Florida Health Sciences Center Institutional Review Board and the Institutional Review Board of Tampa General Hospital. Informed consent was obtained from individuals prior to transplantation or from next of kin (rejected donor hearts). Figures 1A and 1B, and portions of Tables 1 and 2 from *Circulation* 1992;86:426–430, were reproduced with permission of the American Heart Association.

References

1. Burch GE, Tsui CY, Harb JM. Ischemic cardiomyopathy. Am Heart J 1972;83:340–350.
2. Beltrami CA, Finato N, Rocco M, et al. Structural basis of end-stage failure in ischemic cardiomyopathy in humans. Circulation 1994;89:151–163.
3. Gerdes AM, Moore JA, Hines JM, et al. Regional differences in myocyte size in normal rat heart. Anat Rec 1986;215:420–426.
4. Gerdes AM. The use of isolated myocytes to evaluate myocardial remodeling. Trends Cardiovasc Med 1992;2:152–155.
5. Gerdes AM, Kellerman SE, Moore JA, et al. Structural remodeling of cardiac myocytes

in patients with ischemic cardiomyopathy. Circulation 1992;86:426–430.

6. Corya BC, Feigenbaum H, Rasmussen S, et al. Echocardiographic features of congestive cardiomyopathy compared with normal subjects and patients with coronary artery disease. Circulation 1974;49:1153–1159.

7. Grossman W, Jones D, McLaurin LP. Wall stress and patterns of hypertrophy in the human left ventricle. J Clin Invest 1975;56: 56–64.

8. Robinson TF, Cohen-Gould L, Factor SM. Skeletal framework of mammalian heart muscle. Arrangement of inter- and pericellular connective tissue structures. Lab Invest 1983;49:482–498.

9. Terracio L, Borg TK. Factors affecting cardiac cell shape. Heart Failure 1988;4:114–124.

10. Schreiber SS, Oratz M, Rothschild MA, et al. Effect of hydrostatic pressure on isolated cardiac nuclei: stimulation of RNA polymerase II activity. Cardiovasc Res 1978;12:265–268.

11. Weber KT, Pick R, Janicki JS, et al. Inadequate collagen tethers in dilated cardiomyopathy. Am Heart J 1988;116:1641–1646.

12. Schaper J, Froede R, Hein S, et al. Impairment of myocardial ultrastructure and changes of the cytoskeleton in dilated cardiomyopathy. Circulation 1991;83:504–514.

13. Gerdes ÁM, Kellerman SE, Schocken DD. Implications of cardiomyocyte remodelling in heart failure. In: Dhalla NS, Beamish RE, Nagano M, eds. The Failing Heart. New York, NY: Raven Press 1995;197–205.

14. Campbell SE, Gerdes AM, Smith TD. Comparison of regional differences in cardiac myocyte dimensions in rats, hamsters, and guinea pigs. Anat Rec 1987;219:53–59.

15. Kozlovskis PL, Gerdes AM, Smets M, et al. Regional increase in myocyte volume after healing of myocardial infarction in cats. J Mol Cell Cardiol 1991;23:1459–1466.

16. Linzbach AJ. Heart failure from the point of view of quantitative anatomy. Am J Cardiol 1960;5:370–382.

17. Anversa P, Fitzpatrick K, Argani S, et al. Myocyte mitotic division in the aging mammalian heart. Circ Res 1991;69:1159–1164.

18. Olivetti G, Ricci R, Lagrasta C. Cellular basis of wall remodeling in long-term pressure overload-induced right ventricular hypertrophy in rats. Circ Res 1988;63:648–657.

19. Liu Z, Hilbelink DR, Gerdes AM. Regional changes in hemodynamics and cardiac myocyte size in rats with aortocaval fistulas. II. Long-term effects. Circ Res 1991;69:59–65.

Chapter 6

Myocardial Collagenase in the Failing Human Heart

Suresh C. Tyagi, Ph.D., Hanumanth K. Reddy, M.D.,
Scott E. Campbell, Ph.D., Karl T. Weber, M.D.

Introduction

Irrespective of the site of injury, tissue repair and remodeling that follow are broadly referred to as wound healing. Wound healing initially involves collagen degradation, mediated by various proteinases. Ultimately, collagen synthesis determines fibrogenesis. The role of collagen degradation during healing includes the degradation of extracellular matrices, a contribution to new blood vessel formation (angiogenesis), and cell migration.[1,2] The matrix metalloproteinase (MMP) gene family includes multiple proteinases. Particularly relevant to collagen degradation in the heart is interstitial collagenase, which has the unique ability to cleave fibrillar type I and III collagens, the major fibrillar collagens found in the heart, as well as gelatinases.[3-8]

Tyagi et al.[9-11] have demonstrated that the majority of collagenase found in the normal rat myocardium, located in the interstitial space between muscle bundles, is in latent form. Furthermore, latent collagenase is activated by stromelysin,[12] neutrophil elastase,[11] and trypsin.[10] These studies suggest an extracellular regulation of latent collagenase in the myocardium by various proteinases.

The role of MMP in the wound healing response of the myocardium has not been studied extensively. Morphological evidence of fibrillar collagen degradation was observed in postmortem hearts obtained from patients with dilated (idiopathic) cardiomyopathy[13] in keeping with an earlier suggestion that the loss of structural protein scaffolding could represent the anatomical substrate for myocyte slippage and wall thinning.[14] Following myocardial infarction in rats, both morphological and biochemical evidence of collagen degradation[15-18] as well as myocyte slippage[19] have been reported to contribute to ventricular wall remodeling. Cleutjens et al. (see Chapter 13) have further characterized the response of MMP following infarction in the rat heart. MMP activation is also the case in a canine model of dilated cardiomyopathy (DCM) that accompanies rapid pacing (see Spinale, Chapter 8).

To further address the potential importance of collagenase activation in the dilated failing human heart, we determined and compared collagenase activity by zymography in normal and diseased adult human heart tissue obtained either at explant surgery or by endomyocardial biopsy in patients with advanced symptomatic heart failure due to idiopathic DCM or ischemic heart disease (IHD) with previous myocardial infarction(s).

This work was supported in part by NIH Grant GM-48595 (SCT); HL-31701 (KTW), and by a Grant-In-Aid (92–10517) from the American Heart Association, Missouri Affiliate (SCT).

From Weber KT, MD *Wound Healing in Cardiovascular Disease*, Armonk, NY, Futura Publishing Company Inc., © 1995.

Collagenases in Human Heart Tissues

Collagenolytic/Gelatinolytic Activity in Normal Tissue

Collagenolytic activity from normal human left atrial tissue, obtained from donor hearts at the time of transplantation, was compared to left ventricular tissue. Because of difficulties associated with obtaining normal human left ventricular tissue, normal human left atrial tissue was compared to normal rat left atrial tissue. Human left ventricle data were compared with normal rat left ventricle. Results suggested a similar expression of MMP activity on collagen/gelatin gels (zymography) in rat and human tissue.[20] Collagenase activity was 3% ± 1% in normal left atrial tissue, which could be activated to 80%–90% by trypsin or plasmin, indicating that collagenase was normally inactive or in a latent form in normal human heart tissue (Figure 1). Laurent[21] has reported collagen turnover of approximately 3%–5% in rat heart and in other tissues this value reached 10% per day. We found ~3% total collagenase activity, which may be involved in normal collagen turnover.

Several zones of cleavage, representing collagenolytic activity, were seen in these gels. The multiple band pattern after activation reflected the presence of latent and active forms of MMPs in normal human heart tissue (Figure. 1). The band at ~92 kDa is probably due to gelatinase (MMP-2, type IV collagenase) and ~52 kDa is due to interstitial collagenase (MMP-1). This interpreta-

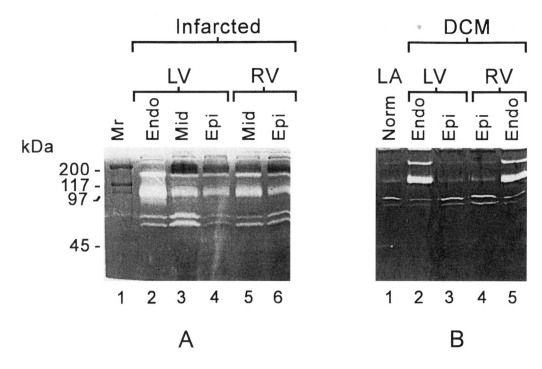

Figure 1. Representative example of collagenase/gelatinase activity in failing human heart. A, ischemic and B, idiopathic cardiomyopathy: zymography (10%) 1 mg/mL gelatin as substrate. A: Lane 1, molecular weight marker; lane 2, left ventricular (LV) endocardium; lane 3, LV midwall; lane 4, LV epimyocardium; lane 5, right ventricular (RV) endocardium; and lane 6, RV epimyocardium. B: Lane 1, normal left atrial tissue; lane 2, LV endocardium; lane 3, LV epimyocardium; lane 4, RV epimyocardium; and lane 5, RV endocardium. All samples were electrophoresed under nonreducing conditions. An extract of 0.2 mL (10 mg/mL of total protein) (pH 7.5) was prepared from 25 mg of tissue and 20 µL of this extract was loaded onto gels.

tion is based on our finding that in fibronectin gels the 92-kDa band was present but the 52 kDa was not. Interstitial collagenase does not cleave or degrade fibronectin in these gels.

Collagenolytic/Gelatinolytic Activity in IHD and DCM

Tissue from IHD and DCM was analyzed for MMP activity by zymography (Figure 1). In endo-and epimyocardium of infarcted left ventricle, collagenase activity was 85%–95% and 10%–20%, respectively, while it was 5%–10% and 3%–5%, respectively, in noninfarcted left ventricle. In DCM, collagenolytic activity in the endocardium and epicardium was 75% ± 5 and 35% ± 5% in the left ventricle and 35% ± 7 and 20% ± 5% in the right ventricle, respectively (Figure 1). Thus, in dilated failing human hearts, and particularly within the endomyocardium, collagenase activity was increased in both the infarcted and noninfarcted portions of either ventricle and in both ventricles in DCM. This suggests a generalized activation of collagenase may contribute to the remodeling of the myocardium and could account for the progressive nature of heart failure that includes ventricular dilatation and wall thinning.

Histopathological Evidence of Fibrillar Collagen Degradation in IHD and DCM

We examined myocardial tissue sections from both ventricles of explanted failing human hearts secondary to IHD or DCM (Figure 2). Tissue sections were stained with collagen-specific picrosirius red and analyzed by light microscopy. In infarcted hearts, extensive myocardial scarring was found. However, focal areas of collagen breakdown were noted in some scars (Figure 2). Also, in some areas of the infarcted heart, inflammatory cells were present. Fibrillar collagen appeared intact elsewhere in the same heart, but in areas remote to these scars. In contrast to infarcted hearts, tissue sections from failing hearts of patients with DCM exhibited less fibrillar collagen than normal, with some focal areas

where collagen was absent (Fig. 2). These histologic findings support our contention that focal and global breakdown of normal fibrillar collagen may occur in failing hearts postinfarction, as well as in association with DCM and could account for an architectural remodeling of the myocardium.

Collagenase in Endomyocardial Biopsies

Collagenolytic/Gelatinolytic Activity in DCM

We examined MMP activity in endomyocardial biopsy specimens obtained from patients with idiopathic DCM and compared these findings to biopsies obtained in patients following transplantation. Post-transplant tissue was considered normal control.[22]

Using echocardiographic guidance, biopsy samples were taken from the same location on the interventricular septum. This enabled us to assess collagenase activity in biopsy samples taken from the same region used for histopathological assessment of collagen morphology. Collagenase activity (63%) was markedly increased in DCM tissue in contrast to normal level of activity (<10%) found in posttransplant controls (Figure 3). Increased collagenase activity observed in the endomyocardial biopsy samples obtained from the DCM hearts may serve as a marker of the severity of the cardiomyopathic process.

Histopathological Evidence of Fibrillar Collagen Degradation in DCM

In DCM, there was echocardiographic evidence of left ventricular chamber dilatation and sphericalization. Histopathological examination by polarized light microscopy revealed areas of scanty myocyte necrosis and absent endomysial and perimysial collagen in areas with intact myocytes in DCM in contrast to normal fibrillar collagen found in posttransplant controls. Areas with little or absent collagen were seen in certain regions of the myocardium associated with markedly increased collagenolytic activity were the cardinal features.

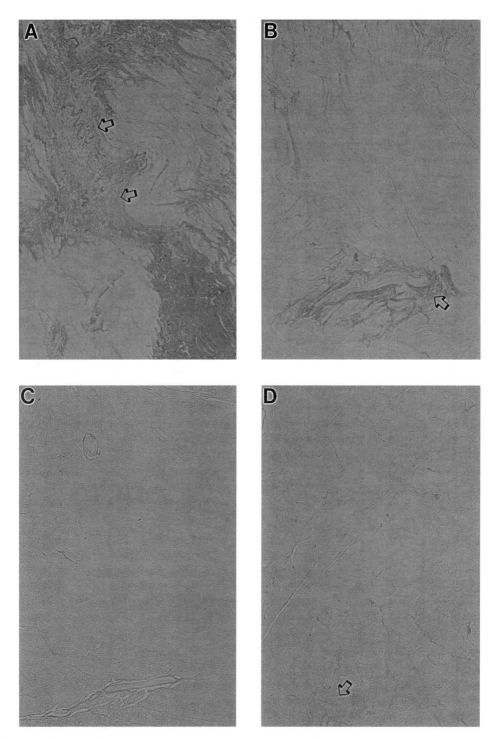

Figure 2. Histopathology of myocardial tissue from explanted human hearts postinfarction (Panels A and B) and following DCM (Panels C and D). Panel A, infarct region in left ventricle of postinfarct patient. Note dense scar in lower right of frame and focal degradation of adjacent region of the same scar (open arrows). Panel B, noninfarcted region of left ventricle. Perivascular fibrosis is evident (open arrow), but interstitial collagen appears normal to below normal. Panel C, left ventricle of DCM patient. Note virtual absence of fibrillar collagen. Panel D, right ventricle from DCM patient. Fibrillar collagen appears relatively normal. Area of perivascular fibrosis (open arrow) appears less dense than expected, possibly indicating some collagen degradation.

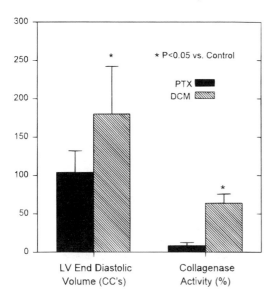

Figure 3. Collagenolytic activity (%) in endomyocardial biopsies and left ventricular (LV) size measured by echocardiography are demonstrated. PTX refers to posttransplant biopsy samples (control tissue); DCM represents patients with idiopathic dilated cardiomyopathy. Values are mean ± SD based on triplicate samples.

Summary

Myocardial collagenase in normal human heart tissue is present in latent form and could be activated by other proteinases. Activation of collagenase may play an important role in the pathophysiology of ventricular remodeling seen in idiopathic DCM and myocardial infarction. In infarcted ventricular tissue, collagenase activity was markedly activated. In noninfarcted tissue, obtained from hearts in which infarction existed, collagenase was also activated, but to a lesser degree. Collagenolytic activity was also increased in ventricular tissue from DCM hearts. Morphological evidence of collagen lysis was found in association with increased collagenase activity. This was particularly the case in idiopathic DCM tissue, where fibrillar collagen was significantly reduced. In endomyocardial biopsy specimens obtained from patients with DCM, collagenase activity was also increased when compared with controls obtained from transplanted hearts. Enhanced collagenolytic activity may contribute to ventricular dilation and wall thinning seen in heart failure.

References

1. Saarialho-Kere UK, Kovacs SO, Pentland AP, et al. Cell-matrix interactions modulate interstitial collagenase expression by human keratinocytes actively involved in wound healing. J Clin Invest 1993;92:2858–2866.
2. Grillo HC, Gross J. Collagenolytic activity during mammalian wound repair. Dev Biol 1967;15:300–317.
3. Welgus HG, Jeffrey JJ, Eisen AZ. The collagen substrate specificity of human fibroblast collagenase. J Biol Chem 1981;256:9511–9515.
4. Welgus HG, Fliszar CJ, Seltzer JL, et al. Differential susceptibility of type X collagen to cleavage by two mammalian collagenases and 72-kDa type IV collagenase. J Biol Chem 1990;265:13521–13527.
5. Matrisian LM. The matrix-degrading metalloproteinases. BioEssays 1992;14:455–463.
6. Hibbs MS, Hasty KA, Seyer JM, et al. Biochemical and immunological characterization of secreted forms of human neutrophil gelatinase. J Biol Chem 1985;260:2493–2500.
7. Murphy GM, Cockett MI, Ward RV, et al. Matrix metalloproteinase degradation of elastin, type IV collagen and proteoglycan. A quantitative comparison of the activities of 95-kDa and 75-kDa gelatinases, stromelysins-1 and -2 and punctuated metalloproteinase (PUMP). Biochem J 1991;277:277–279.
8. Matrisian LM. Metalloproteinase and their inhibitors in matrix remodeling. Trends Genet 1990;6:121–125.
9. Tyagi SC, Matsubara L, Ratajska A, et al. Identification and localization of myocardial collagenase(s). (Abstract) Clin Res 1992;40:757A.
10. Tyagi SC, Matsubara L, Weber KT. Direct extraction and estimation of collagenase(s) activity by zymography in microquantities of rat myocardium and uterus. Clin Biochem 1993;26:191–198.
11. Tyagi SC, Ratajska A, Weber KT. Myocardial matrix metalloproteinases: localization and activation. Mol Cell Biochem 1993;126:49–59.
12. Suzuki K, Enghild JJ, Morodomi T, et al. Mechanisms of activation of tissue procollagenase by matrix metalloproteinase 3 (stromelysin). Biochemistry 1990;29:10261–10270.
13. Weber KT, Pick R, Janicki JS, et al. Inadequate collagen tethers in dilated cardiopathy. Am Heart J 1988;116:1641–1646.

14. Weber KT. Cardiac interstitium in health and disease: the fibrillar collagen network. J Am Coll Cardiol 1989;13:1637–1652.

15. Cannon RO, Butany JW, McManus BM, et al. Early degradation of collagen after acute myocardial infarction in the rat. Am J Cardiol 1983;52:390–395.

16. Sato S, Ashraf M, Millard RW, et al. Connective tissue changes in early ischemia of porcine myocardium: an ultrastructural study. J Mol Cell Cardiol 1983;15:261–275.

17. Takahashi S, Barry AC, Factor SM. Collagen degradation in ischaemic rat heart. Biochem J 1990;265:233–241.

18. Factor SM, Robinson TF, Dominitz R, et al. Alterations of the myocardial skeletal framework in acute myocardial infarction with and without ventricular rupture. Am J Cardiovasc Pathol 1987;1:91–97.

19. Olivetti G, Capasso JM, Sonnenblick EH, et al. Side-to-side slippage of myocytes participates in ventricular wall remodeling acutely after myocardial infarction in rats. Circ Res 1990;67:23–34.

20. Tyagi SC, Reddy HK, Voelker DJ, et al. Myocardial collagenase and tissue inhibitor in dilated, failing human myocardium. (Abstract) Circulation 1993;88:I-407.

21. Laurent GJ. Dynamic state of collagen: pathways of collagen degradation in vivo and their possible role in regulation of collagen mass. Am J Physiol 1987;252:C1-C9.

22. Reddy HK, Tyagi SC, Tjahja IE, et al. Enhanced endomyocardial collagenase activity in dilated cardiomyopathy: a marker of dilatation and architectural remodeling. (Abstract). Circulation 1993;88:I-407.

Chapter 7

Myocardial Collagenase Activity in Experimental Dilated Cardiomyopathy

Joseph S. Janicki, Ph.D., Jeffrey R. Henegar, M.S.,
Scott E. Campbell, Ph.D., Suresh C. Tyagi, Ph.D.

Introduction

Myocyte loss, chronic diastolic ventricular volume overload, and chronic systolic arterial pressure overload are conditions which lead to a structural remodeling of the myocardial muscular, vascular, and interstitial components. However, compensatory cardiac myocyte hypertrophy, capillarization, and increased collagen content ultimately prove insufficient resulting in a failing, dilated, spherical left ventricle with wall thinning and muscle fiber slippage. Myocardial collagen fiber degradation represents a possible common pathway that could lead to these adverse structural and architectural alterations.

Fibrillar collagen provides for muscle fiber and cardiac myocyte alignment. It also imparts a tensile strength to the myocardium which maintains ventricular shape and size and governs tissue stiffness. An anatomical requisite for dilatation, sphericalization, and thinning, therefore, is a disruption of collagen fibers. Morphological evidence of collagen fiber degradation has been found in chronically dilated, thinned-wall, failing ventricles in man,[1] the cardiomyopathic Syrian hamster,[2] and the chronically, rapid paced animal.[3,4] Factors responsible for excessive myocardial collagen proteolysis may include increased synthesis of collagenase, activation of latent collagenase, and progressive myocyte necrosis with accompanying protease release from infiltrating leukocytes. Immunohistochemical labeling indicates the presence of a latent collagenase system which coexists with myocardial fibrillar collagen. Thus, there exists the potential for collagen degradation to exceed synthesis should there be significant activation of this latent collagenase system. In man, with dilated cardiomyopathy (DCM),[5] as well as in the cardiomyopathic hamster,[2] the decompensated state has been found to be associated with collagenase activation. Collagenase activity and its relation to progressive dilatation in DCM will be the subject of this chapter.

Myocardial Collagenase

Once deposited in fibrillar form and subsequently crosslinked, extracellular collagen is extremely stable and not easily degraded. Interstitial collagen consist of three peptide chains which intertwine to form a right handed super helix. This conformation makes interstitial collagens highly resistant to all proteinases except specific collagenases.[6] Because of its stability, the rate-limiting step in the degradation of fibrillar collagen is the catalytic cleavage by interstitial collagenase. Once cleaved, collagen denatures and unwinds to form gelatin. Gelatinase then digests these products into

[1] This work was supported in part by Grants from NHLBI (RO1-HL-46461 and 31701), American Heart Association (901397) and American Heart Association, Missouri Affiliate (93-GS-016).

smaller peptides that are further cleaved by nonspecific proteases.[7]

A collagenase system has been identified within the myocardium by Montfort and Perez-Tamayo[8] using specific antibody and immunofluorescent staining, and by others[9] using immunohistochemical techniques. In the heart the fibroblast is the cellular source of collagenase, which resides in the interstitium mostly in an inactive or latent form.[10] The regulation of this collagenase system remains to be elucidated. Inflammatory cells, leukocytes, and macrophages, add another dimension to collagenolytic activity in that they bring their proteolytic enzymes to the site of wound healing and inflammation.

The synthesis rate of collagen for the right (RV) and left (LV) ventricles has been measured in dogs to be 0.56% of total ventricular collagen per day.[11] If an equilibrium is to exist between collagen synthesis and degradation, then, assuming a similar degradation rate, the half-life of collagen is around 90 days. Thus, the majority of collagenase must be either in its zymogen or pro-enzyme form or bound to a tissue inhibitor of matrix metalloproteinases (MMPs) as was recently demonstrated by Tyagi et al.[10] They found the amount of total collagenase in the rat myocardium to be 5 ± 2 pg/μg of tissue of which 98% was latent.

Myocardial Collagenase Activity and Collagen Degradation

Chakraborty and Eghbali[9] reported that degradation of collagen fibers in rat heart sections, which occurred after 48 hours of incubation under optimal conditions for collagenolytic digestion, was due to activation of myocardial intrinsic collagenase. Studies in rats have indicated rapid collagen degradation within 24 hours after experimental myocardial infarction. In addition, collagen breakdown was significantly greater in infarcted hearts of rats with normal leukocyte response than in rats with experimental leukopenia.[12] In infarcted regions, Takahashi et al.[13] reported decreases of up to 50% in myocardial collagen after 3 hours of infarction. The loss was associated

with a two to threefold increase in activities of tissue collagenase and lysosomal serine proteases. The reader is referred to Chapter 13 for further discussion of collagenolysis postinfarction. While these results suggest a major role of inflammatory cell collagenase in collagen breakdown during myocardial infarction, another consideration is that the increase in the sulfhydryl active compound, oxidized glutathione (GSSG), which is known to occur in the ischemic zone,[14] activates latent collagenase in this area. Glutathione is known to activate mammalian collagenase and has recently been shown to activate myocardial collagenases.[15] This would explain the rapid disruption of collagen struts and loss of collagen weaves in stunned myocardium, where inflammatory infiltrate is not yet present.[16] Similar observations were made by Sato et al.[17] in the infarcted area within 2 to 3 hours after coronary artery occlusion and prior to any appreciable influx of leukocytes. More recently, Charney et al.[18] reported the following in stunned myocardium: (1) a significant expansion of the involved area; (2) a transmural loss of collagen associated with a 74% increase in collagenase activity; and (3) a greater number of exposed N-terminal amino acid residues. Caulfield et al.[19] using an assumed in vivo model of collagen degradation found myocardial hydroxyproline to decrease 50% at which time ultrastructural collagen was markedly reduced.

Myocardial Collagenase Activity and Ventricular Dilatation

Thus, a collagenase system, which normally is almost completely latent has been described in the myocardium. This system when activated as a result of ischemia, with or without the presence of leukocytes, is responsible for rapid collagen degradation in the ischemic area with consequent wall thinning and outward expansion during systole.[3] Before healing, this area devoid of collagen is prone to rupture, particularly if the infarct is transmural (see Chapter 4). Experimentally induced global degradation of myocardial collagen is followed by ventricular dilatation.[19–21] That is, the diastolic

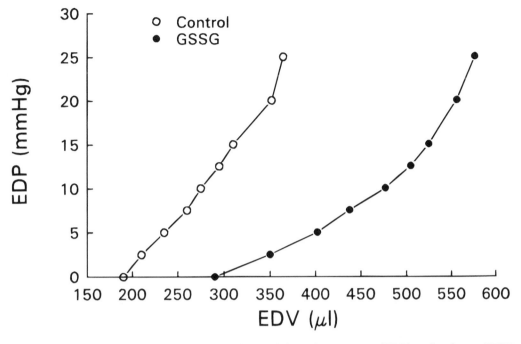

Figure 1. The relation between left ventricular end-diastolic pressure (EDP) and volume (EDV) obtained in isolated rat hearts that were untreated (Control) or treated with oxidized glutathione (GSSG) using the model proposed by Caulfield et al.[19] GSSG results in ventricular dilatation as evidenced by the relation being shifted to the right.

pressure-volume relation of the left ventricles is shifted to the right as demonstrated in (Figure 1).

Preliminary data (Janicki), indicate that an abrupt and sustained increase in ventricle volume (i.e., infrarenal abdominal aorta-vena cava fistula) is associated with a significant activation of the myocardial collagenase system. Using zymographic techniques,[10,15] collagenase activity was found to be significantly increased by 54% relative to control activity as early as 12 hours after initiation of the volume overload condition. Over the next 5 days of volume overload, collagenase activity further increased to levels that were 86% greater than control levels. It then declined over the next 9 days to a level which was 33% above control collagenase activity, and remained at this activity for the duration of the study (i.e., 8 weeks). This increased activity in all likelihood was responsible for the decrease in left ventricular collagen concentration seen in this model of ventricle volume overload.[22] That a remodeling of the myocardium even-

tually occurs with a sustained volume overload is evidenced by a significant shift to the right of the left ventricles diastolic pressure size relationship with respect to the control relationship. In the fistula model of volume overload we found this to occur after 3 weeks of volume overload. That is, for any given diastolic pressure, left ventricular volume 3 weeks after creation of the fistula was significantly greater than that in aged-matched controls.

Collagenase Activity in DCM

In hearts with myocardial damage secondary to myocardial infarction, chronic ischemia, inflammation, or cardiomyopathy, there is a complex sequence of compensatory events that ultimately result in an adversely remodeled myocardium and a dilated, thin-walled, spherical ventricle. For a period of time, a preclinical heart failure state may exist where there is ventricular dysfunction due to myocardial damage but no clinical evidence of cardiac insufficiency, circulatory congestion, or edema. However, in an attempt to maintain this state, there are ongoing myocardial and peripheral adaptations including activation of the renin-angiotensin aldosterone and sympathetic nervous systems, elevations in circulating blood volume and ventricular preload, cardiac myocyte hypertrophy, and progressive heart enlargement. As will be seen, a continual state of remodeling with progressive ventricular dilatation, persistent collagenase activity, inadequate collagen fibrillar matrix, and probably progressive myocyte loss is present. The net effect is loss of reciprocal regulation of collagen synthesis and degradation which leads to progressive ventricular dilatation with wall thinning and sphericalization and eventually congestive heart failure.

Weber et al.[1] documented an inadequate myocardial collagen matrix in postmortem hearts of patients with DCM. Thick coiled perimysial fibers were rare and numerous widened interstitial spaces were present with conspicuous reduction or disruption of lateral connections of collagen between muscle fibers. An absence or disruption of muscle bundle to muscle bundle tethers and other elements of the collagen matrix could lead to ventricular dilation, wall thinning, and possibly interstitial edema. In addition, muscle fiber slippage and a sphericalization of the ventricle are likely to occur. Thus it would appear that collagen breakdown plays a major role in bringing about dilatation, the change in shape, and the increase in distensibility of the cardiomyopathic left ventricle.

Recently Reddy and coworkers[5] used zymography to assess collagenase activity in endomyocardial biopsy tissue obtained from patients with end-stage (ejection fraction = 25% ± 8%) DCM and from posttransplant patients with presumably normal (ejection fraction = 59% ± 5%) hearts. When expressed as percent activity, an eightfold difference between normal and DCM was found. An echocardiographic analysis revealed the DCM left ventricles to be significantly dilated with thinner walls compared to the posttransplant left ventricles. Also, the shape of the DCM LV was more spherical than the normal LV. Thus, there was a correlation between collagenase activity and architectural remodeling of the left ventricles in DCM lending strong support to the hypothesis that enhanced collagenase activity leads to collagenolysis with fibrillar collagen degradation that then leads to progressive ventricular dilatation and sphericalization. The reader is referred to Chapter 6 for a further discussion regarding myocardial collagenase in human ischemic DCMs.

While the above results provide evidence of a possible role for enhanced collagenase activity in the progressive dilatation associated with DCM, they represent data after the fact and shed no insight on the temporal relation between collagenolysis and dilatation. Such information can be acquired from the cardiomyopathic Syrian hamster. This animal model of DCM has the advantages of a predictable pathophysiological course which includes progressive dilatation and failure. The disease process has been described as occurring in four histologic and clinical phases: prenecrotic; necrotic; hypertrophic; and terminal.[23] During the first phase (i.e., <45 days) the animals appear histologically and clinically normal. The necrotic phase is characterized by the incidence of multiple focal areas of myocytolytic necrosis which continues until the age of 120 days. A possible cause of this necrosis may be focal, transient spasms of small blood vessels. Factor et al.[24] found numerous coronary arteriolar constrictions suggestive of microvasculature spasm in the cardiomyopathic hamster during the necrotizing phase of the disease. Such areas were found much less frequently in older cardiomyopathic and golden Syrian hamsters. Figulla et al.[25] observed areas of myocardium with a capillary filling defect in the prenecrotic cardiomyopathic hamster that were not present in age-matched controls. More recently, the coronary vasculature of the young cardiomyopathic hamster has been reported to be significantly more responsive to the endogenous vasoconstrictor, arginine vasopressin, than that of age-matched controls indicating a global vascular defect and further supporting the hypothesis of microvascular spasm as an etiologic factor.[26]

By the end of the necrotic phase healing has occurred with but a few new lesions remaining. The hypertrophic compensated phase continues until the heart begins to dilate with wall thinning at an age around 250 days at which time the fourth stage begins. In this terminal stage all of the clinical signs and constellations of congestive heart failure eventually appear, including a sustained myocardial edema as evidenced by a significant increase in percent myocardial water from 75.3% ± 0.5% to 78.7% ± 0.7%.[23] Myocyte abnormalities such as significant suppression of the Ca^{2+} removal pathways as manifested by slowly decaying intracellular Ca^{2+} transients, prolongation of contraction, the activation of the Na^{+}-Ca^{2+} exchanger,[27] altered pyruvate dehydrogenase control, and mitochondrial free Ca^{2+}[28] are also noted in this final stage.

In addition to the myocytolysis and scarring, there are pronounced alterations in the connective tissue framework surrounding necrotic myocardial lesions which occur at 90 days of age and become progressively larger with age.[29] These alterations consisted of a marked absence of silver stainable connective tissue along the edges of darkly stained lesions and the presence of long, thick fibers apparently tethering necrotic foci to the surrounding normal muscle. Beyond this halo-like, collagen deficient region, the interstitium exhibited a normal pattern of silver staining. Thus, from these observations, one could infer that collagen degradation did not occur globally. Instead, it was a regional phenomenon closely associated with the fibrotic area. This group of investigators speculated that the progressive loss of connective tissue surrounding confluent fibrotic areas may result in myofiber slippage and wall thinning, while the effects of the tethering fibers may lead to an increase in wall stiffness.

To determine the relationship between myocardial collagen concentration, collagenase activity, and ventricular dilatation, myocardial tissue from cardiomyopathic hamsters was examined at ages 150, 180, 210, 240, and 300 days and compared to age-matched golden Syrian hamsters which served as controls.[2] Collagen concentration was determined morphometrically as the collagen volume fraction (CVF) and collagenase activity by zymography. The accumulation of reparative fibrosis as a function of age in the cardiomyopathic hamster is depicted in (Figure 2, see page 86A). At 150 days, the collagen volume fraction (CVF) was found to be 6.3% ± 0.8% (panel A), which was significantly greater than the 1.7% ± 0.3% value obtained in the golden Syrian hamster control (panel E). Collagen volume fraction increased further at 180 days and reached a peak value of 10.3% ± 0.7% at an age of 210 days (panel C). At 240 days (panel D) and 300 days (not shown), the LV wall became notably thinner and CVF began to decline; CVF at 300 days was 6.6% ± 1.5%. Thus up to the age of 210 days, collagen synthesis was greater than degradation leading to a progressive fibrosis. The subsequent decline in CVF with age was due to the collagen degradation rate exceeding the collagen synthesis rate.

Collagen degradation was also seen at the ultrastructural level in nonnecrotic areas of myocardium. A semiquantitative technique to determine the amount of ultrastructural collagen was employed whereby for each heart, 80 fields at a magnification of X4000 were graded as follows: normal amount = 3, above and below normal = 5 and 1, respectively, and no collagen = 0. The average score for the golden Syrian hamster hearts was 2.3 ± 0.1. In the cardiomyopathic hamster hearts the score decreased with age and became significantly different from control for ages >210 days; at 300 days the score was 1.0 ± 0.5.

An example of myocardial collagenase activity at several ages is shown in (Figure 3) for the cardiomyopathic and golden Syrian hamsters. Here the gel lane assignment is random because, at the time of analysis, the investigator was blinded as to the source of tissue. In all cases, the brighter and wider lytic bands were associated with the cardiomyopathic hearts. In contrast to an age invariant collagenase activity in the golden Syrian hamster, the percent of activated collagenase in the cardiomyopathic hamster was found to progressively increase with age. At 150 days it was similar to the control value of 23% ± 2%. At 210 days of age and older, the collagenase activity in the cardiomyopathic hamster was significantly greater than that measured in the control hearts; at 300 days, the activity was increased threefold over that in the control.

Total Protein (SDS PAGE)

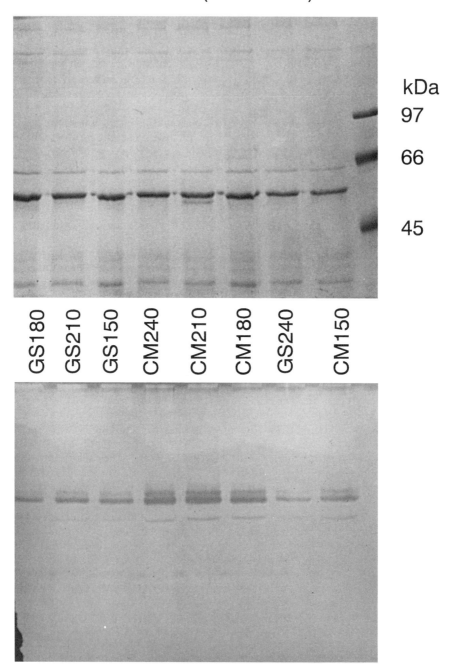

Figure 3. Example of myocardial collagenase activity in 150-, 180-, 210- and 240-day-old cardiomyopathic hamster (CM) and age-matched golden Syrian hamsters (GS). In the lower panel, the zymographic lytic bands for CM are denser and wider indicating enhanced collagenase activity. The SDS-PAGE gel demonstrates that each lane contained similar amounts of protein.

Thus, in the cardiomyopathic hamster, there is a continual increase in collagenase activity with age such that a point is reached where collagen degradation exceeds collagen synthesis. As discussed above, this degradation takes place in and around necrotic areas,[29] as well as remote areas[2] resulting in an inadequate supportive interstitial collagen matrix. This occurs close to the age where significant ventricular dilatation and wall thinning occur, which is indicative of a strong cause and effect relation between collagenase activity and ventricular remodeling.

Future Directions Regarding Potential Therapy

In addition to determining the regulatory mechanisms of myocardial collagenase activity, investigations to determine whether pharmacological inhibition of collagenase will prevent the adverse remodeling associated with cardiomyopathy and heart failure are required. In vitro, a number of compounds have been shown to inhibit collagenase; these include soy bean trypsin inhibitor (SBTI), lima bean trypsin inhibitor (LBTI), nitrophenyl guanidinobenzoate, diisopropyl phosphofluoridate, aprotinin, and tetracycline. Several of these compounds (i.e., SBTI, LBTI, aprotinin and tetracycline) have been used to determine their effects on inflammatory responses or healing following surgery. Aprotinin is produced from bovine lung sources. It has a low molecular weight and moves rapidly from the serum into the extracellular compartment. When given to rabbits prior to and for 3 days after experimental colonic resection and anastomosis, it was found to produce a significant elevation of the bursting pressure and significant improvement in the collagen content of the anastomosis compared to that of anastomotic sites in an untreated group.[30] These efficacious results were attributed to the inhibition of collagenase. Unlike aprotinin, SBTI and LBTI can be administered enterally. When given to rabbits (1 mg/kg), both compounds were found to produce significant reductions (90%) in collagenolytic activity in colonic mucosa within 24 hours of administration.[31]

Recent experiments have shown impressive collagenase inhibitory activity for tetracycline antibiotics independent of its antimicrobial properties.[32] Intramuscular tetracycline (50 mg/kg per day) was administered to rabbits for 10 days to study its effect on the progression of *Pseudomonas aeruginosa* keratitis. Even though the eyes in both groups had intense conjunctival injection, purulent discharge, and diffuse stromal infiltration, the incidence of corneal perforation in the treated group was significantly lower (50%) than that in the untreated group.[33] Thus, this effect appears to be mediated through inhibition of collagenase activity. Another characteristic of tetracycline is its enhanced ability to inhibit neutrophil collagenase (MMP-8). Suomalainen and co-workers[34] found the concentrations of doxycycline and 4-de-dimethylaminotetracycline required to inhibit collagenase activity by 50%, were 15 to 30 μM for human neutrophil and gingival crevicular fluid collagenases. In contrast, the 50% inhibitory concentrations of these compounds were much greater (i.e., 280 and 510 μM, respectively) for fibroblast collagenase. Finally, collagenolysis was prevented in infarcted tissue by effectively removing the source of collagenase. Cannon et al.[12] reported greater preservation of collagen in the 24-hour-old infarcts of irradiated leukopenic rats, compared with those of control rats with normal amount of leukocytes. Thus, while the ability to prevent collagenase activation in the heart has not been studied, feasibility has been demonstrated in vivo in other tissues.

Chronic therapy with an angiotensin-converting enzyme (ACE) inhibitor has been shown to attenuate progressive ventricular enlargement following myocardial infarction.[35] Whether begun at 2 days or 2 weeks following coronary ligation in rats, ACE inhibition prevented ventricular dilatation and there was a significant improvement in survival during a 1-year period postinfarction. Similar efficacious results were obtained in clinical trials with chronic ACE inhibition.[36,37] Patients on active therapy had less ventricular enlargement, fewer manifestations of symptomatic heart failure, reduced number of hospitalizations due to heart failure, and fewer deaths attributed to heart failure. In addition, LV shape of patients at greatest risk for enlargement (i.e., persistently occluded left anterior descending coronary arteries and large infarctions) remained normal with ACE inhibition while placebo-treated patients had progressively more spherical ventricles.[38] Chronic ACE inhibition also favorably altered temporal progression of LV failure and improved mortality in the cardiomyopathic Syrian hamster. Administration of quinapril to the DCM hamster from 180 to 300 days of age prevented the decline of in vitro LV contractile performance, coronary flow and LV dilatation, and increased the median survival time by 33%.[39] The mechanisms responsible for the cardioprotective characteristics of chronic ACE inhibition remain to be determined. Whether myocardial collagenase activity in cardiomyopathy and following myocardial infarction is altered by the chronic administration of an ACE inhibitor needs to be determined.

Summary

Progressive left ventricular dilatation, together with wall thinning and chamber sphericalization, are features of chronic myocardial failure that contribute to its relentless downhill course. Fibrillar collagen provides for muscle fiber and cardiac myocyte alignment. They also impart a tensile strength to the myocardium that maintains ventricular shape, size and governs tissue stiffness. Immunohistochemical labeling indicates the presence of a collagenase system which coexists with myocardial fibrillar collagen; the majority of this collagenase is normally latent. Thus, there exists the potential for collagen degradation to exceed synthesis should there be significant activation of this latent collagenase system. Experimental removal of less than half the normal amount of collagen results in a dilated ventricle with increased compliance. Also, significant collagenase activation and collagen degradation are evident in dilated cardiomyopathy. It is concluded that a dilated, thin wall and spherical ventricle is closely associated with a collagenase-induced degradation of myocardial fibrillar collagen.

References

1. Weber KT, Pick R, Janicki JS, et al. Inadequate collagen tethers in dilated cardiopathy. Am Heart J 1988;116:1641–1646.
2. Janicki JS, Tyagi SC, Henegar JR, et al. Myocardial collagenase activity and ventricular dilatation in cardiomyopathic hamsters. (Abstract) Circulation 1993;88:I-381.
3. Weber KT, Pick R, Silver MA, et al. Fibrillar collagen and remodeling of dilated left ventricle. Circulation 1990;82:1387–1401.
4. Spinale FG, Tomita M, Zellner JL, et al. Collagen remodeling and changes in LV function during development and recovery from supraventricular tachycardia. Am J Physiol 1991;261:H308-H318.
5. Reddy HK, Tyagi SC, Tjahja IE, et al. Enhanced endomyocardial collagenase activity in dilated cardiomyopathy: a marker of dilatation and architectural remodeling. (Abstract) Circulation 1993;88:I-407.
6. Woolley DE. Mammalian collagenases. In: Piez K, Reddi AH, eds. Extracellular Matrix Biochemistry. New York, NY: Elsevier, 1984: 119–158.
7. Woessner JF Jr. Matrix metalloproteinases and their inhibitors in connective tissue remodeling. FASEB J 1991;131:2145–2154.
8. Montfort I, Perez-Tamayo R. The distribution of collagenase in normal rat tissues. J Histochem Cytochem 1975;23:910–920.
9. Chakraborty A, Eghbali M. Collagenase activity in the normal rat myocardium: an immunohistochemical method. Histochemistry 1989;92:391–396.
10. Tyagi SC, Matsubara L, Weber KT. Direct activation and estimation of collagenase(s) activity by zymography in microquantities of rat myocardium and uterus. Clin Biochem 1993;26:191–198.
11. Bonnim CM, Sparrow MP, Taylor RR. Collagen synthesis and content in right ventricular hypertrophy in the dog. Am J Physiol 1981;241:H708-H713.
12. Cannon RO, Butany JW, McManus BM, et al. Early degradation of collagen after myocardial infarction in the heart. Am J Cardiol 1983;52:390–395.
13. Takahashi S, Barry AC, Factor SM. Collagen degradation in ischemic rat hearts. Biochem J 1990;265:233–241.
14. Romero FJ, Montoro A, Saez GT, et al. Myocardial glutathione alterations in acute coronary occlusion in the dog. Free Rad Res Comms 1987;4:27–30.
15. Tyagi SC, Ratajska A, Weber KT. Myocardial matrix metalloproteinase(s): localization and activation. Mol Cell Biochem 1993;126:49–59.

16. Zhao M, Zhang H, Robinson TF, et al. Profound structural alterations of the extracellular collagen matrix in postischemic dysfunctional ("stunned") but viable myocardium. J Am Coll Cardiol 1987;10:1322–1334.

17. Sato S, Ashroy M, Millard RW, et al. Connective tissue changes in early ischemia of porcine myocardium: an ultrastructural study. J Mol Cell Cardiol 1983;15:261–267.

18. Charney RH, Takahashi S, Zhao M, et al. Collagen loss in the stunned myocardium. Circulation 1992;85:1483–1490.

19. Caulfield JB, Norton P, Weaver RD. Cardiac dilatation associated with collagen alterations. Mol Cell Biochem 1992;118:171–179.

20. O'Brien LJ, Moore CM. Connective tissue degradation and distensibility characteristics of the non-living heart. Experimentia 1966;22:845–847.

21. Janicki JS, Matsubara BB. Myocardial collagen and left ventricular diastolic dysfunction. In: Gaasch WH, LeWinter MM, eds. Left Ventricular Diastolic Dysfunction and Heart Failure. Philadelphia,Pa: Lea & Febiger, 1994:125–140.

22. Ruzicka M, Leenen FHH. Renin-angiotensin system (RAS) and volume overload-induced cardiac remodelling. (Abstract) Can J Cardiol 1994;10:57A.

23. Gertz EW. Cardiomyopathic Syrian hamster: a possible model of human disease. Prog Exp Tumor Res 1972;16:242–260.

24. Factor SM, Minase T, Cho S, et al. Microvascular spasm in the cardiomyopathic Syrian hamster: a preventable cause of focal myocardial necrosis. Circulation 1982;66:342–354.

25. Figulla HR, Vetterlein F, Glaubitz M, et al. Inhomogeneous capillary flow and its prevention by verapamil and hydralazine in the cardiomyopathic Syrian hamster. Circulation 1987;76:208–216.

26. Conway RS, Natelson BH, Chen WH, et al. Enhanced coronary vasoconstriction in the Syrian myopathic hamster supports the microvascular spasm hypothesis. Cardiovasc Res 1994;28:320–324.

27. Hatem SN, Sham JSK, Morad M. Enhanced Na^+-Ca^{2+} exchange activity in cardiomyopathic Syrian hamster. Circ Res 1994;74:253–261.

28. Di Lisa F, Fan CZ, Gambassi G, et al. Altered pyruvate dehydrogenase control and mitochondrial free Ca^{2+} in hearts of cardiomyopathic hamsters. Am J Physiol 1993;264:H2188–H2197.

29. Cohen-Gould L, Robinson TF, Factor SM. Intrinsic connective tissue abnormalities in the heart muscle of cardiomyopathic Syrian hamsters. Am J Pathol 1987;127:327–334.

30. Young HL, Wheeler MH. Effect of intravenous aprotinin (Trasylol) on the healing of experimental colonic anastomoses in the rabbit. Eur Surg Res 1983;15:18–23.

31. Lewin MR, Chowcat NL, Jayaraj AP, et al. Collagenase inhibition in colonic mucosa by proteinase inhibitors. J Exp Path 1986;67:523–526.

32. Golub LM, McNamara TF, Angelo GD, et al. A non-antibacterial chemically modified tetracycline inhibits mammalian collagenase activity. J Dent Res 1987;66:1310–1314.

33. Levy JH, Katz HR. Effect of systemic tetracycline on progression of *Pseudomonas aeruginosa* keratitis in the rabbit. Ann Opthalmol 1990;22:179–183.

34. Suomalainen K, Sorsa T, Golub LM, et al. Specificity of the anticollagenase action of tetracyclines. Relevance to their anti-inflammatory potential. Antimicrob Agents Chemother 1992;36:227–229.

35. Pfeffer MA, Pfeffer JM, Lamas GA. Development and prevention of congestive heart failure following myocardial infarction. Circulation 1993;87:IV120-IV125.

36. The SOLVD Investigators. Effect of enalapril on mortality and the development of heart failure in asymptomatic patients with reduced left ventricular ejection fractions. N Engl J Med 1992;327:685–691.

37. Pfeffer MA, Braunwald E, Moye LA, et al. Effect of captopril on mortality in patients with left ventricular dysfunction after myocardial infarction: results of the survival and ventricular enlargement trial. N Engl J Med 1992;327:669–677.

38. Lamas GA, Pfeffer MA. Left ventricular remodeling after acute myocardial infarction: clinical course and beneficial effects of angiotensin-converting enzyme inhibition. Am Heart J 1991;121:1194–1202.

39. Haleen SJ, Weishaar RE, Overhiser RW, et al. Effects of quinapril, a new angiotensin converting enzyme inhibitor, on left ventricular failure and survival in the cardiomyopathic hamster. Circ Res 1991;68:1302–1312.

Chapter 8

The Extracellular Matrix with the Development and Regression from Dilated Cardiomyopathy

Francis G. Spinale, M.D., Ph.D

Introduction

The cardiomyopathies are a constellation of primary myocardial diseases which generally exclude etiologies of vascular, hypertension, and valvular disease. Dilated cardiomyopathy (DCM) is the most common category of the cardiomyopathies and the incidence is increasing.[1] The diagnosis of (DCM) is primarily based upon changes in left ventricular function and geometry. Specifically, left ventricular contractile function is reduced and chamber dimensions are increased without a proportional increase in wall thickness.[2] As a consequence of this disproportionate increase in left ventricular chamber radius to wall thickness, DCM is accompanied by increased myocardial wall stress which in turn promotes further dilation and reduced pump function.[3] This suggests that significant myocardial remodeling must occur within the left ventricular wall to allow for the chamber dilation and wall thinning which accompanies the development of DCM. While a large number of studies have focused upon biochemical changes which occur within the myocyte with development of DCM,[4,5] there have been few studies which have focused upon structural determinants responsible for the myocardial remodeling which accompanies this disease

process. The extracellular matrix is composed of a fibrillar collagen network, a basement membrane, and proteoglycans.[6-12] The extracellular matrix within the heart provides structural integrity of adjoining myocytes, translates myocyte shortening into ventricular pump function, and influence myocardial stiffness properties.[6-9] Thus, changes in the composition and structure of the extracellular matrix may play a contributory role in the development of DCM. In order to address this issue, this laboratory examined changes in extracellular matrix structure and composition with the development and regression from a well-characterized model of DCM.[13-31] The findings from these studies which are reviewed in this chapter, provide evidence to suggest that changes within the extracellular space, play a significant and contributory role towards the changes in left ventricular function and geometry which occur with cardiomyopathic disease.

Left Ventricular Function with the Development and Regression from Tachycardia-Induced Cardiomyopathy

Chronic rapid atrial or ventricular pacing in animals has been shown to cause a

[1] This work was supported by a Grant-in-Aid from the American Heart Association and National Institutes of Health Grant R29-HL-45024.
[2] Dr. Spinale is an Established Investigator of the American Heart Association.

dilated, poorly functioning ventricle.[13-31] In this laboratory, we have employed chronic, pacing-induced supraventricular tachycardia in swine to cause a DCM.[14-22,28] In addition, this model has been employed in order to determine changes in left ventricular function and geometry following regression from this form of cardiomyopathic disease.[16,21,28] The general methods employed to create this model of pacing-induced supraventricular tachycardia and the effects upon left ventricular function have been well described previously[14-22] and are briefly reviewed here. Yorkshire pigs (25 to 35 kg) are instrumented with a stimulating electrode sutured to the left atrium and a modified pacemaker placed in a subcutaneous pocket. Following recovery from surgery, pacing is initiated at 240 bpm and is continued for 21 days. In order to examine changes in left ventricular function and geometry which occur following regression from this form of cardiomyopathy, a second group of pigs undergo rapid atrial pacing for 3 weeks followed by a 4-week recovery period. Finally, a third group of pigs are treated in identical fashion with the exception of rapid pacing and serve as age- and weight-matched controls. At the appropriate intervals, the pigs are instrumented for simultaneous echocardiographic and catheterization study to determine left ventricular pressures and dimensions.[28] Changes in left ventricular function with the development and regression from tachycardia-induced cardiomyopathy are summarized in Table 1. Following 3 weeks of chronic rapid atrial pacing, left ventricular fractional shortening, peak pressure, and peak $+dP/dt$ significantly fell from control values. In the chronic tachycardia group, end-diastolic dimension, peak systolic wall stress, and pressure all significantly increased from controls. Following a 4-week recovery period following the development of tachycardia-induced cardiomyopathy, left ventricular fractional shortening, peak pressure, peak $+dP/dt$, and peak systolic wall stress all returned to control values. However, left ventricular end-diastolic pressure and dimension following a 4-week recovery from pacing-induced cardiomyopathy remained higher than controls. Left ventricular mass or body weight ratio remained unchanged in the tachycardia group, but increased by 58% following a 4-week recovery period from pacing-induced cardiomyopathy. In addition, this laboratory has computed regional myocardial stiffness in these animals based on the analysis of the curvilinear stress strain relation.[21,28] The regional myocardial stiffness constant (K_m) computed at similar end-diastolic pressures by dextran infusion, remained unchanged in the pacing-induced cardiomyopathy pigs compared to control pigs (11.8 ± 2.1 vs. 9.2 ± 1.5; $P > 0.50$). However, K_m significantly increased following a 4-week recovery from

Table 1

Left Ventricular Function with Development and Recovery From Pacing Induced Cardiomyopathy

	Control	SVT-DCM	Post-DCM
Basal Heart Rate (bpm)	98 ± 5	148 ± 7*	96 ± 7
LV Peak Pressure (mmHg)	88 ± 5	76 ± 5*	89 ± 5
LV Peak + dP/dT (mmHg/s)	1464 ± 127	875 ± 185*	1585 ± 130
LV End Diastolic Pressure (mmHg)	5 ± 2	26 ± 4*	12 ± 3*
LC End Diastolic Dimension (cm)	3.8 ± 0.2	5.6 ± 0.8*	5.3 ± 0.4*
LV End Diastolic Wall Thickness (cm)	0.8 ± 0.1	0.6 ± 0.1*	1.2 ± 0.2*
LV Fractional Shortening (%)	33 ± 3	13 ± 5*	35 ± 2
LV Peak Systolic Wall Stress (g/cm²)	45 ± 3	132 ± 7*	47 ± 6
LV Mass/Body Weight (gm/Kg)	2.6 ± 0.2	2.9 ± 0.4	4.1 ± 0.2*
Sample Size	7	7	6

Abbreviations: control, sham operated controls; SVT-DCM, supraventricular tachycardia-induced dilated cardiomyopathy; Post-DCM, SVT-DCM followed by 4-week recovery period.
* Significantly different from control values, $P < 0.05$.

pacing-induced cardiomyopathy (14.6 ± 1.1; $P<0.05$). Thus, chronic pacing-induced tachycardia caused a DCM with no significant change in left ventricular mass or myocardial stiffness. In contrast, termination of rapid pacing and a 4-week recovery period normalized indices of left ventricular systolic function, but was associated with persistent left ventricular dilatation, hypertrophy, and increased myocardial stiffness.

Collagen Remodeling with Tachycardia-Induced Cardiomyopathy and Recovery

In light of the fact that chronic tachycardia caused significant left ventricular dilation with no change in mass, then significant changes in myocardial structure, and composition must have occurred. A series of experiments were performed in order to examine whether changes in fibrillar collagen content, structure and composition accompanied the development and regression from tachycardia-induced cardiomyopathy.[16,21,22] The results from these studies are summarized in Table 2. Myocardial collagen content based upon hydroxyproline assays revealed a significant reduction in collagen within the subendocardial region of the left ventricular free wall with the development of tachycardia-induced cardiomyopathy. With a 4-week recovery period from tachycardia-induced cardiomyopathy, myocardial collagen content was increased in both the subendocardial and subepicardial region of the left ventricular free wall. In order to more carefully quantify changes in fibrillar collagen, collagen cross-linking and the relative content of each collagen type were examined. In these experiments, collagen was extracted using salt precipitation and pepsin digestion and collagen typing was performed using SDS-PAGE.[32] The percent of the total collagen which was salt extractable significantly increased in the tachycardia-induced cardiomyopathy group compared to controls.

Table 2

Myocardial Collagen Biochemistry and Morphometry Following the Development and Recovery from Pacing-Induced Cardiomyopathy

	Control	SVT-DCM	Post-DCM
Biochemical Composition			
Subendocardium			
Collagen (mg/gdwt)	35.6 ± 1.2	27.5 ± 1.7*	42.8 ± 0.3*
Extractable Collagen (%)	24.5 ± 0.7	36.3 ± 1.3*	23.7 ± 1.2
Extractable Collagen Type I (%)	68.3 ± 1.2	57.3 ± 0.9*	65.3 ± 0.8
Extractable Collagen Type II (%)	26.6 ± 0.7	39.6 ± 1.2*	21.4 ± 1.3
Subepicardium			
Collagen (mg/gdwt)	43.4 ± 1.6	36.6 ± 1.5	48.6 ± 0.4*
Extractable Collagen (%)	23.6 ± 0.5	36.8 ± 0.8*	22.1 ± 1.1
Extractable Collagen Type I (%)	67.4 ± 1.0	56.9 ± 1.2*	65.5 ± 1.2
Extractable Collagen Type II (%)	24.3 ± 1.2	40.2 ± 0.6*	22.4 ± 0.8
Collagen Morphometry			
Subendocardium			
Collagen Volume Fraction (%)	7.5 ± 0.8	4.6 ± 0.4*	14.5 ± 0.8*
Collagen Confluence (%)	5.7 ± 0.1	2.8 ± 0.2*	16.7 ± 1.0*
Subepicardium			
Collagen Volume Fraction (%)	9.8 ± 1.1	8.7 ± 0.6*	17.3 ± 0.7*
Collagen Confluence (%)	6.7 ± 0.2	4.1 ± 0.3	24.3 ± 1.2*
Sample Size	7	7	6

Abbreviations: Control, sham operated controls; SVT-DCM, supraventricular tachycardia-induced dilated cardiomyopathy; Post-DCM, SVT-DCM followed by 4-week recovery period.

* Significantly different from control values, $P < 0.05$.

These results suggest that with the development of supraventricular tachycardia cardiomyopathy, the degree of collagen crosslinking is significantly reduced. Following a 4-week recovery from pacing-induced tachycardia, the percent of extractable collagen returned to control values. The relative content of types I and III collagen within the extracted collagen significantly changed with the development pacing-induced cardiomyopathy. In the DCM group, the extracted collagen contained a greater amount of collagen type III and a lesser amount of collagen type I compared to the control group. Results from this analysis suggest that there is a significant reduction in collagen type III covalent crosslinks with the development of tachycardia cardiomyopathy. In addition to biochemical quantitation of fibrillar collagen with the development and recovery from tachycardia-induced cardiomyopathy, collagen structure was also examined and the results from these studies are summarized in Table 2. Using silver impregnation staining, left ventricular myocardial sections were examined by morphometric techniques.[21] The volume fraction of collagen significantly decreased in the tachycardia-induced cardiomyopathy group compared to the control group. Similarly, there was a significant increase in the volume fraction of positive silver staining following a 4-week recovery from tachycardia-induced cardiomyopathy. The confluence of the collagen weave, as quantitated by the percent of continuous, unbroken, collagen fibers, was significantly reduced with tachycardia-induced cardiomyopathy. The percent of interconnected collagen fibers significantly increased following a 4-week recovery from pacing-induced cardiomyopathy. Using scanning electron microscopy, the three-dimensional structure of the fibrillar collagen network could be readily appreciated in control sections (Figure 1A). In these control sections, smaller collagen bundles and fibrils branched off of larger collagen struts. In contrast, the fibrillar collagen weave could not be readily observed in myocardial sections examined after the development of tachycardia-induced cardiomyopathy (Figure 1B). The fine collagen latticework appeared greatly disrupted in sections taken from the cardiomyopathic

group compared to controls. Following a 4-week recovery from pacing-induced cardiomyopathy, an increase in the thickness of the collagen struts was observed between adjacent myocytes (Figure 1C).

The development of tachycardia-induced cardiomyopathy resulted in a reduction in myocardial collagen content, disruption in the continuity of the fibrillar collagen weave, reduced collagen crosslinking, and changes in the relative content of types I and III with collagen extraction. The increased collagen extraction with tachycardia-induced cardiomyopathy suggests diminished covalent intramolecular crosslinking.[32] It has been shown previously that the degree of collagen crosslinking will affect myocardial stiffness properties.[32] These changes in collagen cross-linking may be a contributory factor for the diminished collagen content with tachycardia-induced cardiomyopathy and is discussed later in this chapter. With a one-month recovery following the development of tachycardia-induced cardiomyopathy, collagen deposition within the myocardium significantly increased, collagen extraction normalized, and the ratio of collagen types I and III from the extracted collagen samples returned to control values. The majority of previous studies reporting changes in collagen composition or structure have been following the development of pressure or volume overload hypertrophy.[32-35] For example, Weber et al. reported that increased fibrosis accompanied the development of left ventricular hypertrophy in a primate model of systemic hypertension.[34] In addition, these investigators reported that the relative distribution of collagen types I and III were unchanged from control.[34] Following volume overload hypertrophy in dogs, Iimoto and colleagues reported no overall change in collagen content but significantly increased collagen crosslinking.[32] In this past report, these investigators attributed the increased myocardial stiffness to changes in collagen crosslinking, rather than changes in overall collagen content. While a large number of studies have examined changes in the fibrillar collagen network following the development of myocardial disease, few investigations of collagen content and structure have been performed with recovery

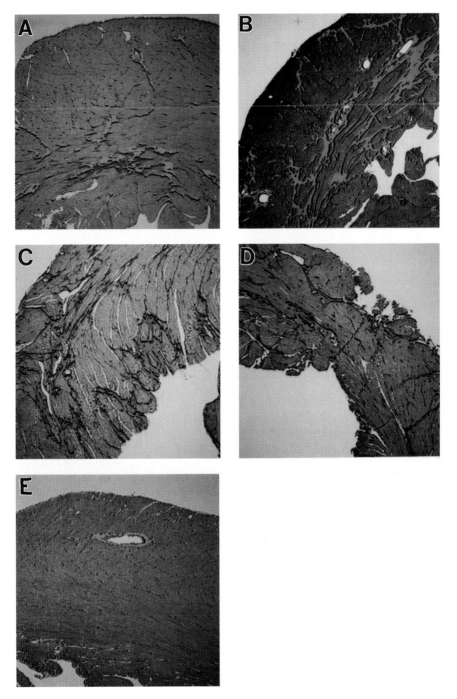

Figure 2. Fibrillar collagen (delineated by orange overlay) in CHF 146 cardiomyopathic hamsters. Panel A: 150 days of age, collagen volume fraction (CVF) = 6.3% ± 0.8%. Panel B: 180 days of age, CVF = 7.6% ± 1.6%. Panel C: 210 days of age, CVF = 10.3% ± 0.7%. Panel D: 240 days of age, CVF = 8.4% ± 2.8%. Panel E: Control golden Syrian hamster, CVF = 1.7% ± 0.3%.

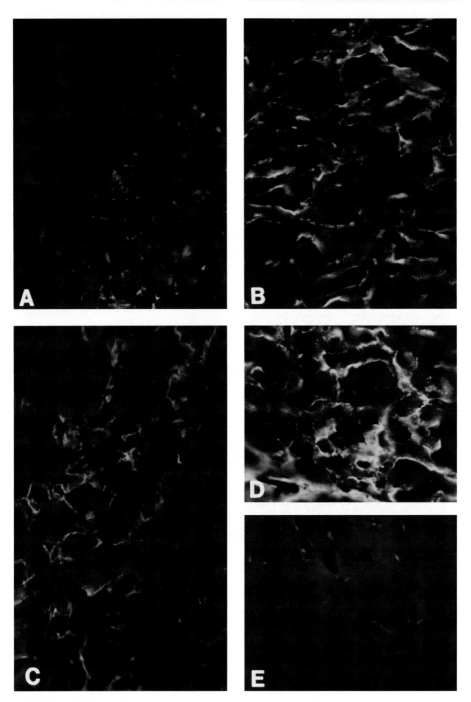

Figure 4. Immunofluorescent staining using a monoclonal antibody against chondroitin sulfate.[39] (A) Sections taken from control myocardium revealed a homogenous, well distributed pattern of staining within the extracellular space. (B) An increased intensity of the immunofluorescent staining pattern was observed in left ventricular sections taken subsequent to the development of tachycardia-induced cardiomyopathy. (C) Left ventricular sections taken from pigs with the development of tachycardia-induced cardiomyopathy followed by a 4-week recovery period. The intensity and distribution of immunofluorescent staining was similar to that observed in control sections. (D) Higher magnification of tachycardia-induced cardiomyopathic myocardium demonstrating intense deposits of chondroitin sulfate within the extracellular space. (E) Substitution of primary antibody with nonimmune mouse sera abolished all staining within the extracellular space. Original magnification of A, B, C, E: x400, D: x600.

86B

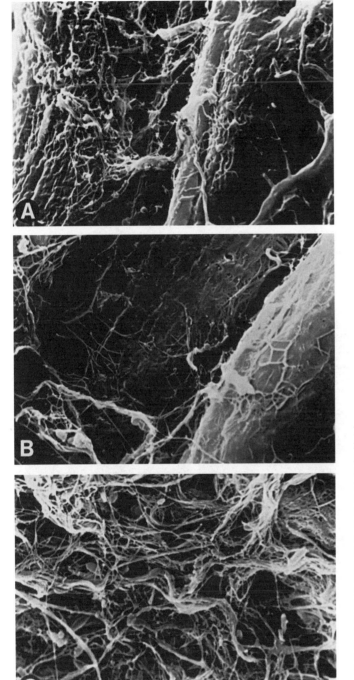

Figure 1. Representative scanning electron micrographs of freeze fractured left ventricular sections taken from control (A), with the development of chronic supraventricular tachycardia-induced cardiomyopathy (B), and with the development of tachycardia-induced cardiomyopathy followed by a 4-week recovery period (C). In control sections (A), a well-defined pattern of invaginations along the outside surface of the myocyte were observed. Collagen fibrils could be clearly seen spanning the extracellular space between adjacent myocytes. (B) In myocardial sections taken with the development of tachycardia-induced cardiomyopathy, a flattening of the sarcolemma was observed. The regular pattern collagen fibril latticework surrounding the myocytes could no longer be seen. The collagen latticework appeared disrupted and disorganized within the extracellular space. (C) Following a 4-week recovery from tachycardia-induced cardiomyopathy, the collagen matrix appeared to increase in density from control sections. The collagen weave appeared thickened and surrounded individual myocytes. Original magnification; x4000.

from the disease process. With a 1-month recovery from tachycardia-induced cardiomyopathy, myocardial collagen content and fibrillar density increased (similar to pressure overload hypertrophy[33,34]), and collagen crosslinking increased from cardiomyopathy values (similar to volume overload hypertrophy[32]).

Myocyte Basement Membrane Adhesion with Tachycardia-Induced Cardiomyopathy and Recovery

This laboratory has developed methods by which to directly examine the effects of tachycardia-induced cardiomyopathy upon myocyte structure and contractile function.[15–18,20,22,36] Specifically, myocytes are enzymatically disassociated from the left ventricular free wall and carefully resuspended in cell culture media and myocyte contractile function examined using computer assisted videomicroscopy.[17,18,20,36] Using these methods, a high yield of viable myocytes from control and cardiomyopathic ventricles have been obtained for study.[15–18,20,22] The advantages of using isolated myocytes for study are that they can be performed independent of loading conditions and neurohormonal influences. Representative photomicrographs of isolated myocytes with the development and regression from tachycardia-induced cardiomyopathy are shown in Figure 2.

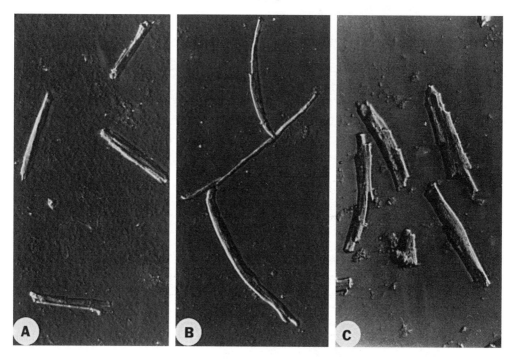

Figure 2. Contrast photomicrographs of myocytes isolated from control (A), after 3 weeks of pacing-induced supraventricular tachycardia (B), and with a 4-week recovery period following the development of tachycardia-induced cardiomyopathy (C). In all isolation procedures, a minimum of 60% rod-shaped, Ca^{+2}-tolerant cells were obtained. With tachycardia-induced cardiomyopathy (B), isolated myocytes were longer than control cells. With a 4-week recovery from cardiomyopathy (C), the length and width of isolated myocytes were greater than controls. Quantitative measurements performed on these isolated myocytes revealed over a 30% increase in myocyte length with the development of tachycardia-induced cardiomyopathy.[15,16] With a 1-month recovery period from this type of cardiomyopathy, both isolated myocyte length and cross-sectional area were increased.[15,16] Original magnification x300.

Tachycardia-induced cardiomyopathy caused over a 30% increase in isolated myocyte length when compared to control values.[15,16] The increased myocyte length persisted following a 4-week recovery period from tachycardia-induced cardiomyopathy.[16] In order to examine whether alterations in myocyte shape were associated with changes in basement membrane adhesion capacity, isolated myocytes were allowed to attach to increasing concentrations of the basement membrane components laminin, fibronectin, and collagen type IV.[22] Myocyte adhesion capacity to the basement membrane substrate laminin is shown in Figure 3. These studies demonstrated that myocytes attach to basement membrane substrates in a time- and concentration-dependent manner. In the pacing cardiomyopathy group, isolated myocyte attachment to laminin was reduced by over 60% for all times and concentrations used. With a 4-week recovery period from pacing-induced cardiomyopathy, isolated myocyte attachment to the laminin substrate returned to control levels. Similar findings were obtained for the basement membrane components fibronectin and collagen IV.

While the fibrillar collagen network provides for structural support within the extracellular space, the basement membrane is responsible for mediating attachment of the collagen fibrils to the cell membrane.[9,10] It has been shown that adult mammalian myocytes adhere to laminin, fibronectin, and collagen IV; all major constituents of the basement membrane.[9,10,37,38] Adherence of the myocyte sarcolemma to the basement membrane provides a means by which myocyte contractile forces are

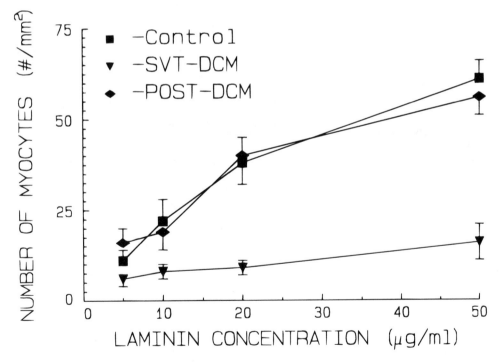

Figure 3. Isolated myocyte binding curves to the basement membrane substrate laminin. The X-axis shows the different concentrations of laminin used in these adhesion studies. The Y-axis represents the number of myocytes which attached to this concentration of laminin following a 60–minute incubation period. Control myocytes bound to laminin in a concentration-dependent manner. With the development of supraventricular tachycardia-induced dilated cardiomyopathy (SVT-DCM), myocyte adhesion was significantly reduced at all laminin concentrations ($P<0.05$). Following a 1-month recovery from tachycardia-induced cardiomyopathy (Post-DCM), myocyte adhesion capacity to laminin had returned to control levels. Bars reflect the standard error of the mean.

transduced into the extracellular matrix.[9,10] Myocyte adhesion capacity to components of the basement membrane has been the subject of several investigations.[9,10,37,38] For example, Terracio and colleagues reported that the development of pressure overload hypertrophy in rats was accompanied by increased myocyte binding capacity to components of the basement membrane.[38] However, prior to the studies outlined in this chapter and reported previously,[22] myocyte adhesion characteristics had not been examined with the development and regression from a cardiomyopathic disease process. The development of tachycardia-induced cardiomyopathy was accompanied by a significant reduction in myocyte adhesion capacity to components of the basement membrane. With a 1-month recovery from tachycardia-induced cardiomyopathy, myocyte adhesion capacity had returned to control levels. These changes in myocyte adhesion capacity with the development and regression from tachycardia-induced cardiomyopathy may have played a contributory role to the changes in the left ventricular dilation and dysfunction which accompanied this disease process and are discussed in a following section.

Myocardial Proteoglycan Content with Tachycardia-Induced Cardiomyopathy and Recovery

In order to examine whether alterations in proteoglycan composition occurred within the extracellular space with the development and recovery from tachycardia-induced cardiomyopathy, left ventricular myocardial sections were stained with a monoclonal antibody against chondroitin sulfate.[39] Representative immunofluorescent photomicrographs are presented in Figure 4. In control sections, immunofluorescent staining for chondroitin sulfate revealed a homogenous pattern within the extracellular space (Figure 4A, see page 86B). With the development of tachycardia-induced cardiomyopathy, increased intensity and staining density for chondroitin sulfate was observed in all sections examined (Figure 4B). Upon inspec-

tion at higher magnification, a dense positive staining pattern surrounded individual myocytes in the tachycardia-induced cardiomyopathy group (Figure 4C). Following a 4-week recovery from pacing-induced cardiomyopathy, the relative content and distribution of chondroitin sulfate appeared to return to control levels (Figure 4D). In order to ensure specificity of the antibody, normal mouse sera was substituted for the antibody in each staining protocol. Substitution of nonimmune mouse sera abolished all staining within the extracellular space (Figure 4E).

To our knowledge, this is the first study to examine the relative content and distribution of myocardial proteoglycans with the development and recovery from cardiomyopathic disease. The proteoglycan chondroitin sulfate is the most well characterized of these large extracellular molecules.[11,12] This particular proteoglycan consists of a central protein core in which up to 100 chondroitin sulfate chains are covalently bound.[11,12] The abundant binding of negatively charged unbranched glycosaminoglycans within chondroitin sulfate, results in a molecule with a very high osmotic activity.[11,12] Accordingly, changes in the content and distribution of this proteoglycan will affect hydration within the extracellular space. It has been reported previously that tachycardia-induced cardiomyopathy resulted in increased myocardial water content.[16] The results from the present study suggest that the increased myocardial water content with this form of cardiomyopathy may be due, in part, to increased chondroitin sulfate within the extracellular space. This laboratory has demonstrated previously that with a 1-month recovery from tachycardia-induced cardiomyopathy, myocardial water content returned to control values.[16] Similarly, the relative content and distribution of chondroitin sulfate within the extracellular space, normalized with a 1-month recovery from tachycardia-induced cardiomyopathy. In light of the fact that proteoglycan content can significantly influence tissue compliance characteristics,[11,12] the unique finding that changes in proteoglycan content occur within the extracellular space, with the development and recovery from this form of cardiomyopathy, may provide further insight into the structural basis for changes in myocardial stiffness. This issue is discussed in the following section.

Relation Between Left Ventricular Function and the Extracellular Matrix with Tachycardia Cardiomyopathy

It is now well documented that chronic pacing-induced tachycardia causes a DCM with no change in left ventricular mass.[13–31] The changes within the extracellular space which have been outlined in the preceding section provide a potential structural mechanism for how these changes in left ventricular geometry may evolve with chronic tachycardia. With tachycardia-induced cardiomyopathy, a reduction in collagen content and crosslinking and a disruption in the fibrillar collagen network was observed. In addition, tachycardia-induced cardiomyopathy caused reduced myocyte adhesion capacity to components of the basement membrane. This reduction in myocyte extracellular support and tethering with tachycardia-induced cardiomyopathy may cause increased stress upon the myocytes, which in turn, result in cellular realignment within the left ventricular free wall. These results provide insight into structural mechanisms which may play a contributory role for the left ventricular dysfunction with tachycardia-induced cardiomyopathy. First, with a failure of myocyte adhesion to the basement membrane, myocyte shortening will not be transduced into the extracellular matrix and will result in reduced force production. Second, with the loss of myocyte adhesion to the basement membrane, the structural support and interface within the fibrillar collagen network is lost and subjects the myocyte to increased compressive force, stress, and deformation. An illustration of how these changes in myocyte geometry and extracellular structure could potentially influence myocardial remodeling with tachycardia-induced cardiomyopathy, is presented in (Figure 5).

A 1-month recovery period from the development of tachycardia-induced cardiomyopathy, resulted in an increased fibrillar collagen weave surrounding individual myocytes and a normalization of basement membrane adhesion capacity. These changes will provide increased extracellular support and fixation of the myocytes.[9,10] Thus, the persistent left ventricular chamber dilation which was observed following a 1-month recovery period from tachycardia-induced cardiomyopathy is probably due to enhanced extracellular structural fixation, which in turn, maintained the changes in myocyte alignment and orientation which occurred during the development phase of tachycardia-induced cardiomyopathy. An additional contributory factor towards the residual chamber dilation with recovery from tachycardia-induced cardiomyopathy is that isolated myocyte length remained increased from control values. Finally, the increased left ventricular wall thickness observed with recovery from the development of cardiomyopathy was probably due to the augmentation in isolated myocyte width. An illustration which summarizes these changes in myocyte and extracellular remodeling with recovery from tachycardia-induced cardiomyopathy is summarized in Figure 5.

With the development of tachycardia-induced cardiomyopathy, significant alterations in myocardial composition were observed. However, past studies have failed to demonstrate a significant change in left ventricular myocardial stiffness.[21,28] These results suggest that changes in myocardial collagen content and structure are not the sole determinants of myocardial compliance characteristics. For example, changes in myocardial water and proteoglycan content may significantly influence myocardial compliance. The relative content of chondroitin sulfate, an osmotically active proteoglycan, increased in the extracellular space with the development of tachycardia-induced cardiomyopathy. Thus, similar to what has been observed for other tissues,[11,12] increased myocardial proteoglycan content with tachycardia-induced cardiomyopathy may have significantly increased extracellular turgor pressure. In recent reports from this laboratory, the velocity of isolated myocyte lengthening was significantly prolonged with tachycardia-induced cardiomyopathy.[18,20] In addition, indices of active myocardial relaxation have

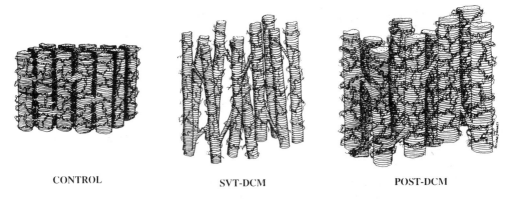

CONTROL   SVT-DCM   POST-DCM

Figure 5. Schematic summary of the changes which occurred within the extracellular space with the development of tachycardia-induced cardiomyopathy and following a 1-month recovery from this form of cardiomyopathic disease. In control myocardium (left), microscopic studies revealed a homogeneous collagen fibrillar network between myocytes. With the development of tachycardia-induced cardiomyopathy (center), myocyte length increased with a concomitant reduction in cross-sectional area. Collagen fibrils were reduced, collagen struts were not well connected to adjoining myocytes, and myocyte adhesion capacity was significantly reduced. These changes in myocyte and extracellular structure most likely contributed to the chamber dilation and orientation of myocytes within the ventricular free wall. With a 1-month recovery from tachycardia-induced cardiomyopathy (right), left ventricular mass, myocyte length, and cross-sectional area were all increased from control values. The fibrillar collagen weave had increased above control levels and myocyte adhesion capacity had normalized. Thus, the remodeling which occurred with a 1-month recovery from this form of cardiomyopathy was accompanied by myocyte hypertrophy and increased collagen content. This myocyte and extracellular remodeling with the regression from tachycardia-induced cardiomyopathy probably played a significant contributory role in the increased myocardial stiffness and persistent left ventricular dilation which was observed.

been shown to be abnormal with tachycardia-induced cardiomyopathy.[28,31] These past findings suggest that impaired myocyte active relaxation may also significantly influence myocardial stiffness with tachycardia-induced cardiomyopathy. Accordingly, the unaltered myocardial stiffness with the development of this form of cardiomyopathy is probably due to opposing changes in the determinants of myocardial stiffness; reduced collagen tethering, cross-linking, and basement membrane adhesion (decreasing myocardial stiffness), and increased proteoglycan content and myocyte relaxation (increasing myocardial stiffness). Following a 1-month recovery from tachycardia-induced cardiomyopathy, myocardial stiffness was significantly increased. The structural basis for increased stiffness with a 1-month recovery period following the development of tachycardia-induced cardiomyopathy was probably due to several factors which include: (1) increased

myocardial collagen content; (2) increased fibrillar collagen weave surrounding myocytes; (3) a normalization of collagen cross-linking and basement membrane adhesion capacity. Thus, the factors which may have contributed to decreased myocardial compliance with the development of tachycardia-induced cardiomyopathy (reduced collagen support, crosslinking, and basement membrane attachment), are reversed following a 1-month recovery. It has been shown previously that increased collagen content and a profuse fibrillar collagen weave surrounding individual myocytes can affect myocardial compliance characteristics.[6–8,33,34] Further, it has been demonstrated that in volume overload hypertrophy, an increase in collagen crosslinking alone can affect myocardial stiffness.[32] The association between increased myocardial stiffness and increased fibrillar collagen weave with a normalization of collagen crosslinking, following a 1-month recovery from tachycardia-induced cardiomyopathy, are consistent with these past reports. With recovery from tachycardia-induced cardiomyopathy, the normalization of basement membrane attachment reestablished the myocyte to collagen interface, and therefore provided the structural means by which the increased fibrillar collagen could exert resistive forces upon the myocyte during diastole. While these changes within the extracellular space probably contributed to myocardial stiffness characteristics, changes in myocyte structure may also have played a role. The results reviewed in this chapter as well as the findings from previous studies by this laboratory and others,[13–31] suggest that the changes in left ventricular function and geometry with the development and regression from tachycardia-induced cardiomyopathy are due to extracellular as well as cellular remodeling within the myocardium. Specifically, abnormalities in myofibril content and structure have been observed within myocytes following the development of tachycardia-induced cardiomyopathy.[14–16] In addition, isolated myocyte contractile function is significantly impaired with the development of tachycardia-induced cardiomyopathy.[17,18,20] Taken together, results from these past studies as well as those reviewed in this chapter suggest that intracellular, cellular, and extracellular processes all significantly contribute to the overall changes in left ventricular function and geometry with tachycardia-induced cardiomyopathy. Furthermore, the results from the present study, suggest that isolated myocyte shortening with tachycardia-induced cardiomyopathy (albeit reduced), will not be effectively transduced into overall force production.

Potential Mechanisms for the Changes Within the Extracellular Matrix with Tachycardia Cardiomyopathy

Using in situ hybridization studies, it has been demonstrated that fibroblasts within the myocardium expressed mRNAs for collagen types I and III; and is the cellular component responsible for synthesis of fibrillar collagens.[40] Following synthesis of

procollagen within the fibroblast, these molecules are extruded into the extracellular space.[41] Once in the extracellular space, procollagen undergoes polymerization into collagen fibrils. The lysyl and hydroxylysyl residues in these collagen fibrils undergo oxidation, providing a substrate for covalent crosslinking between collagen molecules.[41] This posttranslational step which occurs within the extracellular space, significantly contributes to the overall stability of the collagen fiber. Furthermore, collagen turnover can be as high as 5% to 6% in a 24-hour period.[42] Thus, overall changes in collagen content and composition can occur over a fairly short period of time. Significant changes in collagen content and composition occurred with the development of tachycardia-induced cardiomyopathy, and changed in the opposite direction after a 1-month recovery period from this form of cardiomyopathy. These findings suggest that the fibrillar collagen network has a high degree of plasticity and that these changes may have occurred at both the transcriptional and posttranslational level.

In an attempt to examine whether alterations in collagen transcriptional mechanisms occur with the development and recovery from tachycardia-induced cardiomyopathy, the relative mRNA levels for collagen types I and III were measured. The cDNA probes used for these studies localized the mRNA for the respective collagens at the previously reported and validated molecular size.[43,44] Representative Northern blots for collagen type Iα1 and type IIIα1 are shown in Figure 6. Following confirmation of the specificity of the cDNA probes used in this portion of the study, slot-blot and densitometric quantitation were performed and normalized to the mRNA signal of the constitutively expressed glycolytic enzyme; glyceraldehyde 3-phosphate dehydrogenase (GAPDH).[45] The collagen type Iα1 mRNA to GAPDH ratio was 2.68 ± 0.59 in control myocardium and did not significantly change with tachycardia-induced cardiomyopathy (2.42 ± 0.41, $P = 0.85$) or following a 1-month recovery period from the cardiomyopathy (2.58 ± 0.53, $P = 0.70$). The collagen type IIIα1 mRNA to GAPDH mRNA ratio was 0.60 ± 0.15 in control myocardium with a similar value obtained

COLLAGEN Iα1   COLLAGEN IIIα1

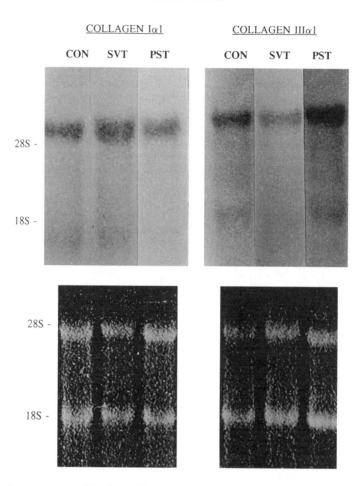

Figure 6. Top: Representative Northern blots using cDNA probes for collagen type Iα1 and type IIIα1. The lanes are marked for control myocardium (CON), with the development of supraventricular tachycardia-induced cardiomyopathy (SVT), and a 4-week recovery period from tachycardia-induced cardiomyopathy (PST). The location of the 28S and the 18S ribosomal subunits are marked respectively. The positive signal for collagen type Iα1 was above the 28S region consistent with for this 4.7-kb mRNA. The positive signal for collagen type IIIα1 was also above the 28S region corresponding to this 5.4-kb mRNA. Bottom: Ethidium bromide stain of the lanes used in the above Northern blot analysis. While similar qualitative results were observed for collagen type Iα1, the relative mRNA signal for collagen type IIIα1 appeared to increase with a 1-month recovery period following the development of cardiomyopathy. Quantitative measurements of the relative content of collagen mRNA for the three groups were performed using slot-blot analysis and two-dimensional densitometry. The collagen mRNA signals were then normalized to the expression of the constitutive enzyme: glyceraldehyde 3-phosphate dehydrogenase. The results from these experiments are summarized in the text.

with the development of cardiomyopathy ($0.64 \pm 0.12, P = 0.90$). However, following a 1-month recovery from tachycardia-induced cardiomyopathy, a significantly higher collagen type IIIα1 mRNA to GAPDH mRNA ratio was observed ($0.85 \pm 0.04, P = 0.035$). These results suggest that alterations in collagen content and structure with the development of tachycardia-induced cardiomyopathy were probably due to posttranscriptional events rather than changes in the transcription of fibrillar collagen. In rats with pressure overload, Eleftheriades and colleagues demonstrated that collagen accumulation was the result of both pretranslational as well as posttranslational mechanisms.[45] In this past study, alterations in the rate of intracellular procollagen synthesis and degradation accompanied the alterations in loading conditions. The reduction in collagen content with tachycardia-induced cardiomyopathy are probably due to these posttranslational mechanisms. The finding that steady state levels of collagen mRNA are increased following a 1-month recovery period from tachycardia-induced cardiomyopathy are consistent with studies demonstrating a concomitant rise in fibrillar collagen mRNA content and accumulation with pressure overload hypertrophy.[45,46] Similar to a recent report which examined the relationship between changes in collagen mRNA content and synthesis with pressure overload hypertrophy, the positive procollagen mRNA levels were normalized to a constitutively expressed mRNA; GAPDH.[44] In this manner, changes in overall regulation in transcription, differences in ribosomal RNA, and total mRNA with the development and recovery from tachycardia-induced cardiomyopathy could be taken into account. This is particularly important since a preliminary report from our laboratory demonstrated that steady state mRNA levels for cytoskeletal proteins (historically used for normalizing mRNA measurements), is increased with tachycardia-induced cardiomyopathy.[47] While steady state mRNA levels for the fibrillar collagens appeared unaltered with the development of tachycardia-induced cardiomyopathy, it remains unknown whether changes in mRNA stability, transcriptional efficiency, or translational capacity for fibrillar collagen occurred with this form of cardiomyopathic disease. With the recovery from tachycardia-induced cardiomyopathy, the increased mRNA levels for collagen type III probably played a contributory role towards the observed changes in collagen content and structure.

The observed changes in extractable collagen with the development and regression from tachycardia-induced cardiomyopathy suggest that alterations in posttranslational events such as collagen crosslinking occurred. It has been demonstrated that

newly synthesized, uncrosslinked collagen molecules are highly susceptible to degradative enzymes such as collagenase.[48] Thus, the reduced collagen crosslinking with the development of tachycardia-induced cardiomyopathy may result in enhanced extracellular degradation of collagen fibrils. Following a 1-month recovery from tachycardia-induced cardiomyopathy, extractable collagen had returned to control values. Thus, the normalization of intramolecular crosslinking with recovery from this form of cardiomyopathy will result in improved stability of newly synthesized collagen fibrils. It has been previously reported by this laboratory and others that the development of tachycardia-induced cardiomyopathy is associated with significant alterations in neurohormonal systems.[19,20,23,24,27,29] These neurohormonal changes with tachycardia-induced cardiomyopathy may significantly influence not only fibroblast synthetic activity but also degradative processes. Specifically, the reduced fibrillar collagen content with tachycardia-induced cardiomyopathy may be secondary to increased collagenase activity. Interstitial collagenase belongs to a large family of metalloproteinases (MMPs) which are now recognized to play a significant role in connective tissue remodeling.[49] Collagenase, also known as MMP-1, is one of the major proteinases responsible for extracellular degradation of the fibrillar matrix and has been shown to increase in activity with myocardial disease such as ischemia.[50] In a preceding chapter by Tyagi and colleagues (Chapter 6), collagenase activity as measured by a sensitive zymographic method, was increased in the endocardial samples taken from human hearts with DCM. Interestingly, these investigators reported a much lower collagenase activity in the subepicardium of samples taken from human cardiomyopathic samples. In our model of tachycardia-induced cardiomyopathy, collagen content was significantly reduced in the subendocardial region but to a much lesser degree in the subepicardium. These findings along with the results from Tyagi and colleagues, suggest that collagenase activation may play a significant role in the development of cardiomyopathic disease and may be locally regulated.

Future Directions

The studies outlined in this chapter have demonstrated that dynamic changes occur within the extracellular matrix with the development and regression from tachycardia-induced DCM. The changes in fibrillar collagen content, steady state mRNA levels, and intramolecular crosslinking which occurred in this model of cardiomyopathy may provide a means by which to identify specific mechanisms which control collagen synthesis and degradation. For example, fibroblast activity is significantly influenced by catecholamines and by angiotensin II,[51-53] and alterations in these neurohormonal systems have been demonstrated to occur in tachycardia-induced cardiomyopathy.[20,23,24,26,29] Modulation of these neurohormonal systems through β-adrenergic receptor blockade or by angiotensin converting enzyme inhibition may identify specific receptor transduction systems which are responsible for alterations in collagen metabolism in the setting of cardiomyopathic disease. As outlined in a preceding chapter, increased expression and activity of interstitial collagenase may have also played a significant contributory role in the decreased fibrillar collagen content, which was observed with the development of tachycardia-induced cardiomyopathy. Thus, this model may provide a means by which to identify specific mechanisms responsible for the induction and modulation of collagenase activity. Additional contributory factors towards the stability of the extracellular matrix within the myocardium are the basement membrane and proteoglycans. This model of DCM may provide a means by which to elucidate important structure/function relationships between changes in basement membrane constituents and integrin expression and function. Proteoglycans have been shown to be important determinants in mechanical properties of several tissues such as cartilage and tendon.[54] However, changes in proteoglycan composition within the myocardial extracellular matrix and the mechanisms which regulate biosynthesis of these noncollagenous glycoproteins has remained largely unexplored. Future studies focused upon proteoglycans within the myocardium may provide new and important insights into how this major constituent of the extracellular matrix may influence mechanical properties of the myocardium as well as other biological processes within the extracellular space with cardiomyopathic disease.

Acknowledgments

The author wishes to thank the dedication and hard work by Diane Eble, Rupak Mukherjee, Wendy Johnson, Paul Munyer, and James Zellner. The author would like to acknowledge the assistance of Michael Zile with respect to the diastolic function studies and to Thomas Borg for his advice and support regarding the basement membrane adhesion assays, as well as the valuable discussions regarding the extracellular matrix.

References

1. WHO:ISFC Task Force. Report on the WHO/ISFC task force on the definition and classification of cardiomyopathies. Br Heart J 1980; 44:672–673.

1a. Manolio TA, Baughman KL, Rodeheffer R, et al. Prevalence and etiology of idiopathic dilated cardiomyopathy (Summary of a National Heart, Lung, and Blood Institute Workshop). Am J Cardiol 1992;69: 1458–1466.

2. Hosenpud JD. The cardiomyopathies. In: Hosenpud JD, Greenberg BH, eds. Congestive Heart Failure. Pathophysiology, Diagnosis, and Comprehensive Approach to Management. New York, NY: Springer-Verlag, 1994:196–222.

3. Grossman W, Jones D, McLaurin LP. Wall stress and patterns of hypertrophy in the human left ventricle. J Clin Invest 1975;56: 56–64.

4. Hasenfuss G, Holubarsch Ch, Just H, et al. Cellular and Molecular Alterations in the Failing Human Heart. New York: Springer-Verlag, 1992.

5. Mercadier JJ, Hatem S, Schwartz K. Dilated cardiomyopathies: molecular changes responsible for altered contraction and relaxation. Heart Failure 1993;9:112–119.

6. Weber KT. Cardiac interstitium in health and disease: the fibrillar collagen network. J Am Coll Cardiol 1989;13:1637–1652.

7. Weber KT, Brilla CG. Pathological hypertrophy and cardiac interstitium. Fibrosis and

renin-angiotensin system. Circulation 1991; 83:1849–1865.

8. Weber KT, Anversa P, Armstrong PW, et al. Remodeling and reparation of the cardiovascular system. J Am Coll Cardiol 1992;20: 3–16.

9. Borg TK, Terracio L. Interaction of the extracellular matrix with cardiac myocytes during development and disease. In: Robinson TF, Kinne RKH, eds. Cardiac Myocyte-Connective Tissue Interactions in Health and Disease. Basel: Karger, 1990:113–130. (Stolte H, Kinne RKH, Bach PH, eds. Issues in Biomedicine; vol 13.)

10. Terracio L, Borg TK. Factors affecting cardiac cell shape. Heart Failure 1988;4:114–124.

11. Kuettner KE, Kimuar JH. Proteoglycans: An overview. J Cell Biochem 1985;27:327–336.

12. Hardingham TE, Fosang AJ. Proteoglycans: many forms and many functions. FASEB J 1992;6:861–870.

13. Coleman HN, Taylor RR, Pool PE, et al. Congestive heart failure following chronic tachycardia. Am Heart J 1971;81:790–798.

14. Spinale FG, Hendrick DA, Crawford FA, et al. Chronic supraventricular tachycardia causes ventricular dysfunction and subendocardial injury in swine. Am J Physiol 1990; 259:H218-H229.

15. Spinale FG, Crawford FA Jr, Hewett KW, et al. Ventricular failure and cellular remodeling with chronic supraventricular tachycardia. J Thorac Cardiovasc Surg 1991;102: 874–882.

16. Spinale FG, Zellner JL, Tomita M, et al. Relationship between ventricular and myocyte remodeling with the development and regression of supraventricular tachycardia induced cardiomyopathy. Circ Res 1991;69: 1058–1067.

17. Spinale FG, Clayton C, Tanaka R, et al. Myocardial Na$^+$,K$^+$-ATPase in tachycardia induced cardiomyopathy. J Mol Cell Cardiol 1992;24:277–294.

18. Spinale FG, Fulbright BM, Mukherjee R, et al. Relationship between ventricular and myocyte function with tachycardia induced cardiomyopathy. Circ Res 1992;71:174–187.

19. Burchell S, Spinale FG, Tanaka R, et al. The alterations in the beta-receptor pathway with tachycardia induced cardiomyopathy. J Thorac Cardiovasc Surg 1992;104:1006–1012.

20. Tanaka R, Fulbright BM, Mukherjee R, et al. The cellular basis for the blunted response to β-adrenergic stimulation in supraventricular tachycardia induced cardiomyopathy. J Mol Cell Cardiol 1993;25:1215–1233.

21. Spinale FG, Tomita M, Zellner JL, et al. Collagen remodeling and changes in LV function during development and recovery from supraventricular tachycardia. Am J Physiol 1991;261:H308-H318.

22. Zellner JL, Spinale FG, Eble DK, et al. Alterations in myocyte shape and basement membrane attachment with tachycardia induced heart failure. Circ Res 1991;69:590–600.

23. Roth DA, Urasawa K, Helmer GA, et al. Downregulation of cardiac guanosine 5'-triphosphate binding proteins in right atrium and left ventricle in pacing induced congestive heart failure. J Clin Invest 1993;91: 939–949.

24. Calderone A, Bouvier M, Li K, et al. Dysfunction of the β- and α- adrenergic systems in a model of congestive heart failure. The pacing-overdrive dog. Circ Res 1991;69:332–343.

25. Armstrong PW, Stopps TP, Ford SE, et al. Rapid ventricular pacing in the dog: pathophysiological studies of heart failure. Circulation 1986;74:1075–1084.

26. Travill CM, Williams TDM, Pate P, et al. Hemodynamic and neurohormonal response in heart failure produced by rapid ventricular pacing. Cardiovasc Res 1992;26:783–790.

27. Cavero PG, Miller WL, Heublein DM, et al. Endothelin in experimental congestive heart failure in the anesthetized dog. Am J Physiol 1990;25:F312-F317.

28. Tomita M, Spinale FG, Crawford FA, et al. Changes in left ventricular volume, mass and function during development and regression of supraventricular tachycardia induced cardiomyopathy: disparity between recovery of systolic vs. diastolic function. Circulation 1991;83:635–644.

29. Riegger GA, Elsner D, Kromer EP, et al. Atrial natriuretic peptide in congestive heart failure in the dog: plasma levels, cyclic guanosine monophosphate, ultrastructure of atrial myoendocrine cells, and hemodynamic, hormonal and renal effects. Circulation 1988;77:398–406.

30. Weber KT, Pick R, Silver MA, et al. Fibrillar collagen and remodeling of dilated canine left ventricle. Circulation 1990;82:1387–1401.

31. Perreault CL, Shannon RP, Komamura K, et al. Abnormalities in intracellular calcium regulation and contractile function in myocardium from dogs with pacing induced heart failure. J Clin Invest 1992;89:932–938.

32. Iimoto DS, Covell JW, Harper E. Increase in cross-linking of type I and III collagens associated with volume-overload hypertrophy. Circ Res 1988;63:399–408.

33. Jalil JE, Doering CW, Janicki JS, et al. Fibrillar collagen and myocardial stiffness in the intact hypertrophied rat left ventricle. Circ Res 1989;64:1041–1050.

34. Weber KT, Janicki JS, Shroff S. Collagen remodeling of the pressure-overloaded, hypertrophied nonhuman primate myocardium. Circ Res 1988;62:757–765.

35. Bishop JE, Greenbaum R, Gibson DG, et al. Enhanced deposition of predominantly type I collagen in myocardial disease. J Mol Cell Cardiol 1990;22:1157–1165.

36. Mukherjee R, Hewett K, Spinale FG. Relation between dynamic cellular and sarcomere contractile properties from the same cardiocyte. Am J Appl Physiol 1993;74:2023–2033.

37. Lundgren E, Gullberg D, Rubin K, et al. In vitro studies on adult cardiac myocytes: attachment and biosynthesis of collagen type IV and laminin. J Cell Physiol 1988;136: 43–53.

38. Terracio L, Gullberg D, Rubin K, et al. Expression of collagen adhesion proteins and their association with the cytoskeleton in cardiac myocytes. Anat Rec 1989;223:62–71.

39. Avnur Z, Geiger B. Immunocytochemical localization of native chondroitin sulfate in tissues and cultured cells, using specific monoclonal antibody. Cell 1984;38:811–822.

40. Eghbali M, Blumenfeld OO, Seifter S, et al. Localization of types I, III, and IV collagen mRNAs rat heart cells by in-situ hybridization. J Mol Cell Cardiol 1989;21:103–113.

41. Davidson JM, Berg RA. Posttranslational events in collagen biosynthesis. Methods Cell Biol 1981;23:119–136.

42. Laurent GJ. Dynamic state of collagen: pathways of collagen degradation in vivo and their possible role in regulation of collagen mass. Am J Physiol 1987;252:C1-C9.

43. Genovese C, Rowe D, Kream B. Construction of DNA sequences complementary to rat α1 and α2 collagen mRNA and their use in studying the regulation of type I collagen synthesis by 1,25-dihydroxyvitamin D. Biochemistry 1984;23:6210–6216.

44. Chu M-L, Weil D, de Wet W, et al. Isolation of cDNA and genomic clones encoding human pro-α1(III) collagen. J Biol Chem 1985;260:4357–4363.

45. Eleftheriades EG, Durand JB, Ferguson AG, et al. Regulation of procollagen metabolism in the pressure-overloaded rat heart. J Clin Invest 1993;91:1113–1122.

46. Chapman D, Weber KT, Eghbali M. Regulation of fibrillar collagen types I and III and basement membrane type IV collagen gene expression in pressure overloaded rat myocardium. Circ Res 1990;67:787–794.

47. Eble DM, McDermott PJ, Zile MR, et al. Effects of chronic supraventricular tachycardia (SVT) on contractile and non-contractile protein mRNA expression: relation to changes in myocyte structure and function.(Abstract) Circulation 1993;88(Suppl. I):I-528.

48. Vater CA, Harris ED, Siegel RC. Native cross-links in collagen fibrils induce resistance to human synovial collagenase. Biochem J 1979;181:639–645.

49. Woessner FJ. Matrix metalloproteinases and their inhibitors in connective tissue remodeling. FASEB J 1991;5:2145–2154.

50. Takahashi S, Barry AC, Factor SM. Collagen degradation in ischaemic rat hearts. Biochem J 1990;265:233–241.

51. Bhambi B, Eghbali M. Effect of norepinephrine on myocardial collagen gene expression and response of cardiac fibroblasts after norepinephrine treatment. Am J Pathol 1991; 139:1131–1142.

52. Jalil JE, Janicki JS, Pick R, et al. Fibrosis induced reduction of endomyocardium in the rat after isoproterenol treatment. Circ Res 1989;65:258–264.

53. Burgess ML, Carver WE, Terracio L, et al. Integrin mediated collagen gel contraction by cardiac fibroblasts. Effects of angiotensin II. Circ Res 1994;74:291–298.

54. Heinegard D, Oldberg A. Structure and biology of cartilage and bone matrix noncollagenous macromolecules. FASEB J 1989;3: 2042–2051.

Chapter 9

Myocarditis

Bernhard Maisch, Ute Schönian, Matthias Herzum,
Günter Hufnagel

"The most important role in the etiology of heart failure is played by inflammatory processes of the myocardium"

(P. von Schroetter, 1899)

Introduction

Historical Retrospective

Almost 100 years after Paget von Schroetter's insight[1] our knowledge on inflammatory and reparative processes of the heart and their etiology and pathogenesis has expanded dramatically. In the 18th and 19th century inflammation was a common cause of disease. Cardiotropic viruses and bacteria, were not yet known as causes of disease. In 1772 Jean Baptiste Senac, private physician of the ordinary to Louis XV[2] described what has been the accepted medical opinion until the midst of our century: "We have examined the course and sequelae of inflammatory processes and abscesses of the heart. But what is the fruit of our investigations? The inflammation of the heart is difficult to diagnose and if we have diagnosed it, we can then treat it better?"

In the 18th and 19th century coronary artery disease was almost unknown, inflammation, was preeminent. As reviewed by Christian (1951)[3] inflammatory and reparative processes in the myocardium, that we know today as viral myocarditis, pericarditis or myopericarditis, have been described as early as 1854 as a clinical syndrome long before virus isolation, viral serology, dot blot techniques or in situ hybridization were available. So Bornholm's disease or pleurodynia[4] was known

long before its viral origin could be ascertained. Myocardial inflammation in mumps[5] in influenza, in coxsackie infections, in cytomegalovirus and Epstein-Barr Virus myocarditis were described in this century (Table 1). Gore and Saphir[55] first classified a large cohort of probably fairly heterogeneous forms of myocarditis patients in 1968 and reviewed it some 20 years later.[65] It wasn't until recently that we appreciated the central role of viruses in originating and in some cases in perpetuating inflammatory heart disease, in the affection of the vascular endothelium and conduction system and in consecutive wound healing and reparative processes, which would result in impaired myocardial function. Thus the attempt to characterize heart muscle diseases by central hemodynamics only, as attempted by the WHO-ISFC task force defining cardiomyopathy[66] as heart muscle disease of unknown cause and classifying cardiomyopathies in hypertrophic, dilated and restrictive forms, can only be considered as an intermediate step to a better understanding of etiology and pathogenesis.

Since then we have come to a new understanding of myocarditis and its interrelationship as virus myocardiopathy,[67] by the evolution and implementation of molecular biology, experimental and clinical immunology, virology and biochemistry with advanced techniques:

A humoral immune response to the virus in myocarditis by antibodies of different isotypes has been known for years.[68,69] Viral persistence, has now been demonstrated in patients who have been clinically classified, either dilated cardiomyopathy or

From Weber KT, MD *Wound Healing in Cardiovascular Disease*, Armonk, NY, Futura Publishing Company Inc., © 1995.

Table 1

Viral Heart Disease in Humans

Classification	Virus	Selected References
1.0 RNA virus		
1.1 Picorna virus (Enterovirus)	Coxsackie A	(6–8);
	Coxsackie B	(9–20);
	Echo	(21–22)
	Polio	(23–27)
1.2 Orthomyxovirus	Influenza A + B	(29–34);
1.3 Paramyxovirus	Mumps	(35);
	Rubeola (measles)	(36)
1.4 Togavirus	Chikunguna	(37, 38);
	Dengue	
	Yellow fever	(38,39)
	Rubella	(40)
1.5 Rhabdovirus	Rabies	(41, 42)
1.6 Arenavirus	Lymphocytic choriomeningitis	(43);
2.0 DNA-virus		
2.1 Herpesvirus	Cytomegalovirus	(44–48)
	Epstein-Barr-virus	(49);
	Varicella-zoster	(50–53);
	Herpes simplex	(54)
2.2 Adenovirus	Adeno	(55–57)
2.3 Poxvirus	Variola	(58, 59)
	Vaccinia	(60–62)
3.0 Unclassified	Hepatitis	(63, 64)
4.0 HTLV	AIDS	(65–67)

Updated from Woodruff, 1980.

myocarditis, by a positive probe of coxsack-ievirus RNA by in situ-hybridization,[16] or dot blot techniques,[15] or with cytomegalovirus being persistent in the myocytes, the endothelial and interstitial cells of the heart[43–45] even when the inflammatory process has subsided.

Evidence of cellular and humoral autoreactivity in myocarditis[70–97] is convincing and is suggestive in about one third of patients with dilated heart muscle disease.[81–102] Mediators and soluble factors of inflammation, de novo expression of major histocompatibility antigens have been demonstrated.[103–105] It is yet unresolved, which definition of myocarditis is most appropriate: the Dallas criteria,[106] or similar definitions[82,84,87–107] or the newly evolving entity of immune mediated heart disease.[85,108] It is still a matter of debate if the virus is only the trigger of myocardial inflammation, which is upheld or expanded by immune cells and antibodies, as derived from some animal models of myocarditis,[74–77,108–113] or

is the virus also the killer of the myocytes and interstitial cells?

Cardiac Inflammation and Reparation: Definition of the Syndrome

If we do not include infective endocarditis deliberately, cardiac inflammation comprises myocarditis, pericarditis or misdiagnosed "cardiomyopathy." Therefore we have adopted the following working definitions:

Histologically validated acute myocarditis can be defined as active, healing or healed myocarditis according to Daly et al.,[114] or the almost identical Dallas criteria[106] (Table 2a). Others have subclassified acute forms of myocarditis, clinically and histologically in fulminant forms with severe acute complications (cardiogenic shock), and either acute death, or almost complete recovery; and separated them

Table 2a

Criteria of Myocarditis and Perimyocarditis

Essential criteria:
1) Inflammation of the myocardium determined by biopsy/necropsy with infiltrate, focal necrosis, interstitial edema) with or without fibrosis. According to Daly et al 1984 and Aretz et al 1987 one can distinguish different forms of *myocarditis:*
   —active myocarditis (prominent infiltrate close to myofibers, necrosis ± fibrosis
   —healing myocarditis (scarce (interstitial) infiltrate, fibrosis, no or very little necrosis)
   —healed myocarditis (2nd biopsy: focal fibrosis, no infiltrate; but in 1st biopsy :active inflammation)
   or
2) Pericardial rubs or pericardial effusion with segmental wall motion abnormality and dysrhythmia after exclusion of coronary artery disease by coronary angiography (= perimyocarditis)

Additional criteria:
   Positive RNA or DNA probe for cardiotropic viruses.
   A more than threefold alteration of titer in complement-fixation or neutralization test against cardiotropic viruses.

Table 2b

Criteria of Dilated Cardiomyopathy

Essential criteria:
   —Cardiomegaly in laevocardiography (left ventricular end-diastolic volume index >100 ml/m^2 and reduced ejection fraction ($<55\%$)
   —Exclusion of coronary artery disease, valvular heart disease, hypertension and other forms of secondary heart muscle diseases (e.g. diabetes mellitus, neuroendocrine disorder, alcohol consumption

Addition criteria:
   —Indicative histomorphology with hypertrophy and branching of myocytes, diffuse or focal fibrosis

Table 2c

Criteria for Postmyocarditic Heart Muscle Disease

Biopsy proven cellular infiltrate in 1st biopsy and missing infiltrate in second biopsy
   or
Perimyocarditis proven by clinical criteria (Table 2a) at first examination; no infiltrate in 2nd biopsy but cardiomegaly with reduced ejection fraction at the 2nd examination.

from more frequent chronic forms with incomplete recovery or poor long term prognosis.[115,116] Interobserver variability[117] and subjective definition of myocarditis are still eminent problems, however, Lie (1988),[118] comparing findings from 13 reports on the incidence of myocarditis over 6 years, gives figures ranging from less than 2.5% to 67% concludes that myocarditis in acute heart failure is as predictable as Russian roulette.

Chronic myocarditis in its histological definition is not yet accepted by many pathologists, who do not hesitate to use the term chronic in hepatitis, glomerulonephritis or appendicitis. Features of chronicity, have been known for long in myocarditis as well. In our experience, studies on the secondary immunopathogenesis in protracted forms of (peri)myocarditis and in enteroviral heart disease with viral persistence, suggest that this term should become accepted once again.[88,115]

We have defined *perimyocarditis* as pericardial effusion, associated with cardiomegaly and/or segmental wall motion abnormality (Table 2a). Pericardial effusion

Table 3

Etiology, Pathophysiology and Pathogenesis of the Acute Pericarditis Syndrome and Present Therapeutical Options

Etiological Classification	Incidence*	Therapeutical Options*
1. Idiopathic pericarditis	26*	physical restraint; aspirin (3 g/d) or corticoids in case of recurrence (initial dose: 100 mg/d) PC or PD for diagn. reasons & in tamponade
2. Infectious pericarditis		PC or PD for diagn. reasons & in tamponade
2.1 Viruses:	10*	physical restraint, immunoglobulins; specific therapy is mostly experimental:
2.1.2 Coxsackie A and B		(interferon (IFN)
2.1.3 Echovirus (e.g. type 4)		
2.1.4 Cytomegalovirus		(hyperimmune sera; gancyclovir)
2.1.5 Ebstein-Barr (posttransfusion syndrome)		
2.1.6 Mumps		
2.1.7 Herpes		
2.1.8 Varicella		
2.1.9 Hepatitis B		(hyperimmune sera, IFN)
2.2 Bacteriae:	8*	
2.2.1 Tuberculosis	4*	PC; tuberculostatic therapy (isoniazid 300 mg/d & rifampicin 600 mg/d for 9 months ethnambutol 25 mg/kg/d for 2 months; prednisone 1 mg/kg/d (2 months), tapered off
2.2.2 Pneumococcus		sensitive antibiotics
2.2.3 Staphylococcus		sensitive antibiotics
2.2.4 Streptococcus		sensitive antibiotics
2.2.5 Gram-negative rods & Haemophilus		sensitive antibiotics
2.2.6 Gonococcus		sensitive antibiotics
2.2.7 Legionella pneumophia		sensitive antibiotics
2.2.8 Rickettsiosis		tetracycline for 3–6 months
2.2.9 Borreliosis		long term antibiotics for 3–6 months
2.3 Fungo-bacterial:	rare	
2.3.1 Actinomyces		selected antimycotic treatment
2.3.2 Nocardia		selected antimycotic treatment
2.4 Fungal:	rare	
2.4.1 Candida		selected antimycotic treatment
2.4.2 Histoplasmosis		selected antimycotic treatment
2.4.3 Blastomycosis		selected antimycotic treatment
2.4.5 Coccidioidomycosis		selected antimycotic treatment
2.5 Parasitic	rare	
2.5.1 Amebiasis		metronidazole 3× 0.5–0.75 mg/d (2 weeks) or dehydroemetin 1 mg/kg 2×/d (max. dose 1 g)
2.5.2 Echinococcosis		no puncture but surgery, if possible, to eliminate the cysts, otherwise poor prognosis
2.5.3 Toxoplasmosis		pyrimetamin & sulfadiazin or spiromycin with limited success, wide pericardiectomy

(continued)

Table 3 (continued)

Etiology, Pathophysiology and Pathogenesis of the Acute Pericarditis Syndrome and Present Therapeutical Options

Etiological Classification	Incidence*	Therapeutical Options*
2.6 Other inflammatory disorders:	rare	
2.6.1 Sarcoidosis		see 1.0 or 3.1
2.6.2 Amyoloidosis,		
2.6.3 Inflammatory bowel disease		see 1.0
2.6.4 Whipple's disease		see 1.0, PC or PD in case of tamponade
2.6.5 Temporal arteritis		see 1.0 or 3.1
2.6.7 Behçet's syndrome		see 1.0 or 3.1
3. Immunologically mediated	30*	
3.1 Postinfectious, secondary autoimmune (often relapsing)	14*	physical restraint; prednisone (initial dose: 1.25 mg/kg/d for 4 weeks, 2–3 months 0.3 mg/kg/d, then tapered off, azathioprin: initial dose 2 mg/kg/d for 4 weeks, 2–3 months 0.85 mg/kg/d) in case of recurrence: Colchicin: initial dose 3 mg for 2 days, then 2 mg for 2 days, 1 mg for 3–12 months
3.2 Postcardiac injury syndromes (delayed hypersensitivity reactions)	16*	
Postcardiotomy syndrome (p10th d) (DD: early booster 3rd-5th day)	–30**	postoperatively; restraint of physical activity, small effusions: antiphlogistics (aspirin 1–3 g/d for 8–12 weeks), larger effusions: prednisone as in 3.1, azathioprin is rarely needed)
3.3 Postinfarction (Dressler's) syndrome (DD: pericarditis epistenocardica)	5**	of infarctions; therapy see 3.2 after 1–2 days of infarct only antiphlogistics
3.4 In systemic connective tissue disease and autoimmune disorders	7*	
3.4.1 Acute rheumatic fever		aspirin 6–8 g/d or 1–2 mg/kg/d prednisone
3.4.2 Systemic lupus erythematosus	35**	see 3.1 or cyclophosphamide
3.4.3 Rheumatoid arthritis	30**	see 3.1
3.4.4 Still's disease	7**	see 3.1
3.4.5 Spondylitis ankylosans	1**	see 3.1
3.4.6 Reiter's syndrome	2**	see 3.1
3.4.7 Systemic sclerosis	56**	see 3.1
3.4.8 Mixed connective tissue disease		see 3.1
3.4.9 Wegner's granulomatosis		cyclophosphamide 2 mg/kg/d & 60 mg prednisone or see 3.1
3.4.10 Churg-Strauss syndrome/ vasculitis		see 3.4.9
Panarteritis nodosa		see 3.4.9
4. Trauma	1*	
Hemopericardium		following trauma, surgery, pacemaker insertion; PC or PD
Pneumopericardium		following trauma, surgery, pacemaker insertion; PC or PD
Postradiation		(with secondary immunopathogenesis) possible

(continued)

Table 3 *(continued)*

Etiology, Pathophysiology and Pathogenesis of the Acute Pericarditis Syndrome and Present Therapeutical Options

Etiological Classification	Incidence*	Therapeutical Options*
5. Uremia untreated renal failure during ineffective hemodialysis	12*	
6. Neoplastic	17*	PC for diagnostic purposes, intrapericardial Cisplatin***
7. Myxedema	0.5*	thyroid hormones
8. Chylopericardium	rare	surgery to ligate thoracic duct
9. Hydropericardium	30*	diuretics and classic heart failure therapy (4 D's) with ACE-inhibitors

(Modified from B. Maisch, 1992)

PC: pericardiocentesis; PD: pericardiectomy.

* Incidence of pericarditis in proportion to the total number of pericarditis patients of the Marburg Registry on pericardial diseases 1980–1992.

** Incidence of pericarditis in the course of the systemic disorders (from Maisch B: The heart in rheumatic disease) 1992.

(in the absence of neoplastic, postradiation or postinjury syndromes or uremia) is indicative of the inflammatory epicardial or pericardial process, cardiac dilatation or wall motion abnormality, suggests the myocardial involvement in such inflammatory heart disease.[84–86] As already pointed out by Woodruff, (1980)[114] viral pericarditis is frequently associated with epicardial and myocardial inflammation. The term myopericarditis or perimyocarditis are almost adequate. Since myocarditis is not necessarily associated with a pericardial effusion, both clinical syndromes overlap but are not identical.

Pericarditis is an increase in pericardial fluid excluding its non inflammatory causes (Table 3). Acute, chronic, chronically recurring and constrictive forms of pericarditis. It may be diagnosed by pericardial rubs or, more frequently, by echocardiography[119,120] (Table 3).

Inflammatory heart muscle disease should be specified in myocarditis, perimyocarditis, and rejection episodes.

Dilated heart muscle disease can either be idiopathic (dilated cardiomyopathy (Table 2b)), or secondary to other causes, one of which may be myocarditis.[124] The diagnostic criteria for perimyocarditis or di-

lated heart muscle disease, are summarized in Table 2a–2c.

Viral heart disease is defined as structural abnormalities in inflammatory or dilated heart disease with the demonstration of viral RNA or DNA in the myocardium. By in situ hybridization of enterovirus RNA in infected cells in endomyocardial biopsies, Kandolf and Hofschneider[16] demonstrated a positive finding in 19 of 81 patients with suspected myocarditis, and in 8 of 27 patients with dilated cardiomyopathy. This amount is about half the percentage that Archard et al. 1988[122] demonstrated with a southern blot technique. Our own data using PCR to a group-specific sequence of enteroviral RNA gives less than 10% of enteroviral myocarditis in the entire group of myocarditis patients. Other cardiopathic agents are cytomegalovirus (CMV) which reaches up to 15% of patients with myocarditis, Influenza A and B, adeno-human, T-cell lymphotropic virus (HTLV), and a bacterial agent that can be treated with antibiotics, i.e., borreliosis (B. Burgdorferi) or Lyme disease, which may be associated in up to 20% of cases with myocarditis in endemic areas.[123] In our own patient cohort this is less than 3%.

Immune mediated heart disease or sec-

Table 4

Immunological Classification of Dilated Heart Muscle Diseases

	Endomyocardial Biopsy			Peripheral Blood			
	Lymphocytic Infiltrate	IgG, M, A, C3 Binding	Class II Expr. on M[1]	Cardio-LC[2]	NK-Cell Act[3]	AMLAs[4] or Anti-ANT ab	AFA[5] ab Matrix ab/AEA[6]
Myocarditis	+ +	+ +	+	+	reduced	+ +	+
Perimyocarditis	+ +	+ +	+	+	reduced	+ +	+
Pericarditis	−	+	±	−*	=	+	−
postmyoc. HMD**	−	+ +	−	+	reduced	+ +/+	+
DCM***	−	±	−	±	reduced/=	+	+

= = unchanged.

− = negative.

+ = postiive finding in more than 50% of patients.

+ + = positive finding in more than 80% of patients.

[1] = myocytes.

[2] = lymphocytotoxicity to isolated rat heart cells by peripheral blood lymphocytes (non-MHC, controlled lymphocytotoxicity).

[3] = Natural killer cell activity to K562 erythroblast cell line (Perlmann & Perlmann 1971).

[4] = antimyolemmal antibodies.

[5] = antifibrillary antibodies mostly from the antimyosin type.

[6] = antiendothelial antibodies.

* no cardiocytotoxicity of peripheral blood lymphocytes but strong lymphocytotoxicity from lymphocytes of the pericardial fluid (unpublished).

** heart muscle disease.

*** dilated cardiomyoapthy.

ondary immunopathogenesis refers to patients having either inflammatory heart disease or dilated heart muscle disease with signs of autoimmunity.[86,90] We recently distinguished several forms of this disorder by immuno- and immunohistopathology, in vitro assays of humoral and cellular autoreactivity (Table 4).

Cardiac *reparation* is a process associated with scarring or *reparative fibrosis* that accompanies myocyte necrosis in wound healing after ischemia or inflammation. Degradation of the extracellular matrix and collagen may in turn give rise to the formation of antibodies to components of the interstitium as can be demonstrated by endomyocardial biopsy of patients with restrictive, postinflammatory or dilated "cardiomyopathy".[88] This should be separated from constitutive or reactive fibrosis which is observed in arterial hypertension and congestive heart failure associated with an activated renin-angiotensin-aldosterone system (RAAS). This type of fibrosis can be reversed best by ACE inhibitors or by aldosterone antagonists. This has not been shown convincingly for reparative fibrosis, however.

Wound Healing in Myocarditis: An Immune Response and its Structural and Hemodynamic Consequences

Virus and Wound Healing

Virus induction of myocardial inflammation was demonstrated in many patients with myocarditis and dilated cardiomyopathy. Viral persistence by itself, does not prove that myocardial inflammation and destruction or the induction of reparative processes are mediated or caused by the virus that may have just left its fingerprints.

Pathogenesis in coxsackievirus induced myocarditis seems to be multifactorial. First of all coxsackieviruses are cytotoxic to susceptible cells. In situ hybridization studies have shown that in myocarditis the virus infects connective tissue cells as well as the myocytes themselves.[16] It remains to be determined, how much the viral infection of the myocyte and its sequela contribute to the clinical picture of the disease. The observation that clinical symptoms of myocarditis are mostly seen after the overt viral disease has subsided, and experimental studies demonstrating humoral and cellular immune reactions toward the myocardium has suggested an important role of the immune system in the mediation of coxsackievirus induced cardiac damage.

Upon viral infection of the host, humoral immune reactions to the virus and to the cardiocytes arise. Antibodies to the virus are formed to fight the infection. However, crossreaction of these antiviral immunoglobulins with cardiac myocytes and sarcolemmal proteins in particular, has been demonstrated by immunoabsorption studies with viral proteins and synthetic peptides[92,124] isolated vital cardiocytes in a complement dependent way, suggesting their pathogenic role for myocyte necrosis seen in histologic specimens. Furthermore anti-idiotypic antibodies to antiviral antibodies may bind to structures belonging to the virus receptor on the myocyte cell surface as has been shown for reovirus.[125] Several autoantigens have been described. In experimental coxsackie B3 myocarditis antibodies to cardiac myosin, seem to play a major role in mediating late phase myocarditis.[126] In humans antimyosin antibodies develop in the course of myocarditis, their incidence and pathogenic role in coxsackievirus induced myocarditis remains to be elucidated. The mitochondrial ADP/ATP translocator is yet another antigenic determinant targeted by humoral immune reactions in human and experimental coxsackievirus myocarditis. A crossreaction with the Ca-channel on the cell surface supports the idea of a pathogenic factor in the pathogenesis of myocarditis.[127] Knowledge of cellular immune reactions towards the myocardium in coxsackievirus induced myocarditis mainly stems from experimental models, because syngeneic myocardial cells as target cells for cellular immune reactions are barely available in humans. In coxsackievirus B3 infected mice depletion of T-lymphocytes by polyclonal and monoclonal an-

tibodies largely abolishes the inflammation in the myocardium.[80] Three distinct epitopes expressed on myocardial cells are recognized by cytolytic T-lymphocytes. First CD4 positive T cells lyse virally infected cardiocytes triggered by antigens belonging to coxsackievirus itself. A second type of T cells also kills virally infected cells. The antigen recognized appears on the cell surface after infection of the cell with many enteroviruses and actinomycin D, a drug known to inhibit cellular protein synthesis. An antigen arising from metabolic disturbances by the viral infection of the cell is suggested by these findings. The third population of cardiocytotoxic T lymphocytes belong to the CD 8 positive cytolytic/suppressor cell class and are activated by a yet undefined antigen on normal uninfected cardiac myocyte.[108] Whether a similar pattern exists in human coxsackievirus, induced myocarditis awaits further investigations.

CMV Myocarditis

As possible direct pathological mechanisms, one may discuss the role of the virus as a mediator for a hyperplasia for the cell by stimulation of growth factors and cytokines. The damage of the myocardial cell by the virus may lead to fibrosis.[128] Indirect mechanisms for virus induced cell damage may be the increased expression of cell surface molecules and Fc-receptors in infected cells[129] and the adhesion of lymphocytes and granulocytes to the cell surface which leads to cell damage and necrosis. Crossreacting antibodies between CMV and human myocardial tissue could attribute to this effect. According to Beck S. & Barrell B.[130] there is a sequence homology of a gene of the human cytomegalovirus to the gene expressing the coding of class I MHC-molecules in vertebrates. MHC-class I-molecules bind covalent to β2-microglobulin, so CMV could bind on the same structure.[131] This corresponds with the assessment of CMV bound to β2-microglobulin in the urine of patients. By the binding of β2-microglobulin to MHC class I-antigens on one side and CMV on the other side CMV there could be an uptake of CMV in the cell. This might lead to a loss of specificity of the immune response, first directed against the virus and leads to a subacute or chronic damage of the myocardial tissue. The expression of antigens or neo-antigens at the endothelium or on the myocyte could lead to a secondary immune pathogenesis.[132]

Inflammation and Induction of Fibrosis in Heart Disease

Myocyte destruction is regularly followed by repair through fibrous tissue (Fig. 1A). This mechanism accounts for focal scars in myocarditis both in man and experimental animal. So one prerequisite for focal fibrosis is myocardial necrosis. This mechanism does not explain diffuse interstitial fibrosis (collagen network) in patients with DCM. Nor does it account for the development of excessive endocardial fibrosis. Hypotheses and limited evidence to explain this focal or diffuse fibrosis include the several possibilities:

1. Constitutive fibrosis induced by paracrine or endocrine mechanisms such as stimulation of the RAAS after/during inflammation.

2. Response of collagen synthesis to mechanical overload and consecutive hypertrophy by yet unknown stimuli, perhaps also via RAAS activation. In nonhuman primate hypertrophy strands and tendons around myocytes were remodeled[133] (*mechanical overload hypothesis*).

3. In experimental myocardial infarction, a necrosis model in rats, the infarct size expansion coincided with a loss of collagen birefringence, indicating damaged collagen structure.[134] Similar changes were accounted for in stunned myocardium[135] (*collagen damage hypothesis*). This collagen damage hypothesis could be extended to damage fibrous tissue not directly involved in scarring.

4. In myocarditis and DCM structural focal and global alterations were

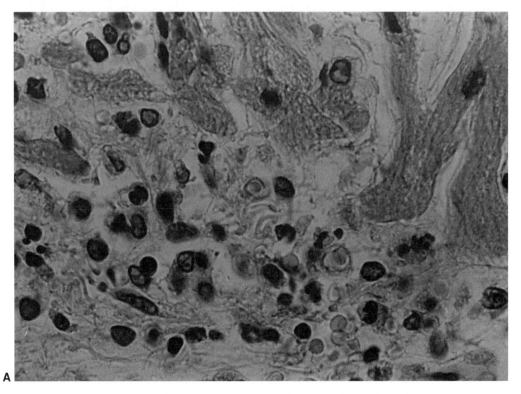

A

Figure 1a. Active myocarditis with an infiltrate of mononuclear cells and myocytolysis.

found in the matrix. In interstitial focal (healing) myocarditis fibroblast reactivity is predominant,[136] but also a global fibroblast response to focal inflammation can be observed in the myocardium, which is probably mediated by growth factors that are liberated in the course of inflammation and may be different from the RAAS activation (*mediator and growth factor hypothesis*).

Mediators and Growth Factors in Fibroblast Activation

A central role has been attributed to the mononuclear phagocyte on the way from tissue injury, which is associated with a loss of endothelial cells and an induction of fibroblast proliferation resulting in facets of inflammation. When mesenchymal cells transform to fibroblasts, chemoattractive factors are secreted.[137] Before proliferation of fibroblasts can take place, an early *competence signal* e.g., by the platelet derived growth factor (PDGF (A) and (B)), about 31 KD disulphide protein, has to be present from m-RNA levels of LPS stimulated tissue macrophages, it can be derived that the B chain genes may be expressed continuously. This gene expression is followed by a *progression signal* e.g., the insulin derived growth factor (IgF1). Both DPGF and IgF1 reside in or stored in macrophages. Fibrosis could therefore be prevented by suppression, the activation for the respective gene, the suppression of the release of the mediator, or by preventing the mediators from triggering proliferation.

The role of cytokines is just emerging in inflammation and reparation and is still speculative in myocarditis. Samsonov et al., 1991 and Klappacher et al., 1991(a,b)[138–140] have demonstrated that in dilated cardiomyopathy as in any other form of congestive failure, neopterin is increased. Neopterin is released by monocytes under control of activated T-lymphocytes via interferon-gamma, thus reflecting T-cell activation. Tumor necrosis factor alpha (TNF$_{alpha}$) was found increased in advanced stages of heart failure independent from their cause. In addition beta 2-microglobulin levels were found increased in sera of patients with dilated cardiomyopathy, both due to impairment of renal function in advanced heart failure and due to T-cell activation. The first data on mediators in possibly postviral dilated heart muscle disease, demonstrate trends similar to those in rejection after heart transplantation.

Some other reparative features, e.g., hypertrophy, may be controlled by proto-oncogenes, such as c-myc and c-fos or by collagen genes, which have been expressed de novo in different forms of heart disease and first described in rejection[141] or by focal stretch or overload.

The Role of T-cells in Myocarditis and Reparative Fibrosis

Lymphocyte Subpopulations and Peripheral Blood Cells

In our own patients,[84,141] white cell blood count did not show significant differences between patients with viral or idiopathic myocarditis, perimyocarditis, pericardial effusion, dilated cardiomyopathy, postmyocarditic heart disease and non cardiac controls. In one-fourth of patients with acute inflammation, only lymphocytosis was observed. Distribution of T-lymphocyte subpopulations in patients with myocarditis were not significantly different from a control population except of an increase in OKlal-positive B cells and activated T-lymphocytes were significantly in perimyocarditis and a marginal decrease in T-suppressor cells in postmyocarditic heart muscle disease, was demonstrated (table 4). In contrast, in primary dilated cardiomyopathy circulating OKMI-positive monocytes were increased.[84]

Lymphocytes from Endomyocardial Biopsies

Lymphocytes can also be outgrown from the biopsies of patients with suspected myocarditis or dilated cardiomyopathy and can be cultured and expanded in the presence of human recombinant interleukin 2. CD4+ cell populations prevailed in 2 thirds of patients when compared to CD8+ cells or a mixed population (142, Schultheiß HP (personal communication)). They may exert natural killer cell activity and produce lymphokines like IL2.

T-suppressor Cell Activity

The reports on changes of T-suppressor cell activity in myocarditis and dilated cardiomyopathy vary considerably. In contrast to others[100] in our patients with myocarditis spontaneous (assessed according to Breshnihan & Jasin 1977[143]) in vivo and Con A generated T-suppressor cell activity (assessed according to Hallgren & Yunis[144]), did not differ from sex- and age-matched controls without heart disease.[94] In postmyocarditic dilated heart disease in selected indicator systems such as the autologous irradiated mixed lymphocyte reaction and the allogenic mitogen stimulation a significant reduction in T-suppressor cell activity was seen. There is, a broad variance in T-suppressor cell activity, both in controls and in patients with acute inflammatory heart disease. Different indicator systems for the assessment of T-suppressor cell activity may not possess the same sensitivity in expressing changes in some of the T-suppressor cell subpopulations. It cannot be ruled out that the antigen-specific T-suppressor cell activity may have been changed, also global changes were not found.

Cellular Effector Mechanisms in Man

Natural Killer Cell Activity

Natural killer cell activity in patients with perimyocarditis was markedly decreased in the acute state in all three lymphocyte/target cell rations examined. In postmyocarditic dilated muscle heart disease, NK cell activity had almost returned to normal (Table 5). In primary dilated cardiomyopathy a significant decrease NK-cell activity was observed again.[84,98]

Target Cell Specific Non MHC Restricted Lymphocytotoxicity

In contrast, in myocarditis, target cell specific non MHC restricted lysis against

Table 5

Immunohistological Findings in Endomyocardial Biopsy. Würzburg Multicentre Study
(% positive titres ≥ +1)

Clinical Diagnosis	N	Trivalent	IgG	IgM	IgA	C3	C3 or IgM
Myocarditis (active/acute)	20	100*†	90*†	55*†	70*†	70*†	85*†
Perimyocarditis (active/acute)	20	100*†	100*†	95*†	90*†	90*†	100*†
Status postmyocarditis (no cardiomegaly)	22	100*†	95*†	32*	32*	36*	45*
Status postperimyocarditis (no cardiomegaly)	15	73*	60*	13	7	33*	40*
Postmyocarditic HMD‡ (cardiomegaly)	28	79*	75*	18	36*	61*†	75*
Dilated cardiomyopathy (idiopathic)	50	60*	56*	48*†	8	12	48*
Dilated HMD‡ with increased alcohol intake	20	60*	60*	15	25*	35*	40*
Noncardiac controls	17	12	12	0	0	0	0
Coronary artery disease	100	43*	41*	11	20*	3	14

*$P < 0.05$ by χ^2 analysis when compared to noncardiac controls.
†$P < 0.05$ by χ^2 analysis when compared to coronary artery disease.
‡ HMD, Heart muscle disease. From Eur Heart J 9, Suppl H, p. 68.

living adult allogenic rat myocytes, is sustained or slightly enhanced (Table 4). This also applies to postmyocarditic dilated heart disease and primary dilated cardiomyopathy in which one third of patients demonstrated an increase of target cells specific cytotoxicity. Analysis of antibody-dependent cellular cytotoxicity (ADCC) showed little variation from normal.[92]

A related aspect can be derived from experimental murine Coxsackie B myocarditis in Balb c mice; when CD8- positive cells are depleted, both the inflammatory reaction and the consecutive diffuse fibrosis are significantly reduced.[145]

The Response of the Fibroblasts in Myocarditis—Mechanisms of Control

The fibroblasts are responsible for collagen synthesis and collagenolysis in the interstitium of the heart.[146] Immune cells release factors, lymphokines and monokines, that stimulate proliferation and matrix synthesis by fibroblasts such as interleukins. They produce alpha- and gamma-interferon, which have been shown to inhibit collagen synthesis by fibroblasts. Activated macrophages produce fibronectin, which stimulates the directed migration of fibroblasts. Macrophages also produce fibroblast growth factor[137] and Il1, which stimulate collagen synthesis. Cytokines, may have diverse effects on different subsets of fibroblasts. Prostaglandin E_2 may inhibit certain gingival fibroblasts. C_{1q} may bind to some fibroblasts, it may stimulate their proliferation and increase their collagen synthesis.[147] Certain viruses e.g., Rous sarcoma virus decreases collagen production,[148] others may stimulate it. The collagenases from macrophages, monocytes and neutrophiles may be involved in collagen degradation, but the most important cells, that secrete and produce collagenases in man are fibroblasts.

Structural Alterations of the Cytoskeleton in Diseased Human Myocardium

In acute myocarditis, hallmarks are focal myocytolysis, cellular infiltrates (fig. 1a) and also alterations of the interstitial tissue (fig. 1a). It is likely, that the inflammatory or the degenerative processes also involve proteins of the sarcolemma and the extracellular matrix. It has been pointed out that this is likely to be due to autoreactive, but can also be due to degenerative processes alone. The histologic characteristics of dilated heart muscle disease during and after myocarditis, are interstitial and subendocardial fibrosis (fig. 2), fiber hypertrophy and mitochondriosis.

Schaper and coworkers[149,150] and ourselves[88,151] have analyzed the microscopic alterations of the cytoskeleton with monoclonal antibodies in myocarditis and dilated cardiomyopathy and described the following observations:

1. Desmin, is normally located at the Z-band and has the function of alignment to adjacent cells. In myocarditis it is decreased in areas of infiltrating lymphocytes, in DCM it may be formed highly irregularly, when probed for with a monoclonal antidesmin antibody.

2. Tubulin, which also belongs to the skeleton, may be decreased during the acute inflammation but diffusely increased or altered in DCM.

3. Vinculin is incorporated into the sarcolemmal membrane and the intercalated discs and has among others the function to bind actin. In acute myocarditis and DCM it may be increased or have an irregular shape in EMB.

4. Laminin, a 220 KDA protein, is closely associated with the basement membrane. It has the function to bind to collagen IV and is in continuous contact with the cytoskeleton. In myocarditis and DCM it has been demonstrated to be irregularly shaped and increased in content.

5. Fibronectin, is another basement protein which binds cells to collagen. In myocarditis and DCM it may also be increased and appear in irregular forms.

6. Vimetin is found in endothelial cells and in fibroblasts. Its monoclonal antibody gives a speckled pattern in the immunofluorescence test. In

chronic myocarditis and DCM it may be increased due to increased fibrosis in EMB.

It is unclear if these alterations are linked to the primary pathogenetic process in myocarditis and dilated heart muscle disease in a cause-consequence relationship or if they are, which is more likely a secondary phenomena of the pathogenic process.

Myocardial Antigens in Inflammatory and Autoimmune Heart Disease

This overview details the still limited knowledge that we possess in response to autoreactive mechanisms to the myocardium, which may involve the myocyte, the endothelial cells and the fibroblasts, their micro-, intermediate- and macrofilaments and their extracellular matrix and the "tissue-specific" sarcolemmal-myolemmal epitopes. Apart from molecularly defined

(neo) antigens this contribution focuses on autoreactive mechanisms involving extracellular matrix and collagen tissue.

Autoantigens of the Myocyte

Antigens that were identified as targets of humoral and cellular autoreactivity include all components that can be identified by light microscopy or with cryostat sections. They can be derived from (Fig. 1b). Some antigens can also be identified further biochemically or defined by monoclonal antibodies. Most important antigens are the following:

1. The *sarcolemma and myolemma*, to which cytolytic complement-fixing antibodies are directed in Coxsackie B, mumps and influenza myocarditis.[83–87,92] Recent evidence has been accumulated that antigenic mimicry may play a role: Epitopes on the sar-

ORGANELLES AND STRUCTURES OF A CARDIOCYTE

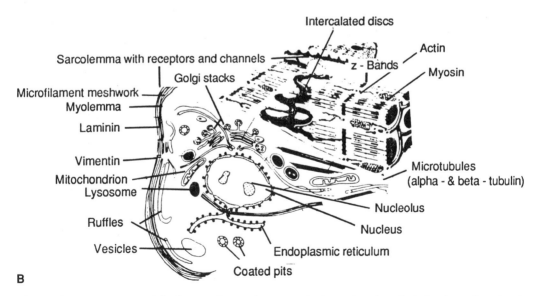

B

Figure 1b. Autoantigens of the heart. The myolemma, which can be identified clearly with isolated human heart cells consists of the plasmalemma, the myolemma and basement membrane and is made up with laminin, proteoglycanes, membrane bound receptors and membrane specific epitopes. The sarcolemma as identified by immunofluorescence techniques includes the endomyosium with fibronectin, type I, III and V collagen. The interstitium comprises the epimyosium with its biochemically defined components.

colemmal surface were found to share antigenic properties with Coxsackie B viruses. The sarcolemmal fluorescence was greatly diminished and the cytolytic serum activity was absorbed by the virus.[83,85,89,97]

2. *Mitochondrial proteins*,[78,79,152,153] which include the antinucleotide translocator (ANT) that has been proposed to cross react to parts of the calcium channel and/or to the gap junction proteins.[152] The anti-M7 antibody(ies) has also been described as a tissue-specific mitochondrial antigen in myocarditis and dilated cardiomyopathy, but it is not positive in all patients.[79,154] It is noteworthy that other mitochondrial antigens may also evoke a humoral immune response. Anti M_1–M_6 antibodies may be found as well, but do not possess tissue specificity.[79] Experimentally induced antibodies to the *antinucleotide translocator* do not necessarily bind complement in order to be of pathogenetic relevance. Since they might crossreact with the *calcium channel* one can speculate, that they may keep the calcium channel open, thus accelerating a deleterious calcium entry into the cell.[152]

3. *Antibodies to fibrils* have been described in DCM[90,93] as in cases with myocarditis[155,156] as antibodies to myosin and actin. In rabbits, sensitized lymphocytes have been demonstrated to respond to purified myosin in a dose-response-like manner.[90,112] Myocardial lesions with larger infiltrates and rarely some focal infiltrates in the skeletal muscle were detected by light microscopy already after the 2nd and 3rd booster injection. Antimyosin antibodies in high titers associated with antisarcolemmal antibodies were the most prominent serological finding (Table 6). In CVB$_3$ myocarditis analysis of genetically different strains of mice revealed that two different forms of myocarditis could be induced:

1. An early (before day 14) virus in-

duced form with a polymorphe infiltrate.

2. A late (after day 14) immunopathic CVB$_3$ induced myocarditis, which is characterized by a mononuclear focal cell infiltrate and circulating antimyolemmal-, antisarcolemmal and antimyosin antibodies.[105,157]

3. The early form found in the susceptible strains A.By, A.Sw demonstrated higher viremia. It seems from the studies of Wolfgram et al.[112] and Beisel et al.[158] that the susceptibility or resistence to infection by Coxsackie B2 viruses is under polygenic control both by non H_2 background genes and MHC genes. The later disease was more severe in animals with heart specific autoantibodies, an observation made for the A.CA strain. High antibody producers were found in certain strains (A.Sw; A.CA) only, indicating the strength of the heart-specific antibody reaction is influenced by the MHC. In man it remains unclear, if antimyosin antibodies are only of biographic relevance, since during infections in childhood they can be induced and may persist. They may also be natural antibodies without significant pathogenetic relevance.[86]

4. Antibodies to the *beta-adrenoceptor* have recently been demonstrated to exist in patients with dilated cardiomyopathy.[159] These antireceptor antibodies may be of pathogenetic relevance in autoreactive, inflammatory myocardial diseases and postmyocarditic disorders of the heart.

5. Further *nonorgan-specific* but defined *antigens* include desmin found in myocytes, vimentin, a marker of fibroblasts and histiocytes and collagen (particularly type III), fibronectin, myosin and actin. Their histologic localization can be derived from Fig. 2. From our own data, monoclonal antibodies to intermediate, micro- and macrofilaments would give the following staining patterns on human adult cardiocytes, rat cardiocytes, cryostat sec-

Table 6a

Circulating Antibodies to the Sarcolemma, the Extracellular Matrix and Intermediate Filaments (% positive) in Myocarditis and Perimyocarditis

References	n	AMLA (homol)	ASA (homol)	ALA	A-Fibron	Z-Bands	A-Actin	A-Myosin	A-Tubulin	AIDA	A-Desmin	A-Vimentin	ANT	A-M7	AEA	A-BAR	A-Collagen Type I	III	IV	V
de Scheerder [16]	12	100	12	nd	nd	nd	58	67	nd	nd	nd	nd	nd	nd	91	nd	35	40	35	35
Klein [42, 43]	nd	nd	nd	nd	nd	nd	nd	nd	nd	nd	nd	nd	nd	13	nd	nd	nd	nd	nd	nd
Maisch [57, 59, 60, 66, 82]																				
Viral myocarditis (adults)	44	79–90	75–90	nd	nd	15	7	10–50	0	0	nd	nd	nd	nd	80	nd	nd	nd	nd	nd
Idiopathic myocarditis	144	59	45	nd	nd	nd	0	23	9	0	nd	nd	nd	nd	40	nd	nd	nd	nd	nd
Maisch et al. [78] in children		100	100	nd	nd	0	0	0	0	0	nd	nd	nd	nd	91	nd	nd	nd	nd	nd
Maisch et al. [80]	132	nd	nd	30–35	nd	nd	nd	nd	nd	nd	nd	nd	nd	nd	nd	nd	nd	nd	nd	nd
Obermayer et al. [84]	25	64	72	nd	nd	16	0	4	0	nd	0	0	nd	nd	72	nd	nd	nd	35	nd
Schultheiß [103, 105]	29	nd	nd	60	20	nd	nd	nd	nd	nd	nd	nd	nd	nd	nd	nd	30	40	35	35

Abbreviations as in Table 2.
(From Maisch B: Autoreactivity to the cardiac myocyte, connective tissue and the extracellular matrix in heart disease and postcardiac injury. In Springer Seminars in Immunopathology 11, p. 377, 384, 388; 1989 (97) with permission).

Table 6b

Circulating Antibodies to the Sarcolemma, the Extracellular Matrix and Intermediate Filaments (% positive) in Pericarditis

References	n	AMLA (homol)	ASA (homol)	ALA (homol)	A-Fibron	Z-Bands	A-Actin	A-Myosin	AIDA	A-Desmin	A-Tubulin	A-Vimentin	ANT	A-M7	AEA	A-BAR	A-Collagen Type			
																	I	III	IV	V
de Scheerder et al. [16]	10	60	60	nd	nd	nd	10	10	nd	nd	nd	nd	nd	nd	70	nd	nd	nd	nd	nd
Maisch et al. [65] Tuberculous pericarditis	10	100	100	nd	nd	0	8	67	0	nd	nd	nd	nd	nd	42	nd	nd	nd	nd	nd
Maisch et al. [69] uremic pericarditis	41	30–83	50–100	nd	nd	0	0	0	0	nd	nd	nd	nd	nd	20–50	nd	nd	nd	nd	nd
Obermayer et al. [84] idiopathic pericarditis	10	80	50	nd	nd	0	nd	nd	nd	0	0	0	0	nd	nd	nd	nd	nd	nd	nd

Abbreviations as in Table 2.

(From Maisch B: Autoreactivity to the cardiac myocyte, connective tissue and the extracellular matrix in heart disease and postcardiac injury. In Springer Seminars in Immunopathology 11, p. 377, 384, 388; 1989 (97) with permission).

Table 6c

Circulating Antibodies to the Sarcolemma, the Extracellular Matrix and Intermediate Filaments (% positive) in Dilated Cardiomyopathy

References	n	AMLA (homol)	ASA (homol)	ALA	A-Fibron	Z-Bands	A-Actin	A-Myosin	AIDA	A-Desmin	A-Tubulin	A-Vimentin	ANT	A-M7	AEA	A-BAR	A-Collagen Type I	III	IV	V
Klein et al. [42]	nd	nd	nd	nd	nd	nd	nd	nd	nd	nd	nd	nd	nd	30	nd	nd	nd	nd	nd	nd
Maisch et al. [67]	79	9	10	nd	nd	nd	4	20	2	nd	nd	nd	nd	nd	13	nd	nd	nd	nd	nd
Maisch et al. [70]	30	33	42	nd	nd	nd	10	33	2	nd	nd	nd	nd	nd	45	nd	12	24	6	24
Schultheiß et al. [104, 105]	51	nd	nd	72	nd	nd	nd	nd	nd	nd	nd	nd	nd	nd	nd	nd	nd	nd	nd	nd
Obermayer et al. [84]	36	42	31	nd	nd	8	0	8	nd	nd	0	0	nd	nd	31	nd	nd	nd	nd	nd

Abbreviations as in Table 2.
(From Maisch B: Autoreactivity to the cardiac myocyte, connective tissue and the extracellular matrix in heart disease and postcardiac injury. In Springer Seminars in Immunopathology 11, p. 377, 384, 388; 1989 (97) with permission).

Table 6d

Circulating Antibodies to the Sarcolemma, the Extracellular Matrix and Intermediate Filaments (% positive) in Healthy Controls

References	n	AMLA (homol)	ASA (homol)	ALA	A-Fibron	Z-Bands	A-Actin	A-Myosin	A-Tubulin	AIDA	A-Desmin	A-Vimentin	ANT	A-M7	AEA	A-BAR	A-Collagen Type I	III	IV	V
Maisch et al. [66, 67]	200	31	35	nd	nd	5	5	5	0	0	0	0	nd	nd	17	nd	nd	nd	nd	nd
Maisch et al. [59, 82]	45	16	18	20	nd	nd	nd	nd	nd	nd	nd	nd	nd	nd	nd	nd	nd	nd	nd	nd
Obermayer et al. [84]	25	20	20	nd	nd	0	nd	nd	0	nd	4	0	nd	nd	nd	nd	nd	nd	nd	nd
de Scheerder et al. [16]	40	10	5	nd	nd	nd	5	3	nd	nd	nd	nd	nd	nd	12	nd	5	5	5	5
Klein et al. [42, 43]	nd	nd	nd	nd	nd	nd	nd	nd	nd	nd	nd	nd	nd	0	nd	nd	nd	nd	nd	nd
Schultheiß et al. [105]	nd	nd	nd	nd	nd	nd	nd	nd	nd	nd	nd	nd	nd	nd	nd	nd	nd	nd	nd	nd

AMLA Anti-myolemmal antibody; *ASA* anti-sarcolemmal antibody; *ALA* anti-laminin antibody; *A-* anti-; *Fibron* fibronectin; *AIDA* anti-intercalated disc antibody; *ANT* anti-nucleotide translocator; *AEA* anti-endothelial antibody; *BAR* beta-receptor.
(From Maisch B: Autoreactivity to the cardiac myocyte, connective tissue and the extracellular matrix in heart disease and postcardiac injury. In Springer Seminars in Immunopathology 11, p. 377, 384, 388; 1989 (97) with permission).

tions of normal human myocardium.[85,86]

6. Stress proteins are synthesized either constitutively or in response to heat shock or other metabolic insults. Stress proteins are immunodominant antigens of mycobacteria and other nonviral mechanisms and have been highly conserved during evolution. Stress proteins therefore have been thought to be involved in the pathogenesis of various autoimmune diseases. In the sera of patients with myocarditis (N = 48) antibodies against hsp27 could be detected in 25%, against hsp60 in 8% and against hsp70/hsc70 in 21%. These results were significantly different from the findings in sera of healthy controls (hsp 27 11%, hsp60 1%, hsp70/hsc70 3%). In DCM (N = 87) antibodies against hsp60 and hsp70/hsc70 were significantly increased compared to controls (I. Portig, unpublished data).

Humoral Autoreactivity in Myocarditis and Perimyocarditis

Circulating Autoantibodies to the Myocardium and its Constituents

Apart from tissue-specific epitopes which may give rise to organ-specific antibodies like the antimyolemmal bodies, the antisarcolemmal antibody (Figure 2a) the anti-ANT carrier antibody or the beta-receptor, a polyclonal immune response takes place which involves (Figure 2b) also cytoskeletal proteins and intermediate filaments to varying degrees[86] (Table 6). It remains unresolved, if these antibodies particularly when they are low in titer, and "natural" antibodies, which had already been present

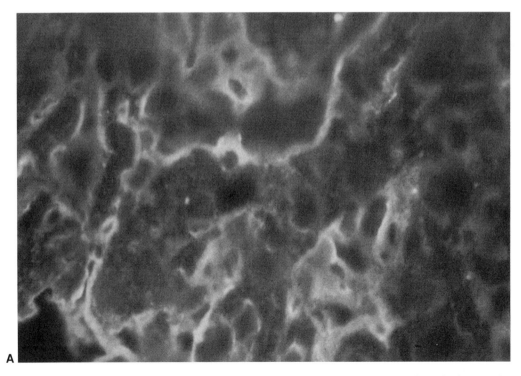

A

Figure 2A. The identity of bound and circulating (FITC-labeled) antisarcolemmal antibodies can be demonstrated in the same patient with a double sandwich technique. ($\times 800$, Anti-human IgG, Medac; dilution 1:1,000; Fab$_2$-fragments; serum dilution 1:320).

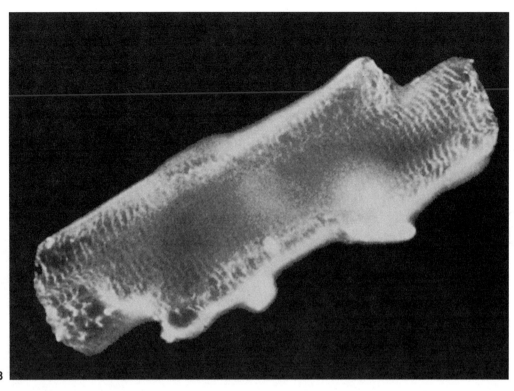

B

Figure 2B. Demonstration of antimyolemmal antibodies of the same patient with an isolated intact human atrial cardiocyte. (×1200, FITC-labeled anti-human IgG, Medac; dilution 1:1000; Fab₂-fragments; serum dilution 1:320).

before the inflammatory disease occurred, and if they are only remnants of former viral infections. For mumps it is known, that an antimyosin antibody, primarily of the IgM-type, later also of the IgG-type may occur. From our control data in children ranging from one month to 16 years of age, we have low but rising incidence of antibodies to the sarcolemma, to the intermediate filaments, to collagen and to the vascular endothelium, even if no myocardial involvement in infections was ever noticed. These antibodies not only circulate in the peripheral blood of the patients, they also bind in varying degrees to the autologous myocardial biopsy specimens. Figure 2b gives an overview on histologic structures that can be identified in endomyocardial biopsies or with the indirect immunofluorescence test on cryostat sections to which these antibodies may be directed. Different from "natural" antibodies are heterophilic antibodies that mostly react with nonhuman tissue and

may also give a sarcolemmal or interstitial staining.[160]

Bound Autoantibodies in Endomyocardial Biopsies (EMB) in Myocarditis

It is of diagnostic importance that IgG antibodies bind to the sarcolemma and interstitial tissue in EMBs in more than 98% of cases (Fig. 2C). This finding lacks specificity, because in other forms of heart disease like coronary artery disease or hypertension as well as in healthy controls IgG may bind to the extracellular matrix and/or the sarcolemma. In the immunofluorescence test this is indistinguishable. IgG-binding ranges in coronary artery disease between 20 to 35% (Fig. 2a). The IgM antimembrane antibody and complement fixation are specific for acute or postacute inflammatory diseases. Particularly when they are found concomi-

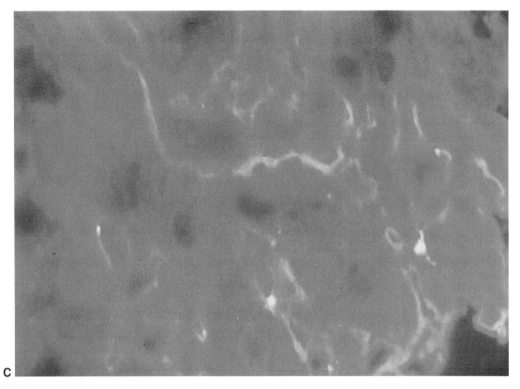

Figure 2C. Demonstration of bound antisarcolemmal antibodies (IgG, C3-fixation, IgA) in the endomyocardial biopsy specimen of a 42 year old male patient with postviral (previous Coxsackievirus-myocarditis) dilated heart muscle disease. The immunoglobulin binds to sarcolemma and interstitial space. ($\times$800; Anti-human IgG, Medac; dilution 1:1000; TRICT-labeled Fab$_2$-fragments).

tanty.[86,87,93] This binding pattern (Fig. 2c) can be attributed both to specific antimyolemmal antibodies, antisarcolemmal antibodies or those directed collagen in the extracellular matrix. Thus more than the hardly identifiable binding site, it is the function of the antibody in myocarditis which is important. Cytolytic antibodies point to an autoreactive mechanism in myocarditis and perimyocarditis, particularly when complement fixation is present. In biopsy specimens the latter may occur only focally, which is then well in accordance with the focal lesions of myocarditis.

Cytolytic and Cytotoxic Serum Activity

The functional properties of the circulating and bound antibodies in inflammatory heart disease may be manifold: In Coxsackie B myocarditis antibodies which are directed to the myolemma and which crossreact with the Coxsackie B virus are primarily cytolytic. Only in the presence of complement the serum exerts a cytolytic effect on isolated vital cardiocytes.[89,155] The titers of these antibodies correlate roughly with their cytolytic properties. This also holds for influenza- and mumps myocarditis, and for some forms of idiopathic perimyocarditis. In idiopathic myocarditis a certain proportion of patients have antibodies which possess only a marginal cytolytic effect but may be cytotoxic: they decrease the number of viral myocardial cells without addition of fresh complement.[86,89] This phenomenon correlates with observations made by Kühl et al.,[161] that some patients with myocarditis, have an antibody directed to the calcium channel which itself may crossreact to the ADP/ATP translocator. It can be speculated that such an antibody may open the calcium channel and induce intracellular calcium accumulation, thus killing the myocyte without need for complement. We have also observed sera which have been AMLA-positive and were not cytotoxic, but protective with respect to the natural decay of myocytes in culture.

The incidence of antibodies to laminin, fibronectin and different classes of collagen,[16,105] to actin and myosin vary in different studies,[83–86,89] particularly because different assays were used to evaluate their incidence. Since antilaminin, antifibronectin, anticollagen, antiactin, antimyosin and even antiendothelial antibodies may also occur in "healthy," normal individuals, it depends largely on the titers in the reference samples if an assay is termed positive or negative with a low titer antibody possibly being present. It is likely that low titers of antilaminin, antifibronectin, anticollagen antibodies and antibodies directed against intermediate and microfilaments circulate in the peripheral blood of many individuals

as natural antibodies. These may have immuno-regulative properties, and may not be a classical organ-specific "autoantibody." For antibodies directed to the beta-receptor both in myocarditis and in dilated cardiomyopathy stimulating and blocking effects have been reported.[159,162] This indicates that in the course of infections of the heart various antibodies exist, that will exert more than one effect. The role of mediators is still poorly understood. Serum inhibiting factors have been demonstrated in patients with myocarditis, but it is unclear if they are regulatory proteins, e.g., heat shock or stress proteins and their antibodies, toxic substances, lymphokines like the interleukins or interferon, TNF alpha or beta or other substances. The de novo expression of major histo-compatibility class I and II antigens (Fig. 2d) and of adhesion molecules is cytokine induced and can be observed in active and chronic myocarditis.

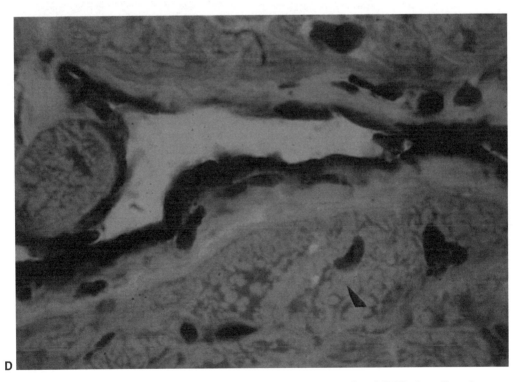

Figure 2D. De novo expression of major histocompatibility complex (MHC) class II antigens at the vascular endothelium in a 29-year-old women with severe heart failure due to lymphocytic myocarditis. CMV-DNA could be demonstrated by in situ hybridization.

Autoreactivity to Cardiocytes and Connective Tissue in Pericarditis

In pericarditis (Table 6b) a shift to antibodies against the extracellular matrix, collagen and intermediate filaments is observed among the circulating antibodies.[85–87] Antiactin and antimyosin antibodies are rare in higher titers, antimitochondrial antibodies have not been investigated further. Data on the beta-receptor antibodies are missing. The incidence of bound antibodies to sarcolemmal proteins in the biopsy studies is reduced in pericarditis[87,89] when compared to myocarditis. Cytotoxic or cytolytic serum activity is less pronounced. No data is known to BAR-antibodies in this group of patients.

References

1. Senac JB: Traité de la structure du coeur, de son action at de ses maladies (1772) quoted by Petra Schramm, Editio rarissima 1986.
2. Schroetter P von: Die Insuffizienz des Herzmuskels. Verh Congr Inn Med 1899;17.
3. Christian HA: Nearly ten decades of interest in idiopathic pericarditis. Am Heart J 1951;42:645.
4. Sylvest E: Epidemic myalgia: Bornholm Disease. London, Oxford 1934.
5. Bengtsson E, Örndahl G: Complications of mumps with special reference to the incidence of myocarditis. Acta Med Scand 1954;149:381.
6. Bell EJ, Grist NR: Coxsackie virus infections in patients with acute cardiac disease and chest pain. Scott Med J 1968;13:47.
7. Grist NR, Bell EJ: Coxsackie viruses and the heart. Am Heart J 1969;77:295.
8. Grist NR, Bell EJ: A six year study of Coxsackie virus B infections in heart disease. J Hyg 1974;73:165.
9. Smith WG: Coxsackie B myopericarditis in adults. Am Heart J 1970;80:34.
10. Kibrick S, Benirschke K: Acute aseptic myocarditis and meningoencephalitis in the newborn child infected with Coxsackie virus group B, type 3. N Engl J Med 1956;255:883.
11. Fletcher E, Brennan CF: Cardiac complications of Coxsackie virus infection. Lancet 1957;1:913.
12. Fletcher GF, Coleman MT, Feorius PM et al: Viral antibodies in patients with primary myocardial disease. Am J Cardiol 1968;21:6.
13. Sainani GS, Krompotic E, Slodki S: Adult heart disease due to the Coxsackie virus B infection. Medicine 1968;47:133.
14. Jennings RC: Coxsackie group B fatal neonatal myocarditis associated with cardiomegaly. J Clin Pathol 1966;19:325.
15. Bowles NE, Ricahrdson PJ, Olsen EGJ et al: Detection of Coxsackie B virus-specific RNA sequences in myocardial biopsy samples from patients with myocarditis and dilated cardiomyopathy. Lancet 1986;1:1120.
16. Kandolf R, Hofschneider PH: Viral heart disease. Springer Semin Immuno Pathol 1989;11:1.
17. Longson M, Cole FM, Davies C: Isolation of a Coxsackie virus group B, type 5, from the heart of a fatal case of myocarditis in an adult. J Clin Pathol 1969;22:654.
18. Russell SJM, Bell EJ: Echoviruses and carditis. Lancet 1970;1:784.
19. Monif GRG, Lee CW, Hsiung GD: Isolated myocarditis with recovery of ECHO type 9 virus from the myocardium. N Engl J Med 1976;277:1353.
20. Ludden TE, Edward JE: Carditis in poliomyelitis: An anatomic study of thirty-five cases and review of the literature. Am J Pathol 1949;25:357.
21. Dolgopol VB, Cragen MD: Myocardial changes in poliomyelitis. Arch Pathol 1948;46:202.
22. Kipkie GF, McAuley JSM: Acute myocarditis occurring in bulbar poliomyelitis. Can Med Assoc J 1954;70:315.
23. Laake H: Myocarditis in poliomyelitis. Acta Med Scand 1951;140:159.
24. Giles C, Chuttleworth EM: Post mortem findings in 46 influenza deaths. Lancet 1957;2:1224.
25. Weinstein L, Shelokov A: Cardiovascular manifestations in acute poliomyelitis. N Engl J Med 1951;244:281.
26. Hamburger WW: The heart in influenza. Med Clin North Am 1938;22:111.
27. Finland M, Parker F Jr, Barnes MW, Joliffe LS: Acute myocarditis in influenza infections: Two cases of non-bacterial myocarditis with isolation of virus from the lungs. Am J Med Sci 1945;209:455.
28. Giles C, Shuttleworth EM 1: Post mortem findings in 46 influenza deaths. Lancet 1957;2:1224.
29. Adams CW: Post viral myopericarditis associated with the influenza virus: Report of eight cases. Am J Cardiol 1959;4:56.
30. Oceasohn R, Adelson L, Kaji M: Clinicopathologic study of thirty-three fatal cases

of Asian influenza. N Engl J Med 1959;260: 509.

31. Coltman Jr CA: Influenza myocarditis: Report of a case with observations on serum glutamic oxaloactic transaminase. JAMA 1962;180:204.

32. Rosenberg GH: Acute myocarditis in mumps (epidemic parotitis). Arch Intern Med 1945;76:257.

33. Giustra FX, Nilsson DC: Myocarditis following measles. Am J Dis Child 1950;79: 487.

34. Gardinger AJS, Short D: Four faces of acute myopericarditis. Br Heart J 1973;35:433.

35. Cannell DE: Myocardial degenerations in yellow fever. Am J Pathol 1928;4:431.

36. Bugher JC: The pathology of yellow fever. In GK Stoker (ed): Yellow Fever. New York, McGraw-Hill, 1951:137.

37. Ainger LE, Lawyer NG, Fitch CW: Neonatal rubella myocarditis. Br Heart J 1966;28:691.

38. Ross E, Amentrout SA: Myocarditis associated with rabies: Report of a case. N Engl J Med 1962;266:1087.

39. Cheetham HD, Hart J, Goghill NF, Fox B: Rabies with myocarditis: Two cases in England. Lancet 1970;1:921.

40. Thiede WH: Cardiac involvement in lymphocytic choriomeningitis. Arch Intern Med 1962;109:50.

41. Ahvenainen EK: Inclusion disease or generalized salivary gland virus infection: Report of five cases. Acta Pathol Microbiol Scand 1952;93(suppl):159.

42. Bodey GP, Wertlake PT, Douglas G, Levin RH: Cytomegalic inclusion disease in patients with acute leukemia. Ann Intern Med 1965;62:899.

43. Maisch B, Crombach C, Schöonian U: Cytomegalovirus infection as a cause of viral myocarditis. Eur Heart J 1991;12(Abstract suppl):1216.

44. Maisch B, Wendl J: Cytomegalovirus DNA in endomyocardial biopsies of patients with (peri)myocarditis (abstract). Eur Heart J 1989;9(Suppl 1):1000.

45. Schönian U, Crombach M, Maisch B: Does CMV infection play a role in myocarditis? New aspects from in-situ hybridization. Eur Heart J 1991;12(Suppl D):65.

46. Hoagland RJ: Cardiac involvement in infectious mononucleosis. Am J Med Sci 1956; 232:252.

47. Hackel D: Myocarditis in association with varicella. Am J Pathol 1953;29:369.

48. Sampson C: Varicella myocarditis: report of case. J Natl Med Assoc 1959;51:138.

49. Tatter D, Gerad PW, Silverman AH, Wang C, Peterson HE: Fatal varicella pancarditis in a child. Am J Dis Child 1964;108:88.

50. Moore CM, Henry J, Benzing G, Kaplan S: Varicella myocarditis. Am J Dis Child 1969; 118:899.

51. Lowry PJ, Thompson RA, Littler WA: Humoral immunity in cardiomyopathy. Br Heart J 1983;50:390.

52. Berkovich S, Rodriguez-Torres R, Lin TS: Virologic studies in children with acute myocarditis. Am J Dis Child 1968;115:207.

53. Henson D, Muffson MA: Myocarditis and pneumonitis with type 21 adenovirus infection: Association with fatal myocarditis and pneumonitis. Am J Dis Child 1971;121:334.

54. Gardiner AJS, Short D: Four faces of acute myopericarditis. Br Heart J 1973;35:433.

55. Gore I, Saphir O: Myocarditis: A classification of 1402 cases. Am Heart J 1947;34:827.

56. Anderson T, Foulis MA, Grist NR et al: Clinical and laboratory observations in a smallpox outbreak. Lancet 1951;1:1248.

57. Dalgaard JB: Fatal myocarditis following smallpox vaccination. Am Heart J 1957;54: 156.

58. Caldera R, Sarrut S, Mallet R et al: Existet-il des complications cardiaques de la vaccine? Sem Hop Paris 1961;37:1281.

59. Maut K: Mort subité due à une myocardité focale suivant une vaccination contre la variole. Ann Med Leg 1963;43:1.

60. Abelmann WH, Kowalski HJ, McNeely WF: Cardiovascular studies during acute infectious hepatitis. Gastroenterology 1954;27: 61.

61. Saphir O, Omromin GD, Yokoo H: Myocarditis in viral (epidemic) hepatitis. Am J Med Sci 1956;231:168.

62. Besterri RB: Cardiac involvement in the acquired immune deficiency syndrome. In J Cardiol, 1989;22:143.

63. Grody WW, Cheng L, Pang et al: Direct infection of the heart by human immunodeficiency virus (HIV). (abstract) Circulation 1989;80(suppl 11):2644.

64. Lewis W: AIDS: Cardiac findings form 115 biopsies. Prog Cardiovasc Dis 1989;32:207.

65. Gore I, Kline IK: Pericarditis and myocarditis. In: Gould SE (ed): Pathology of the heart and blood vessels. 3rd ed Thomas Springfield III 1968:731.

66. Ragosta M, Crabtree J, Sturner WQ, Thompson PD: Report of the WHO/ISFC Task force on the definition and classification of cardiomyopathies. Br Heart J 1980;44:672.

67. Lerner AM, Wilson FM: Virus myocardiopathy. Progr Med Virol 1973;15:63.

68. Banatvala J: Coxsackie B virus infections in cardiac disease. In Waterson AP (ed): Re-

cent Advances in Clinical Virology 3, Churchill Livingstone, Edinburgh 1983:99.

69. Cambridge G, MacArthur CGC, Waterson AP et al: Antibodies to Coxsackie B viruses in congestive cardiomyopathy. Br Heart J 1979;16:692.

70. Alvarez FL, Neu N, Rose NR et al: Heart-specific autoantibodies induced by coxsackievirus B: Identification of heart autoantigens. Clin Immunol Immunopathol 1987; 43:12.

71. Bolte HD, Schultheiss P, Cyran J et al: Binding of immunoglobulins in the myocardium (biopsy). In: Bolte H-D (ed): Myocardial Biopsy, Springer-Verlag Berlin, Heidelberg, New York 1980:85.

72. Beisel KW: Immunogenetic basis of myocarditis: role of fibrillary antigens. Springer Semin Immunopathol 1989;11:31.

73. Bülowius H, Maisch B, Koplf D et al: Lymphozytensubpopulationen bei akuter Perimyokarditis, sekundären und primären dilatativen Herzmuskelerkrankungen, Z Kardiol 1983;72(Suppl I):16.

74. Gauntt CJ, Goeny EK, Lutton CM, Pernandes G: Role of natural killer cells in experimental murine myocarditis. Springer Semin Immunopathol 1989;11:51.

75. Huber SA, Lodge PA: Coxsackie B 3 myocarditis: Identification of different pathogenic mechanisms in DBA/2 and Balb/c mice. Am J Pathol 1984;122:284.

76. Huber SA, Lodge PA: Coxsackievirus B3 myocarditis in BALB/c mice: evidence for autoimmunity to myocyte antigens. Am J Pathol 1984;116:21.

77. Huber SA, Simpson K, Weller A et al: Immunopathogenic mechanisms in experimental myocarditis: evidence for autoimmunity to the virus receptor and antigenic mimicry between the virus and the myocardium. In HP Schultheiß (ed.): New Concepts in Viral Heart Disease. Springer-Verlag Berlin Heidelberg 1988:179.

78. Klein R, Maisch B, Kochsiek K et al: Demonstration of organ specific antibodies against heart mitochondria (anti-M7) in sera from patients with some forms of heart disease. Clin Exp Immunol 1984;58:283.

79. Klein R, Spiel L, Kleemann U et al: Relevance of antimitochondrial antibodies (anti-M7) in cardiac disease. Eur Heart J (Suppl J) 1987;8(Suppl J):223.

80. Lodge PA, Herzum M, Olszewski J et al: Coxsackie B-3 myocarditis: acute and chronic forms of the disease causes by different immunopathogenic mechanisms. Am J Pathol 1987;128:455.

81. Maisch B: Cytolytic serum activity in pa-tients with carditis. In Bolte HD (ed): Viral heart disease. Springer-Verlag, Berlin Heidelberg New York Tokyo 1984:121.

82. Maisch B: Diagnostic relevance of humoral and cell-mediated immune reactions in patients with acute myocarditis and congestive cardiomyopathy. In Chazov EL, Smirnov VN, Organov RG (eds) Cardiology, Plenum Press, London 1984;1327.

83. Maisch B: Surface antigens of adult heart cells and their use in diagnosis. Basic Res Cardiol 1985;80(Suppl 1):47.

84. Maisch B: Immunologic regulator and effector functions in perimyocarditis, postmyocarditic heart muscle disease and dilated cardiomyopathy. Basic Res Cardiol 1986;81: 217.

85. Maisch B: Immunological mechanisms in human cardiac injury. In: Spry JE (ed) Immunology and Molecular Biology of Cardiovascular Disease. In Shillingfort JP (ed): Current status of clinical cardiology. MTP Press, London 1987:225.

86. Maisch B: The sarcolemma as antigen in the secondary immunopathogenesis of myopericarditis. Eur Heart J 1987;8(Suppl J):155.

87. Maisch B: The use of myocardial biopsy in heart failure. Eur Heart J 1988;9(Suppl H): 59.

88. Maisch B: Autoreactivity to the caridac myocyte, connective tissue and the extracellular matrix in heart disease and postcardiac injury. Springer Semin Immunopathol 1989;11:369.

89. Maisch B, Berg PA, Schuff-Werner P, Kochsiek K: Clinical significance of immunopathological findings patients with postpericardiotomy syndrome. II. The significance of serum inhibition and rosette inhibitory factors. Clin Exp Immunol 1979; 38:198.

90. Maisch B, Berg PA, Kochsiek: Immunological parameters in patients with congestive cardiomyopathy. Basic Res Cardiol 1980;75: 221.

91. Maisch B, Trostel-Soeder R, Berg A et al: Assessment of antibody mediated cytolysis of adult cardiocytes isolated by centrifugation in a continuous gradient of Percoll^{TM} in patients with acute myocarditis. J Immunol Methods 1981;44:159.

92. Maisch B, Trostel-Soeder R, Stechermesser E, et al: Diagnostic relevance of humoral and cell-mediated immune reactions in patients with acute viral myocarditis. Clin Exp Immunol 1982;48:533.

93. Maisch B, Deeg P, Liebau G, et al: Diagnostic relevance of humoral and cytotoxic immune reactions in patients with primary

and secondary heart muscle disease. Am J Cardiol 1983;52:1072.

94. Maisch B, Büschel G, Izumi T et al: Four years of experience in endomyocardial biopsy. An immunohistologic approach. Heart and Vessels 1985;1(Suppl I):59.

95. Maisch B, Hauck H, Königer U, et al: Suppressor cell activity in (peri)myocarditis and infective endocarditis. Eur Heart J 1987; 8(Suppl J):147.

96. Maisch B, Weyerer O, Hufnagel G et al: The vascular endothelium as target of humoral autoreactivity in myocarditis and rejection. Z Kardiol 1989;78:95.

97. Maisch B, Bauer E, Cirsi M, et al. Cytolytic cross-reactive antibodies directed against the cardiac membrane of adult human myocytes in Coxsackie B myocarditis—analysis by Western blot, immunofluorescende test and antibody-mediated cytolysis of cardiocytes. Circulation (suppl IV) 1993;4:49.

98. Anderson JL, Carlquist JF, Hammond EH: Deficient natural killer cell activity in patients with idiopathic dilated cardiomyopathy. Lancet II: 1982;2:1124.

99. Das SK, Petty RE, Meengs WA et al: Studies of cell-mediated immunity in cardiomyopathy. In Sekiguchi M, Olsen EGJ (eds) Cardiomyopathy. University of Tokyo Press, Tokyo, Baltimore 1980;375.

100. Fowles KE, Bieber CP, Stinson EB: Defective in vitro suppressor cell function in idiopathic congestive cardiomyopathy. Circulation 1978;59:483.

101. Jacobs B, Matsuda Y, Deodhar S: Cell-mediated cytotoxicity to cardiac cells of lymphocytes from patients with primary myocardial disease. Am J Clin Pathol 1979;72:1.

102. Lowry PJ, Thompson RA, Littler WA: Humoral and cellular mechanisms in congestive cardiomyopathy (Abstr) Br Heart J 1984;51:109.

103. Herngstenberg C, Rose M, Olsen E et al: Immunological parameters in patients with different heart diseases. (Abstract) Eur Heart J 1989;10:27.

104. Hufnagel G, Maisch B: MHC antigen expression in endomyocardial biopsies in patients with myocarditis and dilated cardiomyopathy. (abstract) Eur Heart J (Abstr.-Suppl) 1989;10:28.

105. Rose NR, Wolfram LJ, Herskowitz A, Beisel KW: Postinfectious autoimmunity: two distinct phases of coxsackievirus B 3-induces myocarditis. Ann NY Acad Sci 1986;475:146.

106. Aretz HT, Billingham ME, Edward WD: Myocarditis, a histological definition and classification. Am J Cardiovasc Pathol 1987; 1:3.

107. Mason JW, Billingham ME, Ricci DR: Treatment of acute inflammatory myocarditis assisted by endomyocardial biopsy. Am J Cardiol 1980;45:1037.

108. Buie C, Lodge PA, Herzum M, Huber SA: Genetics of Coxsackie virus B3 and enephalomyocarditis virus-induces myocarditis in mice. Eur Heart J 1987;8(Suppl J):389.

109. Godeney EK, Gauntt CJ: Murine natural killer cells limit Coxsackie B 3 replication. J Immunol 1987;139:913.

110. Herzum M, Huber SA, Maisch B: Coxsackie B 3 myocarditis: genetic aspects of different immunopathogenic mechanisms in Balbic and DBA/2 mices. Antigenic specificity of heart-reactive antibodies in DBA/2 mices. In HP Schultheiß (ed.): New Concepts in Viral Heart Disease, Springer-Verlag Berlin Heidelberg 1988;188.

111. Neu N, Beisel K, Traystman M et al: Autoantibodies specific for the cardiac myosin isoform are found in mice susceptible to coxsackie virus B3-induced myocarditis. J Immunol 1987;138:2488.

112. Wolfgram LJ, Beisel KW, Rose NR: Heart-specific autoantibodies following murine coxsackievirus B3 myocarditis. J Exp Med 1985;161:1112.

113. Wong Y, Woodruff JJ, Woodruff JF: Generation of cytolytic T-lymphocytes during Coxsackie virus B3 infection. I. Model and viral specificity. J Immunol 1977;118:1159.

114. Woodruff JF: Viral myocarditis. A review article. Am J Pathol 1980;101:425.

115. Fenoglio JJ Jr, Ursell PC, Kellogg CF et al: Diagnosis and classification of myocarditis by endomyocardial biopsy. N Engl J Med 1983;308:12.

116. Kawai S, Okada R: A histopathological study of dilated cardiomyopathy: With special reference to clinical and pathological comparisons of the degeneration-predominant type and fibrosis-predominant type. Jap Circulation J 1987;51:654.

117. Shanes Gahli J, Billingham ME, Ferrans VJ, Fenoglio JJ, Edwards WD, Tsai CC, Saffitz JE, Isner J, Furner S, Subramanian R: Interobserver variability in the pathologic interpretation of endomyocardial biopsy results. Circulation 1987;75:401.

118. Lie

119. Feigenbaum H: Echocardiographic diagnosis of pericardial effusion. Am J Cardiol 1970;26:475.

120. Horowitz MS, Schultz CS, Stinson EB et al: Sensitivity and specificity of echocardio-

graphic diagnosis of pericardial effusion. Circulation 1974;50:239.

121. Deck WG, Palacios IF, Fallon JT et al: Active myocarditis in the spectrum of acute dilated cardiomyopathies. Engl J Med 1985; 342:885.

122. Archard LC, Bowles NE, Cunningham L et al: Molecular probes for detection of persisting enterovirus infection of human heart and their prognostic value. Eur Heart J 1989;12(Suppl D):56.

123. Klein J, Stanek G, Bittner R et al: Lyme borreliosis as a cause of myocarditis and heart muscle disease. Eur Heart J 1991;12(Suppl D):73.

124. Schwimmbeck PL, Schultheiß HP, Strauer BE: Identification of a main autoimmunogenic epitope of the adenine nucleotide translocator which cross-reacts with coxsackie B3 virus: use in the diagnosis of myocarditis and dilatative cardiomyopathy. Circulation 1989;80(Suppl II):2642.

125. Noseworthy JH, Fields BN, Dichter MA et al: Cell receptor for the mammalian reovirus: I. Syngeneic monoclonal anti-idiotype antibody identifies a cell surface receptor for reovirus. J Immunol 1983;131:2533.

126. Rose NR, Wolfgram LJ, Herskowitz A et al: Coxsackievirus B3 murine myocarditis: a pathologic spectrum of myocarditis in genetically defined inbred strains. J Am Cell Cardiol 1987;9:1311.

127. Ulrich G, Kühl U, Melzner B et al: Antibodies against the ADP/ATP carrier crossreact with the Ca-channel-function and biochemical data. In HP Schultheiß (ed): New Concepts in Viral Heart Disease. Berlin, Springer-Verlag 1988:225.

128. Gönczöl E, Plotkin SA: Cells infected with human cytomegalovirus release a factor(s) that stimulates cell DNA synthesis. Gen Virol 1987;68:793.

129. Ryan US, Schultz DR, Ryan JW: Fc-receptors on pulmonary endothelial cells: induction by injury. Science 1981;214:557.

130. Beck S, Barrell BG: Human cytomegalovirus encodes a glycoprotein homologous to MHC class I-antigen. Nature 1988;331:269.

131. Grundy JE, McKeating JA, Ward PJ et al: β2-microglobulin enhances the effectivity of cytomegalovirus and when bound to the virus enables class I HLA molecules to be used as virus receptor. J Gen Virol 1987;68:793.

132. Fujinami R, Nelson JA, Walker L et al: Sequence homology and immunologic cross-reactivity of human cytomegalovirus with HLA-DR β-chain: a means for graft rejec-

tion and immunosuppression. J Virol 1988; 62:100.

133. Weber KT, Janicki JS, Shroff SG et al: Collagen compartment remodeling in the pressure overloaded left ventricle. J Appl Cardiol 1988;1:37–46.

134. Willingham MC, Pastan I: An atlas of immunofluorescence in cultured cells. Academic Press London, 1985.

135. Zhao M, Zhang H, Robinson TF et al: Profound structural alterations of the extracellular collagen matrix in postischemic dysfunctional ("stunned") but viable myocardium. J Am Coll Cardiol 1987;1322:10.

136. Yu Z, Sekiguchi M, Hiroe M, et al: Histopathological findings of acute and convalescent myocarditis obtained by serial biopsy. Jpn Cir J 1984;48:1368.

137. Wahl SM: Host immune factors regulating fibrosis. In D Evered, J Whelan (eds): Fibrosis. Pitnam, London 1985;175.

138. Samsonov M, Nassonov E, Kostin S et al: Serum neopterin-possible immunological marker of myocardial inflammation in patients with dilated heart muscle disease. Eur Heart J 1991;12(Suppl D):147.

139. Klappacher G, Pacher R, Woluszczuk W et al: Increased release of neopterin and tumor necrosis factor alpha into the serum of patients with primary dilated cardiomyopathy. Eur Heart J 1991;12(Abstr Suppl):315.

140. Klappacher G, Pacher R, Woluszczuk W et al: Elevated circulating levels of β2-microglobulin in primary dilated cardiomyopathy. Eur Heart J 1991;12(Abstr Suppl):316 (A 1620).

141. Kysal A, Haverich A, Heublein B et al: C myc-oncogene expression in myocytes in heart allografts. 7th International Congress of Immunology, Berlin, 10/7-5/8. Book of Abstracts 1989:814.

142. Kurnick JT, Leary C, Palacios IF et al: Culture and characterization of lymphocytic infiltrates from endomyocardial biopsies of patients with idiopathic myocarditis. Eur Heart J 1987;8(Suppl J):135.

143. Bresnihan B, Jasin ME: Suppressor function of peripheral blood mononuclear cells in normal individuals and in patients with systemic lupus erythematosus. J Clin Invest 1977;59:106.

144. Hallgren HM, Yunis EJ: Suppressor lymphocytes in young and aged humans. J Immunol 1977;59:106.

145. Eckstein R, Mempel W, Bolte H-D: Reduced suppressor cell activity in congestive cardiomyopathy and in myocarditis. Circulation 1982;65:1224.

146. Krane SM: The turnover and degradation

of collagen. In D. Evered, J Whelan (eds): Fibrosis. Pitnam, London, 1985:97.

147. Leroy EC: Collagen deposition in autoimmune disease: the expanding role of the fibroblast in human fibrotic disease. In D. Evered, J Whelan (eds): Fibrosis. Pitnam, London 1985:196.

148. De Crombrugghe B, Liau G, Setoyama C, et al: Structural and Foundational Studies on Interstitial Collagen Genes in D. Evered, J Whelan (eds): Fibrosis. Pitnam, London 1985:20.

149. Schaper J: Ultrastructural feaetures and damage of the cytoskeleton in dilated cardiomyopathy. In H-P Schultheiss: New concepts in viral heart disease. Springer Heidelberg, Berlin, New York, Tokyo, 1988.

150. Schaper J, Froede R, Bleese N et al: Veränderungen der Ultrastruktur und des Zytoskeletts in explantierten menschlichen Herzen. Z Kardiol Suppl 1 (A285) 1987; 77(Suppl 1):82(A285).

151. Maisch B, M Crombach, U Schönian. Änderung zytoskelettaler Proteine bei akuter und chronischer Myokarditis. Z Kardiol (suppl 1) 1994;83(suppl 1):232 (A285).

152. Schultheiss HP: The mitochondrium as antigen in inflammatory heart disease. Eur Heart J 8 1987;8(Suppl J):203.

153. Schultheiss HP, Bolte HD: Immunological analysis of auto-antibodies against the adenine nucleotide translocator in dilated cardiomyopathy. J Mol Cell Cardiol 1985;17: 601.

154. Reinauer KM, Klein R, Seipel L et al: Heart-specific antimitochondrial antibody (anti-M7) in a patient with virus-associated perimyocarditis. Eur Heart J 1987;8(Suppl J): 227.

155. Maisch B, Trostel-Soeder R, Stechemesser E et al: Diagnostic relevance of humoral and cell-mediated immune reactions in patients with acute viral myocarditis. Clin Exp Immunol 1982;48:533.

156. Obermayer U, Scheidler J, Maisch B: Antibodies against micro- and intermediate filaments in carditis and dilated cardiomyopathy—are they a diagnostic marker? Eur Heart J 1987;8(Suppl J):181.

157. Herskowitz A, Beisel KW, Wolfgram LJ et al: Coxsackievirus B3 murine myocarditis: wide pathologic spectrum in genetically defined inbred strains. Hum Pathol 1985;16: 671.

158. Beisel K, Wolfgram ML, Hershkowitz A, Rose N: Differences in severity of Coxsackievirus B3-induced myocarditis among H-2 congenic mouse strain. In S. Skameme (ed): Genetic Control of Host Resistance to Infection and Malignancy, vol 3, Alan R. Liss, New York, p 195.

159. Limas CJ, Goldenberg IF: Autoantibodies against cardiac β-adrenoceptors in human dilated cardiomyopathy. Circulation 1987; 76(Suppl 4):262(A1042).

160. Yamada K, Akiyama S, Hasegawa T et al: Recent advances in the research on fibronectin and other cell attachment proteins. J Cell Biochem 1985;28:79.

161. Kühl U, Ulrich G, Schulteiß H-P: Cross-reactivity of antibodies to the ADP/ATP translocator of the inner mitochondrial membrane with the cell surface of cardiac myocytes. Eur Heart J 1987;8(Suppl J):219.

162. Wallukat G, Boewer V: Stimulation of chronotropic β-adrenoceptors of cultures neonatal rat heart myocytes by the serum of gammaglobulin fraction of patients with dilated cardiomyopathy and myocarditis. Internationales Symposium: Herzinsuffizienz, Pathogenese und Differentialtherapie, Berlin 28.2–2.3 1988, Book of abstracts A 24.

Chapter 10

Endomyocardial Fibrosis

C. Chandrasekharan Kartha, M.D.

Introduction

Among the different morphological expressions of wound healing in the endocardium, endomyocardial fibrosis has characteristic clinical and pathological features. The large patches of fibrosis without appreciable inflammation, involving specific regions of either or both ventricles of the heart was initially discovered in Africans.[1,2] Soon it became known that the disease is also prevalent in other countries in the tropical belt.[3] Morphologically indistinguishable is the late stage of Loeffler's endomyocardial disease, more common in the temperate zone.

Since the term endomyocardial fibrosis (EMF) only describes the nature of the lesion, to comprehend what constitutes the distinctive pathological entity, it is essential to distinguish it from the structural variations of the normal endocardium and other conditions in which the endocardium is thickened and fibrotic.

Normal Endocardium

Ventricular endocardium is thin, and glistening with a high ratio of internal surface area to ventricular volume because of the trabeculae and papillary muscles. In different regions of the ventricle, the thickness varies between 50 to 200 microns. In the inflow portions the endocardium is thin. In the outflow tract where it has to withstand greater turbulence and higher pressures, the endocardium is thicker. Histologically, five layers have been identified.[4] The cavity is lined by a layer of endothelial cells which have an underlying basal lamina. These cells are continuous with the lining cells of the blood vessels. The subendothelial space contains fibroblasts, smooth muscle cells, fibrillar collagen, elastic fibers, and other components of the extracellular matrix (Figure 1). There is also an elastic layer which supports elastic recoil during relaxation and may prevent cardiac overdistension.[5]

Mural Endocardial Thickening

Structural variations (Table 1) of the mural endocardium in disease states have been extensively studied.[6,7] However, there is little information regarding their functional sequelae.

Isolated endocardial thickening, seen as whitish opacities, is frequent in autopsy specimens and is due to stresses of abnormal pressures or frictional effects. A common cause for such patches is valvular incompetence. High pressure jets can produce small pockets (Zahn's pockets). An example of frictional stresses producing fibroelastosis is the lesion in the outflow region of the left ventricle in subaortic hypertrophic cardiomyopathy. The thickened endocardium is composed of fibrous and elastic tissue. Muscle damage and inflammatory infiltrates are not seen.

Diffuse fibroelastosis composed of several layers of parallelly arranged thick and continuous elastic fibers is associated with a variety of congenital heart defects and certain metabolic disorders.[8] There is sharp de-

From Weber KT, MD *Wound Healing in Cardiovascular Disease*, Armonk, NY, Futura Publishing Company Inc., © 1995.

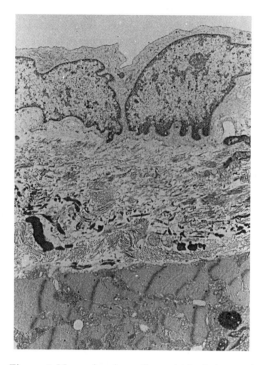

Figure 1. Normal endocardium. A single layer of endothelial cells and subendothelial space with collagen and elastic fibers are seen (Kajikawa stain ×2500).

marcation between the thickened endocardium and underlying myocardium. Inflammation is absent and myocardial lesions are seen only when there is associated coronary artery disease.

Table 1

Different Types of Mural Endocardial Thickening

A] Fibroelastosis
   —isolated pockets
   —diffuse and hyperplastic
B] Elastomyofibrosis
C] Mural endocarditis
D] Mural fibrin thrombi
   —Non specific
   —Becker's cardiomyopathy
E] Endomyocardial fibrosis
   —associated with hypereosinophilia
   —of the tropics
   —adriamycin toxicity
   —methysergide induced

In dilated hearts, cellular response in the endocardium is different; hypertrophy of the smooth muscle layer being the striking feature. Secondary fibroelastosis may be present, resulting in elastomyofibrosis. A similar reaction, but with a typical morphology and formation of thick plaques, is the hallmark of carcinoid heart disease.[9]

Endocardial thickening can also be due to deposition of fibrin, either in areas of mural endocarditis or over myocardial infarcts. Fibrin deposits with mucinous edema of the endocardium and degeneration of myofibers is also a feature of a specific form of cardiomyopathy (Becker's disease) reported from South Africa.[10]

Circumscribed patches of endocardial fibrosis are common in the late stages of Chagas' disease in which a parasitic pancarditis is also present.[11]

Another form of severe endocardial thickening is a scar of reparative processes sequel to destruction of the endocardium. A classic example is Loeffler's endomyocardial disease in which the initial lesions of eosinophilic endomyocarditis heal to form a thick fibrous scar.[12] An identical morphological lesion is seen in endomyocardial fibrosis which otherwise is clinically distinguishable and has an overwhelming tropical prevalence.

What Constitutes Endomyocardial Fibrosis?

Pathological Anatomy

The characteristic feature is the severe, massive, focal, or diffuse endocardial thickening, often up to 1 to 2 millimeters, in either one or both the ventricles of the heart.[13–15], Focal lesions are localized to either the apex, base of the papillary muscles, or posterior wall of the left ventricle behind the posterior cusp of the mitral valve. In the diffuse type, the ventricular chamber is obliterated by an opaque and whitish thick plaque involving the entire inflow and apex of the ventricle, resulting in effacement of the normal trabecular pattern (Figures 2 and 3). The papillary muscle may remain as short fibrotic stumps. Atrioventricular valve involvement is not a common

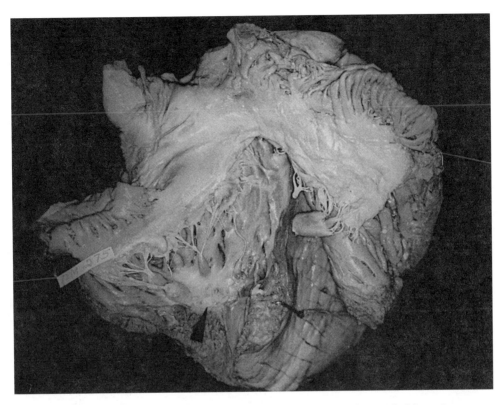

Figure 2. Endomyocardial fibrosis of the right ventricle with apical obliteration.

finding though associated rheumatic type of deformity has been reported.[16] Endocardial fibrosis in the right ventricle can result in apical retraction externally visible as a notch on the right border of the heart. Atria may enlarge aneurysmally and their walls become translucent (Figure 4).

The thickened endocardium consists of a superficial compact layer of collagen which is occasionally hyalinized and calcified. A deeper layer has loose fibrous tissue with numerous capillary channels and scant chronic inflammatory cells. Strands of connective tissue with dilated lymphatics often extend into the inner myocardium (Figure 5). Degenerative changes are frequently seen in myofibers of the subendocardial region. Focal scars, particularly in perivascular regions are visualized elsewhere in the myocardium. Intramyocardial arteries infrequently have occlusive changes due to either mucinous edema or luminal thrombus. Media may be atrophic and fibrosed.

Ultra-structural findings are those of accumulation of cellular and extracellular elements of connective tissue in the endocardial layer (Figure 6), atrophic or hypertrophic changes in myocytes, and thickening or reduplication of the capillary basement membrane.[17]

Extracardiac lesions, except those due to cardiac failure, are not consistently found. Large and medium sized blood vessels also do not have lesions.

A striking similarity in cardiac pathological anatomy is seen in all the cases of endomyocardial fibrosis reported from various regions of the tropical zone. There are also anecdotal reports of endomyocardial fibrosis associated with methysergide or adriamycin toxicity.[18,19]

Functional Features

Severe degree of endocardial thickening and obliteration of the ventricular cavity leads to restriction of diastolic filling of the

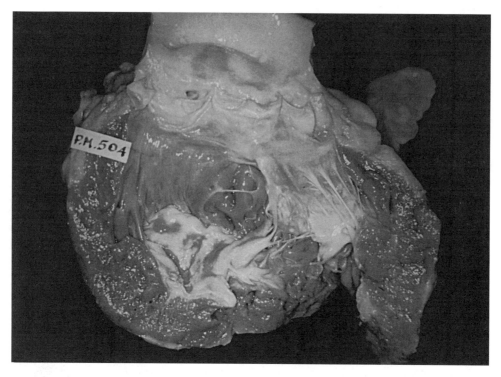

Figure 3. Endomyocardial fibrosis of the left ventricle with thick plaque at the apex.

ventricle. Depending on the extent of involvement of chordae tendineae and papillary muscles in the fibrotic process, there is also incompetence of the atrioventricular valve and valvular regurgitation. Systolic function of the ventricle is relatively well preserved till the late stages of the disease. Endocardiectomy and valve replacement improve functional status and prolong survival of the patients.[20,21]

It is not known whether there is any primary defect of relaxation at the myocyte level in endomyocardial fibrosis. Quantitative studies are also not available to show whether myocardial interstitial fibrosis contributes to the restriction in ventricular filling and reduced myocardial compliance. However, the intensity of myocardial fibrosis is considered to be an important determinant of survival.[21]

In patients with disease of the left ventricle, progressive increase in the severity of valve regurgitation leads to pulmonary venous hypertension. Right atrial enlargement, massive pericardial effusion, systemic venous hypertension and ascites are the outcome when the disease affects the right ventricle.

Clinical Profile

Clinical features which deserve emphasis are the insidious onset and nonepisodic nature of the illness. Patients always present with features of established heart disease and can rarely recall how and when their illness started.[22] There is also lack of evidence of infection, allergy, or poisoning and any consistent association with parasitism.[7]

The clinical signs reflect the hemodynamic alterations.[23–25] Right ventricular EMF may mimic constrictive pericarditis or Ebstein's anomaly.[23,26] Left ventricular endomyocardial fibrosis can simulate rheumatic mitral regurgitation.[27] Impaired ventricular compliance and elevated atrial filling pressures explain the loud third heart sound, a consistent auscultatory finding. Murmurs of valvular regurgitation seldom exceed grade 3 in intensity since the leaflets are neither thickened nor deformed. Echocardiogram is diagnostic of EMF[28] while

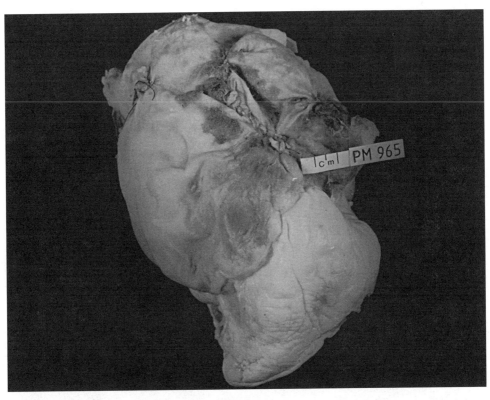

Figure 4. The enlarged right atrium and notch in right ventricular border in a specimen of endomyocardial fibrosis of the right ventricle.

confirmation is obtained by selective cineangiography which reveals the varying degrees of obliteration of ventricular cavity.[29]

Causation

Many theories (Table 2) were advanced in the past but none of them has yet found confirmatory evidence.[30] Malnutrition, vitamin E deficiency, viral infection, parasitic myocarditis, cardiac lymphatic obstruction, and serotonin toxicity from consumption of banana were some of the theories vigorously pursued by earlier investigators. A tuberous diet rich in vitamin D is also proposed to lead to endomyocardial fibrosis.[31]

Another view holds that endomyocardial fibrosis is an immunological variant of hypersensitivity to streptococcal infection.[32] Proponents of this view argue that manifestation as endomyocardial fibrosis is determined by what constitutes a tropical immunological syndrome characterized by presence of high levels of IgM, auto antibodies to the heart, and bound IgG to myofibers and endocardium.[33]

The hypothesis which gained wide attention in the 1980s claims that endomyocardial fibrosis in the tropics and Loeffler's endomyocardial fibrosis are different stages of a spectrum of cardiac responses to injury by eosinophils.[34] Except for a solitary report,[35] observations by tropical investigators suggest that there is a need for a reappraisal of the unitarian concept.[36,37] A comparison of endomyocardial fibrosis and Loeffler's endomyocardial disease reveals that the two entities are dissimilar not only in their eosinophilic profiles but also in epidemiologic and clinical features.[37,38]

The fact that 730 out of 779 cases of endomyocardial fibrosis reported during the last two decades belong to countries within 15° of the equator is a strong pointer to geographical factors in the causation of the dis-

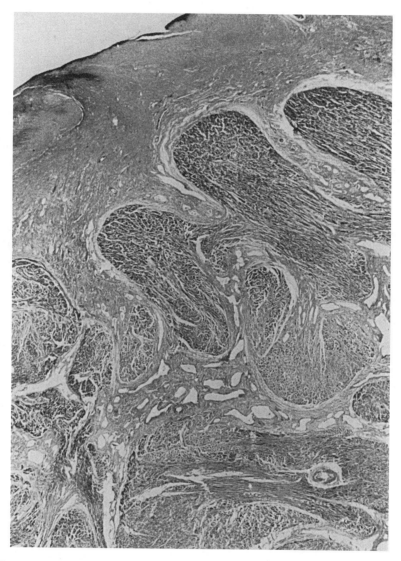

Figure 5. Photomicrograph of thickened endocardium in endomyocardial fibrosis. Strands of vascularized connective tissue are seen extending into myocardium (Masson Trichrome × 20).

ease. Emphasizing the prevalence of endomyocardial fibrosis in regions with latosolic soils with abundant monazite and the striking preference for malnourished children, a geochemical basis for the disease has recently been suggested.[39,40] The early observations raise the possibility that endomyocardial fibrosis is the cardiac expression of a synergistic effect of magnesium deficiency, which commonly accompanies malnutrition in the tropics, and toxicity of cerium, the major elemental component of mona-

zite.[41] Cerium has been shown to stimulate collagen synthesis in cultured cardiac fibroblasts,[42] an observation relevant to the hypothesis. Be that as it may, confirmatory evidence for the hypothesis rests on case control studies and animal experiments.

Pathogenesis

A generally accepted scheme for the evolution of endomyocardial fibrosis is a sequence starting with an acute endomyocar-

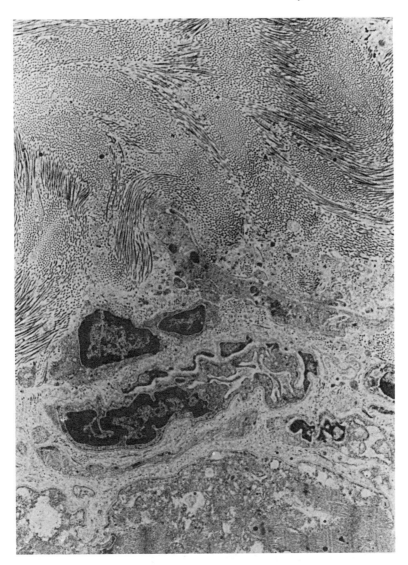

Figure 6. A superficial layer of wavy bundles of collagen fibrils and deeper layer of blood vessels in thickened endocardium (uranyl acetate-lead citrate × 2500).

ditis, with overlying fibrin deposits which heal with incorporation of the thrombus into a fibrosed and contracted ventricle.[34] This concept is based on studies in Loeffler's endomyocardial disease in which hypereosinophilia, circulating eosinophilic proteins, and deposition of eosinophilic proteins in cardiac tissues are evident.[43,44] The mechanism of eosinophil-mediated myocardial injury has been elucidated.[45–47] However, in the tropics eosinophilic endomyocarditis has not been observed in patients.

Another opinion regards endomyocardial fibrosis as a degenerative process and an involvement of metabolic factors is suggested.[7] In animals subjected to chronic mineralocorticoid excess, endomyocardial fibrosis has been produced.[48]

A suggestion based on observations in biopsy material from contralateral ventricle when there is univentricular involvement, is that endomyocardial fibrosis is an interstitial heart disease rather than a reparative process.[49] When fullblown endomyocardial fibrosis is present in one ventricle, the other

Table 2

Factors Implicated in the Causation of
Endomyocardial Fibrosis

—Malnutrition
—Consumption of bananas and serotonin toxicity
—Tuberous diet and vitamin D toxicity
—Viral infections
—Parasitic infections
—Obstruction to cardiac lymphatics
—Tropical immunologic syndrome
—Hypersensitivity to streptococci
—Eosinophil toxicity
—Geochemical factors—cerium toxicity in magnesium deficiency.

ventricle with either focal lesions or no visible lesions, has interstitial fibrosis associated with increase in interstitial cellularity. Studies in African patients have also reported freshly fibrosing endomyocardium with active fibroblasts in the early stages.[50,51]

Any explanation for the pathogenesis has to account for the subendocardial distribution of fibrosis in endomyocardial fibrosis. In other morphological types of healing response to either myocarditis or ischemic injury, the fibrosis is generalized and lacks any characteristic pattern of distribution. In endomyocardial fibrosis, the heart is contracted and small with obliterated ventricular cavities and the systolic function is preserved. This is easily distinguished from the large heart with dilated ventricular cavities and poor contractility observed in reparative processes that are sequel to ischemic, metabolic or infectious injury to the myocardium.

An attractive view on pathogenetic events that could lead to endomyocardial fibrosis has recently been proposed.[52] The primary target of injury is speculated to be the endocardial endothelium. Factors responsible for the activation of matrix producing cells could reach the subendothelial space following altered permeability of endocardial endothelium or be derived from the endocardial endothelial cells as a result of metabolic injury (Figure 7). The hypothesis is consistent with the observations that the endocardial endothelium regulates exchange of substances between blood in ventricular cavities and subendocardial inter-

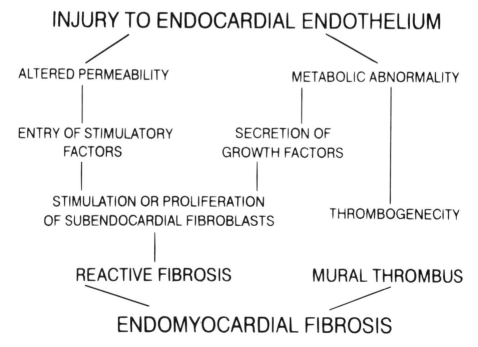

Figure 7. Potential mechanisms for endomyocardial fibrosis.

stitium and that the endothelial cells have secretory properties.[5]

Conclusions

Selective involvement of the heart, severity of fibrosis, preference for malnourished children, predominant tropical prevalence, and diastolic dysfunction are the cardinal features of endomyocardial fibrosis. There is enough evidence to consider EMF of the tropics as separate from other endocardial diseases. While studies related to clinical phenomena and treatment have made considerable progress, investigations on pathogenetic mechanisms have lagged behind. Speculative arguments on mechanisms will continue therefore until direct evidence for injury to the endocardium is obtained and cellular mechanisms are delineated. Search for an etiologic agent for tropical endomyocardial fibrosis should focus on geographical factors which could produce selective injury to the endomyocardium.

References

1. Bedford DE, Konstam GLS. Heart failure of unknown aetiology in Africans. Br Heart J 1946;8:236–237.
2. Davies JNP. Endocardial fibrosis in Africans. East Afr Med J 1948;25:10–14.
3. Hutt MSR. Epidemiology aspects of endomyocardial fibrosis. Postgrad Med J 1983;59: 142–146.
4. Ferrans VJ, Rodriguez ER. Ultrastructure of the normal heart. In: Silver MD, ed. Cardiovascular Pathology. New York, NY: Churchill Livingstone, 1991:43–101.
5. Brutsaert DL. The endocardium. Ann Rev Physiol 1989;51:263–273.
6. Okada R. Clinicopathological study of the thickening of parietal endocardium in the adult heart. Jpn Heart J 1961;2:220–255.
7. Davies JNP, Coles RM. Some considerations regarding obscure diseases affecting the mural endocardium. Am Heart J 1960;59: 600–631.
8. Fishbein MC, Ferrans VJ, Roberts WC. Histological and ultrastructural features of primary and secondary fibroelastosis. Arch Pathol Lab Med 1977;101:49–54.
9. Ferrans VJ, Roberts WC. The carcinoid endo-

10. Becker BJP, Chatgidakis CB, Van Lingen B. Cardiovascular collagenosis with parietal endocardial thrombosis. Circulation 1953;7: 345–352.
11. Laranja FB, Dias E, Norbrega G, et al. Chagas' disease. A clinical, epidemiological and pathologic study. Circulation 1956;14: 1035–1060.
12. Brockington IF, Olsen EGJ. Loeffler's endocarditis and Davies' endomyocardial fibrosis. Am Heart J 1973;85:308–322.
13. Davies JNP, Ball JD. The pathology of endomyocardial fibrosis in Uganda. Br Heart J 1955;17:337–359.
14. Connor DH, Somers K, Hutt MSR, et al. Endomyocardial fibrosis in Uganda (Davies' disease: an epidemiologic, clinical and pathologic study-Part II). Am Heart J 1968; 75:107–124.
15. Kartha CC, Sandhyamani S. An autopsy study of tropical endomyocardial fibrosis in Kerala. Indian J Med Res 1985;82:439–446.
16. Shaper AG, Hutt MSR, Coles RM. Necropsy study of endomyocardial fibrosis and rheumatic heart disease in Uganda 1950–1965. Br Heart J 1968;30:391–401.
17. Kartha CC, Valiathan MS. Cardiac ultrastructure in tropical endomyocardial fibrosis. Indian J Med Res 1988;87:275–282.
18. Harbin AD, Gerson MC, O'Connell JB. Simulation of acute myopericarditis by constrictive pericardial disease with endomyocardial fibrosis due to methysergide therapy. J Am Coll Cardiol 1984;4:196–199.
19. Fitter W, De Sa DJ, Pai KRM. Adriamycin cardiotoxicity: report of an unusual case with features resembling endomyocardial fibrosis. J Clin Pathol 1981;34:602–605.
20. Gupta PN, Valiathan MS, Balakrishnan KG, et al. Clinical course of endomyocardial fibrosis. Br Heart J 1989;62:450–454.
21. Barretto ACP, da Luz PL, Oliveira SA, et al. Determinants of survival in endomyocardial fibrosis. Circulation 1989;80:I-177-I-182.
22. Somers K, Brenton DP, Sood NK. The clinical features of endomyocardial fibrosis of the right ventricle. Br Heart J 1968;30:309–321.
23. Somers K, Brenton DP, D'Arbela PG, et al. Haemodynamic features of severe endomyocardial fibrosis of right ventricle, including comparison with constrictive pericarditis. Br Heart J 1968;30:322–332.
24. Guimaraes AC, Fillio AS, Esteves JP, et al. Haemodynamics of endomyocardial fibrosis. Am Heart J 1974;88:294–303.
25. Puigbo JJ, Combellas I, Acquatella H, et al. Endomyocardial fibrosis in South Amer-

ica—report on 23 cases in Venezuela. Postgrad Med J 1983;59:162–169.

26. Balakrishnan KG, Sapru RP, Sasidharan CK, et al. A comparison of the clinical, haemodynamic and angiographic features in right ventricular endomyocardial fibrosis and Ebstein's anomaly of the tricuspid valve. Cardiology 1982;69:265–275.

27. Metras D, Coulibaly AO, Ouattara KJ, et al. Endomyocardial fibrosis masquerading as rheumatic mitral incompetence. A report of 6 surgical cases. J Thorac Cardiovasc Surg 1983;86:753–756.

28. Venkitachalam CG, Balakrishnan KG, Jagan Mohan Tharakan. Echocardiographic findings in endomyocardial fibrosis. In: Valiathan MS, Somers K, Kartha CC, eds. Endomyocardial Fibrosis. New Delhi: Oxford University Press, 1993:153–167.

29. Jagan Mohan Tharakan, Venkitachalam CG, Balakrishnan KG. Angiographic features of endomyocardial fibrosis. In: Valiathan MS, Somers K, Kartha CC, eds. Endomyocardial Fibrosis. New Delhi: Oxford University Press, 1993:168–184.

30. Falase AO. Endomyocardial fibrosis in Africa. Postgrad Med J 1983;59:170–178.

31. Davies H. Endomyocardial fibrosis and the tuberous diet. Int J Cardiol 1990;29:3–8.

32. Shaper AG. Endomyocardial fibrosis and rheumatic heart disease. Lancet 1966;i: 639–641.

33. Vander Geld H, Peetom F, Somers K, et al. Immuno histological and serological studies in endomyocardial fibrosis. Lancet 1966;ii: 1210–1213.

34. Olsen EGJ, Spry CJF. The pathogenesis of Loeffler's endomyocardial disease and its relationship to endomyocardial fibrosis. In: Yu PN, Goodwin JF, eds. Progress in Cardiology, Vol 8. Philadelphia, Pa: Lea and Febiger, 1979:281–303.

35. Andy JJ, Bishara FF, Soyinka OO. Relation of severe eosinophilia and microfilariasis to chronic African endomyocardial fibrosis. Br Heart J 1981;45:672–680.

36. Patel AK, D'Arbela PG, Somers K. Endomyocardial fibrosis and eosinophilia. Br Heart J 1977;39:238–241.

37. Valiathan MS, Kartha CC. Endomyocardial fibrosis—the possible connection with myocardial levels of magnesium and cerium. Int J Cardiol 1990;28:1–5.

38. Davies J, Spry CJF, Vijayaraghavan G, et al. A comparison of the clinical and cardiological features of endomyocardial disease in temperate and tropical regions. Postgrad Med J 1983;59:179–185.

39. Valiathan MS, Kartha CC, Panday VK, et al. A geochemical basis for endomyocardial fibrosis. Cardiovasc Res 1986;20:679–682.

40. Valiathan MS, Kartha CC, Eapen JT, et al. A geochemical basis for endomyocardial fibrosis. Cardiovasc Res 1989;23:647–648.

41. Valiathan MS, Kartha CC, Renuka Nair R, et al. Geochemical basis of tropical endomyocardial fibrosis. In: Valiathan MS, Somers K, Kartha CC, eds. Endomyocardial Fibrosis. New Delhi: Oxford University Press, 1993: 98–110.

42. Shivakumar K, Renuka Nair R, Valiathan MS. Paradoxical effect of cerium on collagen synthesis in cardiac fibroblasts. J Mol Cell Cardiol 1992;24:775–780.

43. Olsen EGJ, Spry CJF. Relation between eosinophilia and endomyocardial disease. Prog Cardiovasc Dis 1985;27:241–254.

44. Tai PC, Ackerman SJ, Spry CJF, et al. Deposits of eosinophil granule proteins in cardiac tissues of patients with eosinophilic endomyocardial disease. Lancet 1987;i:643–647.

45. Tai PC, Hayes DJ, Clark JB, et al. Toxic effects of human eosinophil secretion products on isolated rat heart cells in vitro. Biochem J 1982;204:75–80.

46. Spry CJF, Tai PC, Davies J. The cardiotoxicity of eosinophils. Postgrad Med J 1983;59: 147–153.

47. Shah AM, Brutsaert DL, Meulemans AL, et al. Eosinophils from hypereosinophilic patients damage endocardium of isolated feline heart muscle preparations. Circulation 1990;81:1081–1088.

48. Selye H. Experimental production of endomyocardial fibrosis. Lancet 1958;i: 1351–1353.

49. Kartha CC. Endomyocardial fibrosis is possibly an interstitial heart disease. Curr Sci 1993;64:598.

50. Parry EHO, Abrahams DG. The natural history of endomyocardial fibrosis. Q J Med 1965;34:383–408.

51. Somers K, Hutt MSR, Patel AK, et al. Endomyocardial biopsy in diagnosis of cardiomyopathies. Br Heart J 1971;33:822–832.

52. Weber KT, Brilla CG. Cardiopathies and fibrillar collagen. In: Opie LH, Sugimoto T, eds. Metabolic and Molecular Aspects of Cardiomyopathy. Tokyo: University of Tokyo Press, 1991:167–186.

Chapter 11

Vascular Wound Healing and Restenosis Following Revascularization

Paul R. Myers, Ph.D., M.D., FACC

Introduction

Occlusive coronary artery disease secondary to atherosclerosis is widely recognized as the primary cause of morbidity and mortality worldwide. Its consequences include sudden death, myocardial infarction and congestive heart failure. Despite a thorough knowledge of the histopathology of atherogenesis, the exact mechanisms responsible for primary atherosclerosis remain largely unknown. In response to the need to safely and effectively reestablish adequate coronary blood flow, and as a consequence of remarkable advances in materials technology, a large array of catheter based devices and procedures to treat the diseased vessel responsible for patient symptoms have been developed.

The impact of coronary artery disease in the United States is enormous. In 1991 heart and blood vessel diseases killed more than 923,000 Americans, and more than 6 million Americans alone have coronary heart disease. More than 2 of every 5 Americans die of cardiovascular disease. More than 1 in 5 Americans have some form of cardiovascular disease.[1] Since it is clear that we are not able to readily eliminate the adverse outcomes posed by atherosclerosis, the application of mechanical and surgical revascularization to the treatment of coronary artery disease has markedly increased. Consequently, the complications and costs of these procedures, coupled with the long-term outcomes, have become a subject of increasing importance.

Historically, coronary artery bypass grafting to treat occlusive coronary artery disease was first applied to large populations of patients beginning in the 1970s. Indeed, the large trials such as the European Coronary Surgery Study,[2] the Veterans Administration Coronary Artery Bypass Surgery Cooperative Study Group,[3] and the Coronary Artery Surgery Study (CASS)[4] provided important guidelines regarding the beneficial effects of medical management versus bypass grafting.

In 1977, however, Gruentzig and coworkers performed the first balloon angioplasty on a patient and pioneered a new era in cardiology, that of catheter based mechanical revascularization.[5,6] In 1989 alone, over 300,000 balloon angioplasty procedures were done in the United States,[7] surpassing the number of bypass surgery procedures in 1990.[8] More recent statistics do not account for the numbers of revascularization procedures done using other newer catheter based devices such as directional coronary atherectomy, laser angioplasty, and the rotablader. Thus it is natural that the focus of therapeutic strategies has shifted from the consideration of medical versus surgical bypass to now include mechanical revascularization. However, all three treatment modalities are beset by: (1) progression of the primary atheroma, in the case of medical therapy; (2) graft occlusion, in the case of bypass surgery; and (3) luminal narrowing secondary to the accumulation of intimal extracellular matrix during

From Weber KT, MD *Wound Healing in Cardiovascular Disease*, Armonk, NY, Futura Publishing Company Inc., © 1995.

the healing response, in the case of mechanical revascularization.

This chapter will concentrate on the latter therapeutic dilemma: luminal narrowing following mechanical revascularization, commonly termed "restenosis." Restenosis is the single factor limiting a favorable long-term outcome of mechanical revascularization, and has increasingly become the focus of criticism regarding the expanding and widespread application of the techniques. As the technology and variety of devices has increased, an increasing number of lesions and more complex lesions are becoming candidates for mechanical, catheter based devices. Experience has now shown, however, that the rate of restenosis is not clearly affected by the type of device used to achieve luminal patency.[7] The focus of this discussion will not be on the many modalities, both pharmacological as well as mechanical, currently under investigation to prevent or limit restenosis, all of which have been exhaustively reviewed.[9,10] Instead, emphasis will be placed upon mechanisms of homeostasis in the vascular wall as part of the wound healing response, and pathological mechanisms that could provide insight regarding therapeutic approaches to the problem.

Restenosis: The Clinical Problem Defined

Multiple studies have shown a variety of restenosis rates following balloon angioplasty, but vary between 25% to 55%, depending upon the endpoints and follow-up to assess restenosis.[11–14] Important to note is that despite newer devices, restenosis rates remain largely unchanged. One commonly utilized pragmatic definition of restenosis is >50% luminal narrowing at follow-up angiography; however, multiple methodologies have been developed, and have become the focus of considerable controversy regarding uniformity of assessing therapeutic outcome. Other studies have utilized noninvasive assessment to longitudinally follow the functional benefit of revascularization. Because of the lack of uniform agreement on methodologies to quantitate lumen diameter, the inherent errors in angiographic assessment, and the nonuniformity in reporting restenosis rates, it is often difficult to assess the success or failure of a treatment modality.[7] Another complicating factor in assessing long-term outcome is changing technology. For example, the recent results of trials utilizing directional coronary atherectomy suggested restenosis rates not unlike that reported for balloon angioplasty.[15,16] However, the endpoint for an acceptable result (i.e., early gain in luminal diameter assessed angiographically as described by Kuntz and Baim[13]) has changed since these trials were published and may call into question the conclusions of these trials. Other reports assessing restenosis following laser angioplasty and rotablader have indicated that restenosis is a significant limitation to a favorable long-term outcome, necessitating either a repeat procedure and/or surgical bypass. In routine clinical practice apart from clinical trials to ascertain efficacy of a treatment modality, the need to reexamine a previously revascularized artery is largely symptom driven and relies heavily upon noninvasive assessment. If there is not hemodynamic compromise of blood flow and if the lumen does not present significant resistance to an increase in blood flow during exercise, then the patient has not symptomatically and clinically experienced restenosis. This method of clinical assessment, of course, is complicated by other factors such as development of collaterals. Of importance, as noted by Califf et al.,[7] it is unusual for pure restenosis lesions to clinically present with acute myocardial infarction. Abrupt occlusion secondary to thrombosis apparently does not occur since the fibrous intimal lesion does not result in a ruptured, ulcerated plaque.

The consequence of restenosis, and the necessity to prevent it, has been the widespread application and testing of myriad therapeutic modalities with little knowledge of the pathogenesis of restenosis. Not surprisingly, pharmacological approaches to restenosis in humans have uniformly failed.[9,10,17] The problem is compounded by the lack of adequate animal models. No currently available animal model, including the rabbit, rat, porcine, and nonhuman primate, provides an economically feasible model that meets all pathophysiological criteria in a realistic experimental time frame. Additionally, multiple promising treatment modalities in the rabbit and rat models have failed to carry over to humans.[18,19] Despite these drawbacks, tissue culture and animal models, or a combination of multiple models, is currently the best option available to test hypotheses on the pathophysiology of restenosis.

The Pathophysiology of Restenosis

The process of restenosis is a very complex response to injury in a blood vessel wall already damaged during the atherosclerotic process (Figure 1). The interventional device removes a variable amount of endothelium and, in the case of balloon angioplasty, causes aneurysmal dilation and rupture of the plaque. With any of the currently available devices, there is damage to the internal elastic lamina and medial layer injury, either through mechanical stretch or tissue removal. Central to this process is the exposure of collagen fibrils to the vessel surface, which is an initiating step in platelet deposition and thrombus formation. Studies have indicated that the process occurs in the vast majority of cases within 6 months of revascularization.[20,21] Restenosis is a healing response that occurs following mechanical injury, and thus, not surprisingly, involves multiple complex, interactive, and interdependent factors. Mechanical revascularization constitutes an insult to a tissue whose homeostatic mechanisms have already been disrupted. The pathological hallmark of restenosis is the gradual accumulation of a fibrous intimal mass in the initial setting of subintimal thrombus and platelet adhesion[22] that is of sufficient magnitude to encroach upon the lumen of the blood vessel to be of hemodynamic conse-

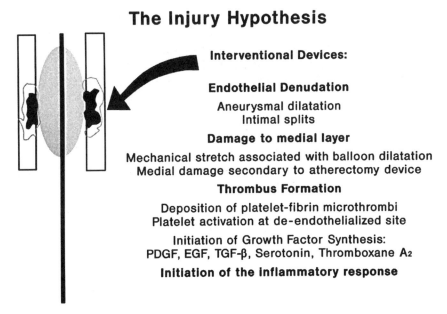

The Injury Hypothesis

Interventional Devices:

Endothelial Denudation
Aneurysmal dilatation
Intimal splits

Damage to medial layer
Mechanical stretch associated with balloon dilatation
Medial damage secondary to atherectomy device

Thrombus Formation
Deposition of platelet-fibrin microthrombi
Platelet activation at de-endothelialized site

Initiation of Growth Factor Synthesis:
PDGF, EGF, TGF-β, Serotonin, Thromboxane A₂

Initiation of the inflammatory response

Figure 1. The injury hypothesis states that restenosis occurs secondary to endothelial cell damage and disruption of the internal elastic lamina. Interventional devices such as angioplasty balloons, atherectomy devices, and lasers yield aneurysmal dilation and/or intimal tears and splits. These are associated with mechanical damage to the medial layer and the subsequent initiation of thrombus formation, growth factor synthesis, and smooth muscle cell migration. The final common denominator in restenosis is the synthesis of sufficient extracellular matrix to impinge upon the lumen of the blood vessel to a degree that is limiting to blood flow at rest or during periods of increased myocardial demand.

quence. Research into restenosis to date has primarily focused upon 1 of 3 general areas: (1) platelet deposition and the coagulation cascade; (2) smooth muscle dedifferentiation, migration, and proliferation; and (3) the secretion and effects of a large array of growth factors. Furthermore, these three areas have been the focus of attempts to arrive at a therapeutic modality. To date, all attempts to modulate these three factors have failed.[9,10] The extracellular matrix has received only secondary attention, with primary emphasis on the longitudinal biochemical characterization of the extracellular matrix following balloon injury, and little emphasis on what controls its synthesis or composition. To place the pathophysiology of restenosis in perspective, we will discuss the blood vessel during health and review evidence to emphasize that the pathology of primary atherosclerosis is significantly different from restenosis pathology, despite the fact that primary atherogenesis and restenosis may share some common characteristics.

The Blood Vessel in Health

In the normal, nondiseased blood vessel, there is homeostasis characterized by a stable intimal extracellular matrix underlying a functionally intact single layered endothelium. The intimal matrix is characterized by a thin, circumferentially intact internal elastic lamina. The underlying media is characterized by smooth muscle cells in a stable supporting extracellular matrix whose primary function is to establish vascular tone in response to local paracrine agents, circulating endocrine agents, and neural influences. The adventitia of epicardial coronary arteries is characterized by an intact neural network and normal appearing vasa vasorum. What is striking about histologic examination of the normal vessel are the features of homeostasis: the absence of mitogenicity; relatively little synthetic activity; and the absence of formed blood elements and inflammatory cells. During health, the vessels are functionally intact, and their functional integrity parallels their structural integrity. Recently, however, there is evidence that functional vascular abnormalities may precede structural abnormalities, and may be an early indicator of disease.[23,24] Increasing evidence strengthens the thesis that the functional and structural integrity of the vascular endothelium is a critical, key element to homeostasis of the vascular wall of the coronary artery.

The Blood Vessel in Disease: The Primary Atheroma

The exact initiating causes of atherosclerosis are currently unknown, however it is generally accepted that as an initiating event damage occurs to the endothelium.[25] Potential causes of endothelial cell damage include oxidation and free radical damage related to lipid metabolism, and shear stress damage at vessel branch points. Whatever the cause, the endothelium is altered in such a fashion as to permit attachment and migration into the subintimal region of inflammatory cells. The early atheroma is characterized by mononuclear cell infiltration. These cells eventually become transformed into macrophages and accumulate lipid to become the characteristic foam cell. There is smooth muscle cell dedifferentiation with transformation of these cells from a quiescent contractile state to a synthetic state, and migration of these cells into the subintimal area of the vessel. These transformed cells, as in the restenosis lesion, are largely responsible for the synthesis of the extracellular matrix found in the atheroma. Other evidence suggests that the endothelium may secrete some collagen, especially types I and VIII, into the subintimal area.[26] As the atheroma enlarges, it is characterized by an extracellular matrix consisting of a complicated mixture of cholesterol and calcium deposits in a complex array of collagens types I and III (primarily type I in the mature atheroma).[27] The collagens comprise approximately 60% of the protein bulk, with progressively less elastin, proteoglycans, and glycoproteins as the atheroma matures.[28] This may or may not be associated with central necrosis and internal hemorrhage. As the atheroma enlarges, it initially impinges upon the vascular wall but later expands into the vessel lumen. If the ulceration and necrosis extends into the luminal surface of the atheroma, exposed collagen and fibrin in an ulcerated plaque become the nidus for platelet aggregation and consequent thrombus formation secondary to activation of the coagulation cascade. The atherosclerotic site becomes the focus of a dynamic "formation and lysis" of thrombus complicated by vasospasm, clinically manifested as unstable, preinfarction angina. The vasomotor actions are primarily secondary to platelet-derived vasoactive agents such as thromboxane, adenosine diphosphate (ADP), and serotonin functioning in an environment devoid of opposing endothelium-derived vasoactive factors such as prostacyclin and endothelium-derived relaxing factor (EDRF). If the thrombus enlarges sufficiently to occlude the lumen, then blood flow ceases and a myocardial infarction ensues. The primary atheroma, characterized by its prominent inflammatory component, is to be distinguished from the pathological characteristics of restenosis lesions.

The Blood Vessel in Disease: Restenosis

Following mechanical revascularization, there is not only partial denudation of the endothelium, but also disruption of the internal elastic lamina and stretch/mechanical injury to the media, often in the nonatherosclerotic portion of the vessel wall. In the balloon injury porcine model of restenosis, the intimal hyperplasia response is dependent upon disruption of the internal elastic lamina. Early in the course of healing, there is rapid endothelial cell proliferation and formation of an endothelial cell sheet over the wound,[29,30] although not all studies agree with this assessment regarding the degree of endothelial cell regeneration. Importantly, balloon angioplasty removes only 30%–35% of the endothelium and does not necessarily cause widespread endothelial cell denudation (unpublished observation). The disruption of the internal elastic lamina and physical removal of the endothelium occurs in a vascular lesion whose endothelium is already dysfunctional in its ability to produce beneficial vasoactive factors such as EDRF and other potentially beneficial key regulator compounds such as

heparin.[31–33] On the other hand, the endothelium in an atherosclerotic lesion could conceivably synthesize and release compounds that exert regulatory effects on the intima and promote restenosis through enhanced extracellular matrix production and smooth muscle cell proliferation. The exact sequence of events that occurs following balloon injury are, in many cases, controversial, and are largely derived from animal models, since human data are difficult to obtain.

Platelet Deposition and the Coagulation Cascade Phase

Following angioplasty, histologic studies have demonstrated that there is platelet adherence to the disrupted intimal surface consequent to exposure of collagen and other fibrous proteins. Subsequent to the adherence, the platelets degranulate and release their contents, including vasoactive factors such as thromboxane, adenosine diphosphate, histamine, and serotonin, and mitogens such as platelet derived growth factor, thrombospondin, and transforming growth factor-β.[34] Animal studies have shown that platelet adherence and thrombus formation have subsided by 48 hours.[35] Associated with platelet adherence is the formation of thrombus in the subintimal areas exposed to the vascular lumen through the dissection or cut surface created by the device.[36] Since thrombin is a potent mitogen, this compound has been implicated in the process of smooth muscle cell migration and proliferation.[37,38] Because of these events, numerous drug trials designed to prevent platelet adherence and/or thrombus formation have been reported, all without effect at the drug concentrations and types of drug delivery methods utilized. However, there are promising reports that proper dosing via local application resulting in decreased thrombus burden may affect the intimal reaction to injury.[39,40]

Smooth Muscle Cell Phase

Smooth muscle cell migration and proliferation has been the subject of intense study trials in restenosis. Because of its perceived central role in restenosis, numerous drug trials have targeted modulation of smooth muscle cell proliferation and/or migration. Most of what we know is derived from the rat model, and has been recently reviewed.[36,41] Early in the course of the injury response, and generally thought to be closely associated with platelet deposition and thrombus burden, there is smooth muscle cell migration into the intima. This chemikinetic response appears to be directed by local factors that attract the cells to the subintimal layer via migration through the ruptured internal elastic lamina. At present, there is substantial evidence that thrombus burden may be critical in determining the degree of smooth muscle cell reaction and resultant intimal burden, despite the relatively small amount of thrombus observed in a mature restenosis lesion and the curtailment of thrombus formation early in the course of the injury response (see ref. 62 for a detailed review). These data suggest that thrombin may be an important initiator, however the presence of other agonist stimuli or the absence of antagonists to smooth muscle cell migration/proliferation/secretion may likely persist after resolution of the thrombus. Certainly multiple growth factors that could conceivably be synthesized by inflammatory cells, smooth muscle cells themselves, and endothelium could propagate the synthetic phase of restenosis (see ref. 82 for a detailed review of growth factors implicated in restenosis). There is some evidence that smooth muscle cells from patients who experience restenosis migrate at a faster rate than smooth muscle cells from patients who do not restenose.[42] The small fraction of smooth muscle cells that do migrate assume a synthetic state and secrete multiple compounds, including the proteins elastin, collagens, and proteoglycans.

Additionally, studies examining DNA synthesis in the smooth muscle cells have demonstrated that some of the cells divide, although the cellularity of the mature restenosis lesion is relatively low at ~15%. Currently it is assumed that proliferation occurs in response to one or more of the numerous growth factors reported relevant to restenosis. Alternatively, there is some evidence that in restenosis patients the smooth mus-

cle cell sensitivity to locally released antimitogens such as heparin is decreased.[43] Once the smooth muscle cell assumes residence in the subintimal area, regulatory events that control synthesis and eventual quiescence following the wound healing response are virtually unknown. It is logical to conclude that at some point in time, cellular signals decline and the secretory/proliferative stimuli are removed. The nature and source of these signals are also unknown, however it is interesting to note that an early study by Fishman et al. reported that smooth muscle cell proliferation is greatest at sites denuded of endothelium.[44]

Secretory Phase

The secretory phase, or laying down of the extracellular matrix, in the restenosis process is concurrent with, and integrally related to, the smooth muscle cell synthetic phase. Relative to the amount of research on platelet deposition, the coagulation process, growth factors, and smooth muscle cell physiology and biochemistry, little is known about the regulation of synthesis and composition of the extracellular matrix. However, it is the extracellular matrix that comprises the bulk of the restenosis lesion and accounts for encroachment on the lumen of the blood vessel. Available evidence indicates that the extracellular matrix is primarily synthesized by the transformed smooth muscle cell that takes up residence in the subintimal layer in response to rupture of the internal elastic lamina.[45] The extracellular matrix appears to be dynamic, with a transition in the chemical makeup of the intimal plaque over the course of several weeks following balloon injury. In the immediate period following injury, the laying down of proteoglycans and elastin predominate, along with synthesis and release into the extracellular matrix of collagen type I. In the weeks following injury, the intimal lesion bulk consists of collagen type III, not unlike the transition seen in primary atherosclerosis but on an accelerated basis (months versus years). The regulatory events of the maturation are not known, however one could postulate this occurs in association with either the alteration of synthetic signals to secretory cells and/or the occurrence of events (such as reestablishment of the internal elastic lamina) that signal the end of the reparative process. Indeed, the composition of the extracellular matrix itself can influence endothelial cell migration and the reendothelialization process.[45] At this point in time, a new homeostasis is achieved, however with a large intimal collagen burden which presumably is stable with time. In patients who experience clinical restenosis, it is unclear if this process would continue, or, if given the opportunity, would be self terminated. Clinical symptoms usually mandate removal or bypass of the occlusion. Once formed, there is currently no evidence that the intimal plaque burden regresses.

The Wound Healing Process: Normal or Abnormal

There may be valuable parallels with the wound healing process in the injured artery and that which occurs normally in skin, especially as it relates to the integrity of the basal lamina (skin) and internal elastic lamina (blood vessel). In the skin, wound healing follows orderly repair and invokes many mechanisms commonly associated with restenosis, i.e., signaling mechanisms, cell migration, matrix formation, growth factors, and epithelialization.[46] Healing processes considered aberrant, such as the hypertrophic scar in the skin, is of no functional consequence. However, aberrant healing with an exaggerated matrix deposition in the coronary artery with the synthesis of an abnormally large bulk of extracellular matrix would have serious functional consequences through encroachment into the lumen of the vessel. Hypertrophic scars have some characteristics common to restenosis lesions by virtue of increased extracellular matrix, collagen deposition, and increased synthetic activity.[47] It is unclear what the "end" signal mechanisms are which modulate synthesis and deposition of extracellular matrix, and if there are close parallels between these signals in skin and those in blood vessels. Some data, however, support the postulate that reestablishment of the integrity of the basal lamina/internal elastic lamina may be a critical step.

Normal skin wound healing, as in the early phases of vascular injury, is characterized by early activation of the coagulation cascade associated with platelet deposition in response to exposure of collagen fibers at the cut edge. The release of vasoconstrictors, along with formation of the platelet plug, functions in the cessation of hemorrhage. In settings of this degree of skin trauma extending through the basal lamina, there is also migration of fibroblasts into the wound associated with the secretion of growth factors. Once the secretory cells take up residence, they synthesize fibrous compounds that eventually seal the wound. The wound contracts and the healing process is terminated along with reestablishment of the basal lamina. All of these processes have common elements with wound healing following injury to an artery through mechanical revascularization. One striking difference, however, is that the coronary artery is already diseased through the process of atherosclerosis, whereas skin wound healing does not occur in this setting.

Multiple studies have attempted to correlate restenosis with clinical factors such as the type of lesion, postpercutaneous transluminal coronary angioplasty (PTCA) results, presence of calcification, unstable versus stable angina, presence of dissection, and others. These extensive studies have failed to clearly delineate risk factors that are predictable and prognostic from one patient, or one study, to another,[48] except perhaps in patients with diabetes and in patients with abnormalities in specific classes of lipoproteins.[49,50] If these results are coupled with the multiple pharmacological failures that have addressed various specific phases of restenosis, it appears that restenosis occurs independently of any of the factors considered to date. This raises the possibility, as is well established in the case of hypertrophic scar formation in the skin, that clinically significant restenosis patients potentially have a genetic basis of, or predisposition toward, restenosis. The aberrant healing process which accumulates a large bulk of extracellular matrix is aberrant simply because it has a functional clinical outcome.

The Role of the Vascular Endothelium in Restenosis

The Endothelium During Health

Prior to the landmark observation by Furchgott and Zadwaski[51] that the endothelium synthesizes and releases endothelium derived relaxing factor (EDRF) and prostanoids, the endothelium was, by in large, thought to primarily function in a "protective and nutritive" role; it was assumed to be primarily a passive border between the vascular lumen and the underlying media. It is now clear that this is not the case. The vascular endothelium is a totipotent cell capable of synthesizing and releasing numerous compounds that have diverse effects via autocrine, paracrine, and endocrine mechanisms (Figure 2). The general classes of compounds include not only vasoactive factors, but also mitogens, antimitogens, modulators of coagulation and platelet adherence, modulators of inflammation, growth factors, and chemotactic factors. A question of critical importance: is there evidence to support the postulate that the endothelium plays a key regulatory role in maintaining homeostasis in the vascular wall, especially with regard to the extracellular matrix? Furthermore, does the endothelium synthesize and release compounds which have opposite actions with regard to vasomotion, mitogenicity, inflammation, and coagulation that could importantly influence the wound healing response? Conceivably, if the hypothesis is correct, a dysfunctional or damaged endothelium could actually promote aberrant healing such as occurs during restenosis through the failure to regulate in an integrated fashion various aspects of coagulation, smooth muscle cell migration and proliferation, growth factor secretion, and extracellular matrix deposition, all thought to be central aspects of restenosis.

There is accumulating evidence that the endothelium has the ability to synthesize compounds with multiple actions, and effects which oppose one another. For example, EDRF is now thought to be either nitric oxide (NO)[52] or a nitric oxide containing compound.[53,54] Not only is EDRF/NO a potent vasodilator,[51,55-60] it also importantly modulates platelet aggregation,[61-69] functions as an antiinflammatory agent[66,70,71] through modulation of neutrophil adherence,[72-75] and has antimitogenic

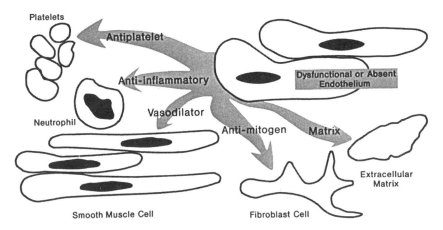

Figure 2. Schematic diagram indicating the multifarious capacity of the vascular endothelium through the synthesis and release of compounds that affect numerous functions via a paracrine mechanism. Several key compounds that may play a critical regulatory role in vascular homeostasis, such as EDRF, prostaglandins, and endothelin, modulate several different activities that are operative during restenosis. It is important to note that some of these compounds have opposite actions, i.e., vasodilation vs. vasoconstriction or one may be a mitogen (endothelin) and the other an anti-mitogen (EDRF). The impairment of one compound could conceivably result in unopposed action of the other compound, resulting in disruption of homeostasis.

properties.[76,77] Prostacyclin is synthesized by the endothelium and is a vasodilator as well as an inhibitor of platelet aggregation.[62,65,67] Heparin synthesized by the endothelium modulates not only coagulation, but also exerts potent antimitogenic activity on the underlying smooth muscle cell and modulates the extracellular matrix composition.[78,79]

Opposing the actions of these compounds are endothelium-derived substances such as endothelin and angiotensin II. For example, endothelin is a potent vasoconstrictor[80-83] and possesses mitogenic properties,[84] and may be subject to autocrine feedback regulation by NO.[85,86]

In addition to synthesizing compounds that have multiple, but opposite actions, there is evidence that the endothelium can modulate the extracellular matrix through its effects on collagen synthesis. Guarda et al. have demonstrated that endothelin can stimulate fibroblast collagen synthesis and downregulate fibroblast collagenase activity via the release of an unidentified soluble factor.[87] Angiotensin II has been shown to be a mitogen, and has been implicated in vascular remodeling following injury,[88,89] perhaps through a signaling mechanism common with endothelin.[90] Angiotensin II has also been implicated in the injury response through its effects on migration of the endothelium following balloon injury.[45] Heparin has been reported to decrease collagen and elastin synthesis in rats.[79] Thus, an imbalance or disruption of normal reciprocal regulation by endothelium-derived compounds during disease could precipitate an aberrant wound healing response and exaggerated intimal fibrous hyperplasia characteristic of restenosis (Figure 3).

The issue of altered homeostasis secondary to endothelial cell dysfunction is complicated by the myriad number of growth factors that appear to function as important determinants of the healing process. A review of growth factors that have been implicated in the restenosis response is beyond the scope of this chapter, and have been recently reviewed.[41,91] Indeed, these growth factors can be synthesized and released by the endothelium itself. How these growth factors relate to other potentially key regulatory endothelium-derived ele-

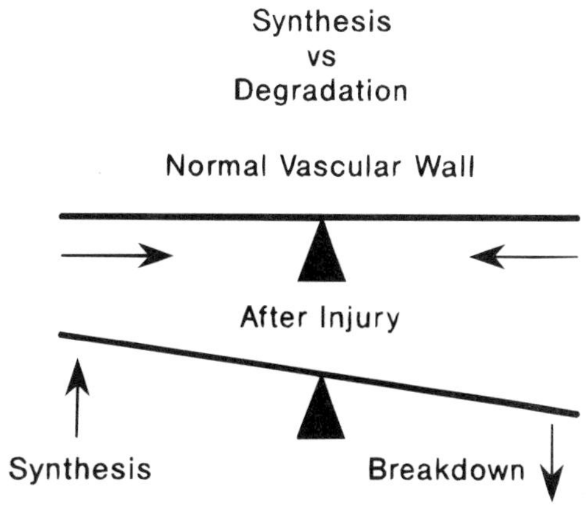

Figure 3. Normal blood vessels are in a state of homeostasis where synthesis of the extracellular matrix is balanced by degradation. The vascular endothelium exerts important paracrine effects via the release of regulatory compounds. Following injury such as occurs during balloon angioplasty, the synthesis of extracellular matrix may override breakdown, resulting in a sufficiently large intimal burden as to encroach upon the vascular lumen.

ments such as EDRF, prostanoids, endothelin, and angiotensin II that have multiple functions in vasomotion, inflammation, mitogenesis, and regulation of platelet function remains to be seen.

The Endothelium During Disease

Experiments from both animal model and humans have shown that during atherosclerosis the endothelium is dysfunctional in its ability to synthesize and release critical factors that are important during health. For example, endothelium-dependent vasomotion secondary to the actions of EDRF is impaired in atherosclerosis.[23,92-100] This observation has now been extended to abnormal control of platelet adhesion.[31,101,102] More recently, it is clear that EDRF/NO may be a critical second messenger mediating inflammation and that during periods of endothelial cell dysfunction, inflammatory cell adherence may increase via the expression of adherence molecules. The consequence of the adherence of inflammatory cells to the endothelium is migration of these cells into the subintimal layer. This is a key primary event thought to occur in early atherogenesis. The exact mechanisms for impaired synthesis or release of EDRF/NO during atherosclerosis is not clear, however altered metabolism of endogenous nitrosovasodilators by compounds such as superoxide and other free radical has been implicated[103] as has inactivation by lipids.[104,105]

There is now evidence that endogenous heparin metabolism by the endothelium is altered during atherosclerosis.[106] The increased metabolism of heparins, along with alterations in other endothelium-derived substances most likely results in the decreased ability to maintain the smooth muscle cell in a quiescent, contractile state, as well as alter the endothelium's ability to modulate local coagulation. Heparin modulates the composition of the extracellular matrix,[79] and during disease alterations in heparin metabolism could have significant effects on the extracellular matrix.

Alternatively, compounds such as endothelin may actually increase during atherosclerosis.[31,107] In the face of impaired synthesis of vasodilators, antimitogens, antiinflammatory, and anticoagulant compounds, such increases in the local paracrine effect of a compound such as endothelin could have marked effects on vascular wall homeostasis and wound healing responses.

The critical question, however, remains to be answered: are there key endothelium-derived regulatory compounds that exert fundamental control over a variety of elements operative during restenosis such as growth factor synthesis (by smooth muscle cells in a "synthetic" state via paracrine mechanisms, and injured endothelium via autocrine mechanisms), coagulation, and the extracellular matrix at the local, paracrine level? Of note, in restenosis the inflammatory process appears to play a relatively insignificant role. If there is/are fundamental key regulatory aspects to the healing response, then pharmacological regulation of these key elements may provide some pragmatic solution to attenuating the extracellular matrix response (hemodynamically significant restenosis) and offer a unifying explanation concerning the multitude of processes that have been implicated following mechanical revascularization, many of which are simply part of a normal wound healing response.

Summary

Restenosis, characterized by the accumulation of a subintimal fibrous plaque that compromises the vascular lumen, is the single most important factor limiting a favorable long-term outcome of mechanical revascularization. The process of intimal hyperplasia as part of the wound healing response is extraordinarily complex and involves both cellular and biochemical/hormonal signals. Restenosis shares many common characteristics with the normal wound healing response seen in, for example, the skin. The difference lies in localization of the wound in an already abnormal atherosclerotic vascular segment, and the impingement of the "scar" on the vascular lumen. Despite advances in technology, the rate of clinically significant restenosis remains at a stubbornly fixed prevalence. It remains to be seen if the intimal hyperplasia following vascular injury simply represents a "normal" wound healing response and that restenosis occurs if there is a functional consequence to repair in a limited space. To adequately arrive at a pragmatic clinical solution to modulation of the degree of intimal hyperplasia in an environment that allows adequate repair of the vessel following mechanical injury will require a much more systematic approach to the problem than has occurred in the past.

References

1. Heart and Stroke Facts: 1994 Statistical Supplement, American Heart Association, Dallas. 1994;99:1–2.
2. Varnaukas E. Twelve-year follow-up of survival in the randomized European Coronary Surgery Study. N Engl J Med 1988;319:332–337.
3. The Veterans Administration Coronary Artery Bypass Surgery Cooperative Study Group. Eleven-year survival in the Veterans Administration randomized trial of coronary bypass surgery for stable angina. N Engl J Med 1984;311:1333–1339.
4. Killip T, Passamani E, Davis K. Coronary

artery surgery study (CASS): a randomized trial of coronary artery bypass surgery: eight years follow-up and survival in patients with reduced ejection fraction. Circulation 1985;72(Suppl. V):V102-V109.

5. Gruentzig A. Transluminal dilatation of coronary artery stenosis. (Letter) Lancet 1978;1:263.

6. Gruentzig A, Senning A, Siegenthaler W. Nonoperative dilation of coronary artery stenosis: percutaneous transluminal coronary angioplasty. N Engl J Med 1979;301:61–68.

7. Califf R, Fortin D, Frid D, et al. Restenosis after coronary angioplasty: an overview. J Am Coll Cardiol 1991;17:2B-13B.

8. Lau K, Sigwart U. Restenosis after PTCA: risk factors and pathophysiology. J Myocard Ischemia 1992;4:15–33.

9. Herrman J, Hermans W, Vos J, et al. Pharmacological approaches to the prevention of restenosis following angioplasty—the search for the Holy Grail? (Part I). Drugs 1993;46:5–18.

10. Herrman J, Hermans W, Vos J, et al. Pharmacological approaches to the prevention of restenosis following angioplasty—the search for the Holy Grail? (Part II). Drugs 1993;46:249–226.

11. Meier B. Restenosis after coronary angioplasty: review of the literature. Eur Heart J 1988;9(Suppl. C):1–6.

12. Holmes D, Vlietstra R, Smith H, et al. Restenosis after percutaneous transluminal coronary angioplasty (PTCA): a report from the PTCA registry of the National Heart, Lung, and Blood Institute. Am J Cardiol 1984;53:77C-81C.

13. Kuntz R, Baim D. Defining coronary restenosis: newer clinical and angiographic paradigms. Circulation 1993;88:1310–1323.

14. Detre D, Holubkov R, Kelsey S, et al. One-year follow-up results of the 1985–86 National Heart, Lung, and Blood Institute's Percutaneous Transluminal Coronary Angioplasty Registry. Circulation 1989;80:421–428.

15. Fishman R, Kuntz R, Carrozza J, et al. Long-term results of directional coronary atherectomy: predictors of restenosis. J Am Coll Cardiol 1992;20:1101–1110.

16. Hinohara T, Robertson G, Selmon M, et al. Restenosis after directional coronary atherectomy. J Am Coll Cardiol 1992;20:623–632.

17. Weintraub W. Clinical trials in interventional cardiology. J Invasive Cardiol 1993;5:6–16.

18. Muller D, Ellis S, Topol E. Experimental models of coronary artery restenosis. J Am Coll Cardiol 1991;19:418–432.

19. Ferrell M, Fuster V, Gold H, et al. A dilemma for the 1990s: choosing appropriate experimental animal model for the prevention of restenosis. Circulation 1992;85:1630–1631.

20. Val P, Bourassa M, David P. Restenosis after successful PTCA: the Montreal Heart Institute experience. Am J Cardiol 1987;60:50B-55B.

21. Serruys P, Luijten H, Beatt K. Incidence of restenosis after successful coronary angioplasty: a time-related phenomenon. Circulation 1988;77:361–371.

22. Ip J, Fuster V, Israel D, et al. The role of platelets, thrombin and hyperplasia in restenosis after coronary angioplasty. J Am Coll Cardiol 1991;17:77B-88B.

23. Werns S, Walton J, Hsia H, et al. Evidence of endothelial dysfunction in angiographically normal coronary arteries of patients with coronary artery disease. Circulation 1989;79:287–291.

24. Ludmer P, Selwin A, Shook T, et al. Paradoxical vasoconstriction induced by acetylcholine in atherosclerotic coronary arteries. N Engl J Med 1986;315:1046–1051.

25. Schwartz C, Valente A, Sprague E, et al. The pathogenesis of atherosclerosis: current concepts. In: Schwartz C, ed. Am J Cardiol Cont. Education Series. 1993:11–17.

26. Rauterberg J, Jaeger E. Collagen and collagen synthesis in the atherosclerotic vessel wall. In: Robenek H, Severs N, eds. Cell Interactions in Atherosclerosis. Boca Raton, Fla: CRC Press; 1992:101–135.

27. Tan E, Uitto J. Pathology of the extracellular matrix in atherosclerosis: in vivo and in vitro models. In: White R, ed. Atherosclerosis and Arteriosclerosis: Human Pathology and Experimental Animal Methods and Models. Boca Raton, Fla: CRC Press, 1989:87–110.

28. Thie M. Regulation of biosynthetic activity in aortic smooth muscle cells by extracellular matrix components. In: Robenek H, Severs N, eds. Cell Interactions in Atherosclerosis. Boca Raton, Fla: CRC Press, 1992:137–163.

29. Madri J. The extracellular matrix as a modulator of neovascularization. In: Gallo M, ed. Cardiovascular Disease: Molecular and Cellular Mechanisms, Prevention, Treatment. New York, NY: Plenum Press, 1987:177.

30. Madri J, Pratt B, Yanniarello-Brown J. Matrix-driven cell size changes modulate aor-

tic endothelial cell proliferation and sheet migration. Am J Pathol 1988;132:18.

31. Tanner F, Boulanger C, Luscher T. Endothelium-derived nitric oxide, endothelin, and platelet vessel wall interaction: alterations in hypercholesterolemia and atherosclerosis. Semin Thromb Hemos 1993;19:167–175.

32. Marcum J. Heparin-like molecules with anticoagulant activity are synthesized by cultured endothelial cells. Biochem Biophys Res Comm 1985;126:365.

33. Preissner K. Physiological role of vessel wall related antithrombotic mechanisms: contribution of endogenous and exogenous heparin-like components to the anticoagulant potential of the endothelium. Haemostasis 1990;20:30–49.

34. Houston D, Shepherd J, Vanhoutte P. Aggregating human platelets cause direct contraction and endothelium-dependent relaxation of isolated canine coronary arteries: role of serotonin, thromboxane A2 and adenine nucleotides. J Clin Invest 1986;78:539–544.

35. Clowes A, Reidy M. Prevention of stenosis after vascular reconstruction: pharmacologic control of intimal hyperplasia. J Vasc Surg 1991;13:885–891.

36. Casscells W. Migration of smooth muscle and endothelial cells: critical events in restenosis. Circulation 1992;86:723–729.

37. Thyberg J, Hedin U, Sjolund M, et al. Regulation of differentiated properties and proliferation of arterial smooth muscle cells. Arteriosclerosis 1990;10:966–990.

38. Cassells W. Smooth muscle cell growth factors. Prog Growth Factor Res 1991;3:177–206.

39. Sarembock I, Gertz S, Gimple L, et al. Effectiveness of recombinant desulphatohirudin in reducing restenosis after balloon angioplasty of atherosclerotic femoral arteries in rabbits. Circulation 1991;84:232–243.

40. Wilcox J. Thrombin and other potential mechanisms underlying restenosis. Circulation 1991;84:432–435.

41. Cercek B, Sharifi B, Barath P, et al. Growth factors in pathogenesis of coronary arterial restenosis. Am J Cardiol 1991;68:C24-C33.

42. Bauriedel G, Windstetter U, DeMaio S Jr, et al. Migratory activity of human smooth muscle cells cultivated from coronary and peripheral primary and restenotic lesions removed by percutaneous atherectomy. Circulation 1992;85:554–564.

43. Chan P, Patel M, Betteridge L, et al. Abnormal growth regulation of vascular smooth muscle cells by heparin in patients with restenosis. Lancet 1993;341:341–342.

44. Fishman J, Ryan G, Karnovsky M. Endothelial regeneration in the rat carotid artery and the significance of endothelial denudation in the pathogenesis of myointimal thickening. Lab Invest 1975;32:339–351.

45. Madri J, Bell L. Vascular cell responses to injury: modulation by extracellular matrix and soluble factors. In: Robenek H, Severs N, eds. Cell Interactions in Atherosclerosis. Boca Raton, Fla: CRC Press, 1992:165–179.

46. Clark D. Wound healing. J Dermatol Surg Oncol; In press.

47. Murray J. Keloids and hypertrophic scars. Clin Dermatol 1994;12:27–37.

48. Bourassa M, Lesperance J, Eastwood C, et al. Clinical, physiologic, anatomic and procedural factors predictive of restenosis after percutaneous transluminal coronary angioplasty. J Am Coll Cardiol 1991;18:368–376.

49. Hearn J, Donohue B, Baalbaki H, et al. Usefulness of serum lipoprotein(a) as a predictor of restenosis after percutaneous transluminal coronary angioplasty. Am J Cardiol 1992;69:736–739.

50. Shah P, Amin J. Low high density lipoprotein level is associated with increased restenosis rate after coronary angioplasty. Circulation 1992;85:1279–1285.

51. Furchgott R, Zadwaski J. The obligatory role of endothelial cells in the relaxation of arterial smooth muscle by acetylcholine. Nature 1980;288:373–376.

52. Palmer R, Ferrige A, Moncada S. Nitric oxide release accounts for the biological activity of endothelium-derived relaxing factor. Nature 1987;327:524–526.

53. Myers P, Guerra R, Harrison D. Release of NO and EDRF from cultured bovine aortic endothelial cells. Am J Physiol 1989;256:H1030-H1037.

54. Myers P, Minor R, Guerra R, et al. Vasorelaxant properties of the endothelium-derived relaxing factor more closely resemble S-nitrosocysteine than nitric oxide. Nature 1990;345:161–163.

55. Griffith T, Henderson A. EDRF and the regulation of vascular tone. Int J Microcirc Clin Exp 1989;8:383–396.

56. Furchgott R. Role of endothelium in responses of vascular smooth muscle. Circ Res 1983;53:557.

57. Luscher T. Endothelium-derived vasoactive factors and regulation of vascular tone in human blood vessels. Lung 1990;168:27–34.

58. Tolins J, Shultz P, Raij L. Role of endothelium-derived relaxing factor in regulation of vascular tone and remodeling: update on

humoral regulation of vascular tone. Hypertension 1991;17:909–916.

59. Furchgott R. The discovery of endothelium-dependent relaxation. Circulation 1993; 87(Suppl. 5):3–8.

60. Griffith T, Edwards D, Lewis M, et al. The nature of endothelium-derived vascular relaxant factor. Nature 1984;308:645–647.

61. Cohen R, Shepherd J, Vanhoutte P. Inhibitory role of the endothelium in response of isolated coronary arteries to platelets. Science 1982;221:273–274.

62. Forstermann U, Mugge A, Bode S, et al. Response of human coronary arteries to aggregating platelets: importance of endothelium-derived relaxing factor and prostanoids. Circ Res 1988;63:306–312.

63. Vanhoutte P, Houston D. Platelets, endothelium, and vasospasm. Circulation 1985; 72:728–734.

64. Sneddon J, Vane J. Endothelium-derived relaxing factor reduces platelet adhesion to bovine endothelial cells. Proc Natl Acad Sci USA 1988;85:2800–2804.

65. Radomski M, Palmer R, Moncada S. The anti-aggregating properties of vascular endothelium: interactions between prostacyclin and nitric oxide. Br J Pharmacol 1987; 92:639–646.

66. Dinerman J, Mehta J. Endothelial, platelet and leukocyte interactions in ischemic heart disease: insights into potential mechanisms and their clinical relevance. J Am Coll Cardiol 1990;16:207–222.

67. MacDonald P, Read M, Dusting G. Synergistic inhibition of platelet aggregation by endothelium-derived relaxing factor and prostacyclin. Thromb Res 1988;49:437–439.

68. Pohl U, Busse R. EDRF increases cyclic GMP in platelets during passage through the coronary vascular bed. Circ Res 1989; 65:1798–1803.

69. Siney L, Lewis M. Endothelium-derived relaxing factor inhibits platelet adhesion to cultured porcine endocardial endothelium. Eur J Pharmacol 1992;229:223–226.

70. Kawabe T, Isobe K, Hasegawa Y, et al. Immunosuppressive activity induced by nitric oxide in culture supernatant of activated rat alveolar macrophages. Immunology 1992; 76:72–78.

71. Bath P, Hassal D, Gladwin A, et al. Nitric oxide and prostacyclin: divergence of inhibitory effects on monocyte chemotaxis and adhesion to endothelium in vitro. Arterioscler Thromb 1991;11:254–260.

72. Cooke J, Tsao P. Cytoprotective effects of nitric oxide. Circulation 1993;88:2451–2454.

73. Gaboury J, Woodman R, Granger D, et al.

Nitric oxide prevents leukocyte adherence: role of superoxide. Am J Physiol 1993;265: H862-H867.

74. Arndt H, Russell J, Kurose I, et al. Mediators of leukocyte adhesion in rat mesenteric venules elicited by inhibition of nitric oxide synthesis. Gastroenterology 1993;105: 675–680.

75. Kubes P, Suzuki M, Granger D. Nitric oxide: an endogenous modulator of leukocyte adhesion. Proc Natl Acad Sci USA 1991;88:4651–4655.

76. Assendere J, Southgate K, Newby A. Does nitric oxide inhibit smooth muscle proliferation? J Cardiovasc Pharmacol 1991;17: S104-S107.

77. Kariya K, Kawahara Y, Araki S, et al. Antiproliferative action of cyclic GMP-elevating vasodilators in cultured rabbit aortic smooth muscle cells. Atherosclerosis 1989; 80:143–147.

78. Herrmann H, Okada S, Hozakowska E, et al. Inhibition of smooth muscle cell proliferation and experimental angioplasty restenosis by beta-cyclodextrin tetradecasulfate. Arterioscler Thromb 1993;13:924–931.

79. Snow A, Bolender R, Wight T, et al. Heparin modulates the composition of the extracellular matrix domain surrounding arterial smooth muscle cells. Am J Pathol 1990;137: 313–330.

80. Luscher T, Boulanger C, Yang Z, et al. Interactions between endothelium-derived relaxing and contracting factors in health and cardiovascular disease. Circulation 1993; 87(Suppl. V):V36-V44.

81. Pernow J, Modin A. Endothelial regulation of coronary vascular tone in vitro: contribution of endothelin receptor subtypes and nitric oxide. Eur J Pharmacol 1993;243: 281–286.

82. Luscher T, Boulanger C, Dohi Y, et al. Endothelium-derived contracting factors. Hypertension 1992;19:117–130.

83. Yanagisawa M, Kurihara H, Kimura S, et al. A novel potent vasoconstrictor peptide produced by vascular endothelial cells. Nature 1988;332:411–415.

84. Weissberg P, Witchell C, Davenport A, et al. The endothelin peptides ET-1, ET-2, ET-3 and sarafotoxin S6b are co-mitogenic with platelet-derived growth factor for vascular smooth muscle cells. Atherosclerosis 1990; 85:257–262.

85. Boulanger C, Luscher T. Release of endothelin from the porcine aorta: inhibition by endothelium-derived nitric oxide. J Clin Invest 1990;85:587–590.

86. Ito S, Juncos L, Nuschiro N, et al. Endothe-

lium-derived relaxing factor modulates endothelin action in afferent arterioles. Hypertension 1991;17:1052–1056.

87. Guarda E, Myers P, Katwa L, et al. Effects of endothelins on collagen turnover in cardiac fibroblasts. Cardiovasc Res 1993;27: 2130–2134.

88. Prescott M, Sawyer W. ACE inhibition versus angiotensin II, AT1 receptor antagonism: a review of effects on intimal lesion formation in animal models of vascular injury, restenosis, and atherosclerosis. Drug Develop Res 1993;29:88–93.

89. Powell J, Muller R, Baumgartner H. Suppression of the vascular response to injury: the role of angiotensin-converting enzyme inhibitors. J Am Coll Cardiol 1991;17: 137B-142B.

90. Fagin J, Forrester J. Growth factors, cytokines, and vascular injury. Trends Cardiovasc Med 1992;2:90–94.

91. Weber H, Webb M, Serafino R, et al. Endothelin-1 and angiotensin-II stimulate delayed mitogenesis in cultured rat aortic smooth muscle cells: evidence for common signaling mechanisms. Mol Endocrinol 1994;8:148–158.

92. Jayakody L, Senaratne M, Thomson A, et al. Endothelium-dependent relaxation in experimental atherosclerosis in the rabbit. Circ Res 1987;60:251–264.

93. Forstermann U, Mugge A, Alheid U, et al. Selective attenuation of endothelium-mediated vasodilation in atherosclerotic human coronary arteries. Circ Res 1988;62: 185–190.

94. Lopez T, Armstrong M, Piegors D, et al. Effect of early and advanced atherosclerosis on vascular responses to serotonin, thromboxane A2, and ADP. Circulation 1989;79: 698–705.

95. Chilian W, Dellsperger K, Layne S, et al. Effects of atherosclerosis on the coronary microcirculation. Am J Physiol 1990;258: H529-H539.

96. Guerra R, Brotherton A, Goodwin P, et al. Mechanisms of abnormal endothelium-dependent vascular relaxation in atherosclerosis: implications for altered autocrine and paracrine functions of EDRF. Blood Vessels 1990;26:300–314.

97. Nabel E, Selwyn A, Ganz P. Large coronary

arteries in humans are responsive to changing blood flow: an endothelium-dependent mechanism that fails in patients with atherosclerosis. J Am Coll Cardiol 1990;16: 349–356.

98. Verbeuren T, Jordaens G, Vanhove C, et al. Release and vascular activity of endothelium-derived relaxing factor in atherosclerotic rabbit aorta. Eur J Pharmacol 1990;191: 173–184.

99. Cohen R, Zitnay K, Haudenschild C, et al. Loss of selective endothelial cell vasoactive functions caused by hypercholesterolemia in pig coronary arteries. Circ Res 1988;63: 903–910.

100. Freiman P, Mitchell G, Heistad D, et al. Atherosclerosis impairs endothelium-dependent vascular relaxation to acetylcholine and thrombin in primates. Circ Res 1986;58: 783–789.

101. Fuster V. Pathogenesis of atherosclerosis: the role of platelets and thrombosis. In: Kwaan H, Bowie E, eds. Thrombosis. Philadelphia, Pa: Saunders, 1982:57–81.

102. Shimokawa H, Aarhus L, Vanhoutte P. Porcine coronary arteries with regenerated endothelium have a reduced endothelium-dependent responsiveness to aggregating platelets and serotonin. Circ Res 1987;61: 256–270.

103. Mugge A, Elwell J, Peterson T, et al. Chronic treatment with polyethylene-glycolated superoxide dismutase partially restores endothelium-dependent vascular relaxations in cholesterol-fed rabbits. Circ Res 1991;69: 1293–1300.

104. Chin J, Azhar S, Hoffman B. Inactivation of endothelial derived relaxing factor by oxidized lipoproteins. J Clin Invest 1992;89: 10–18.

105. Galle J, Mulsch A, Busse R, et al. Effects of native and oxidized low density lipoproteins on formation and inactivation of endothelium-derived relaxing factor. Arterioscler Thromb 1991;11:198–203.

106. Engelberg H. Heparin and the atherosclerotic process. Pharmacol Rev 1984;36: 91–110.

107. Lerman A, Edwards B, Hallett J, et al. Circulating and tissue endothelin immunoreactivity in advanced atherosclerosis. N Engl J Med 1991;325:997–1001.

Chapter 12

The Regulation of Collagen Turnover in the Normal, Hypertrophying, and Fibrotic Heart

Jill E. Bishop, Ph.D., Geoffrey J. Laurent, Ph.D.

Introduction

Collagens are the major extracellular matrix proteins in the heart, contributing to the mechanical properties and maintaining the functional integrity of the tissue. In addition to their structural role, collagens regulate nutrient supply and growth factor presentation, and determine cell phenotype. A host of collagen genes are actively expressed throughout life and the propeptides they generate turn over at rapid rates. Indeed the maintenance of a balance between the synthetic and degradative processes is critical for the continued normal function of the myocardium. The mechanisms that regulate cardiac collagen gene expression and metabolism are ill defined. Here we describe the cardiac collagens; the pathways and rates of collagen synthesis and degradation in normal and diseased heart; and key regulatory mechanisms under investigation.

The Structure of Cardiac Collagens and Their Roles in the Heart

Eighteen collagen types have been identified, coded by at least 30 genes widely distributed throughout the genome (see refs. 1 and 2 for reviews). These collagens have a diverse range of physical and biolog-ical properties such that variations in their relative abundance results in heterogeneous extracellular frameworks that satisfy the diverse range of functional requirements of all tissues in the body. Common to all collagens is a triple-helical domain, composed of three α-chains. Each α-chain consists of a central left handed helical region with the repeating sequence Gly-X-Y (where approximately every third X is proline and every third Y is hydroxyproline), and short non-helical regions at the N- and C-terminal ends. The Gly-X-Y sequence is essential for folding the molecule into a right handed triple helix, stabilized by interchain hydrogen bonds.

Six collagen types have been identified thus far in the cardiovascular system. The most abundant are the fibrillar collagens, types I and III, produced principally by fibroblasts,[3] accounting for over 90% of the total collagen. Types I and III collagen are the major structural collagens, forming the weaves and struts of the collagen network of the heart originally described by Borg and Caulfield.[4] The relative proportion of these collagen types may influence the physical properties of the myocardium. In the adult rabbit heart there is 34% type III, compared to types I plus III collagen.[5] Immunohistochemical evidence suggests that type I collagen molecules assemble into thick fibers which convey tensile strength and thus provide structural support. Type

From Weber KT, MD *Wound Healing in Cardiovascular Disease*, Armonk, NY, Futura Publishing Company Inc., © 1995.

I collagen is most abundant in tissues such as bone and tendon. Type III collagen forms a fine network of fibrils and is associated with highly elastic tissues such as dermis, blood vessels, and lung. The relative amount of these collagens changes during development and aging, with an increase in the proportion of type III occurring from 1 week to 6 months in the rat.[6] Other collagens associated with cardiovascular tissue are types IV, V, VI, and VIII. These collagens (described below) represent a comparatively small proportion of total heart collagen (an estimated 10% in total), the relative proportion of each varies during development and in disease. In addition to their structural role they also regulate cell phenotype and the size of interstitial collagen fibers.

Type IV is a basement membrane protein produced by most cardiovascular cells, particularly myocytes[3] and endothelial cells, and contains segments of nonhelical protease sensitive regions (noncollagen domains). The molecule is laid down directly as an open network with no evidence of extracellular processing.[7] It produces a three-dimensional "chicken wire" network which acts as the skeleton for basement membrane, interacting strongly with other basement membrane components such as laminin, nidogen, and heparan sulphate proteoglycans.[8] As part of the basement membrane, type IV collagen influences cell adhesion, cell spreading and cell proliferation, and acts as a filter of nutrients and growth factors from the circulation to the underlying mesenchymal cells of the vessel wall and myocardial interstitium.

Type V collagen coexists with type IV in the basement membrane and is interspersed with types I and III in the interstitium,[9] where, in addition to its structural role, it modulates fibril diameter.[10] It is associated with blood vessels, being synthesized by most vascular cells, and is present with types I and III in heart valves.[11] Structurally type V is similar to the interstitial collagens. It is closely associated with the cell surface where it contributes to cell shape by forming an exocytoskeleton,[12] as well as binding to other connective tissue components. Type VI collagen forms thin beaded filaments and is associated with hyaluronan to

which it has a high affinity.[13] It is produced by fibroblasts and endothelial cells and is found in the cardiac interstitium, the endomysium and in the media and adventitia of muscular blood vessels, associated with other fibrillar collagens.[14] It coats the surface of collagen fibers,[9] possibly regulating fiber size. Type VIII is a short chain collagen which was first isolated as a product of cultured endothelial cells. It is thought to play a role in angiogenesis[15] and cardiac morphogenesis, being present in the fetal heart, with only very low levels being detected in the neonate or adult heart.[16] In the adult it is associated with blood vessels[16] forming a component of the intimal basement membrane and co-localizing with elastic components of the extracellular matrix.[17]

Changes in Collagen Deposition During the Development of Cardiac Hypertrophy and Fibrosis

Collagen content increases (mg collagen per ventricle) in all forms of cardiac hypertrophy and disease; in man and experimental models of ventricular hypertrophy. If the myocardial contractile component and the extracellular matrix increase in a coordinate fashion, there is no change in collagen concentration (mg collagen per unit mass of tissue), possibly reflecting a common stimulatory mechanism. This may occur during the compensatory phase of hypertrophy due to pressure overload or following volume overload. Although an increase in collagen deposition in the compensatory stage of cardiac hypertrophy may be beneficial as the collagen matrix grows to accommodate the increase in muscle mass, excessive deposition leads to an increase in diastolic stiffness which may contribute to eventual heart failure.[18] Collagen concentration tends to increase, i.e., cardiac fibrosis develops, in the later stages after pressure overload,[19,20] or where the hypertrophy is associated with an inflammatory response.[21] Similarly the cause of hypertrophy determines the effect on collagen concentration in humans.[22] Changes also occur in the relative proportion of types I and III collagen during the development of cardiac hypertrophy. Type III appears to increase in the early stages,[20] but the later stages show an increase in type I,[5,23,24] a sustained increase in type III,[25–27] or a return to normal levels,[20] in both human disease and animal models. These differences are related to the animal model used, the species and age, and the time at which the measurements are made after the stimulus for hypertrophy.

Pathways of Collagen Metabolism and Sites of Regulation During the Development of Cardiac Hypertrophy and Fibrosis

Collagen is synthesized as the precursor molecule, procollagen, following many transcriptional and posttranslational steps, and is degraded both intra- and extracellularly. Thus there are numerous steps in the pathway of collagen metabolism that may be the target for regulation of collagen deposition. Here we describe the pathways of collagen metabolism, and how they are altered during the development of cardiac hypertrophy and fibrosis.

Transcription

Collagen gene transcription and its regulation is described in detail in Chapter 22. Procollagen genes coding for the pro-α_1(I) and the pro-α_2(I) chains consist of about 18 and 38 kb, respectively. Both genes contain approximately 50 introns, the larger size of the α_2(I) gene being due to the larger sized introns. The exons consist of predominantly 54 or 108 base pairs, a feature common to all fibrillar collagen genes. Promoters of the type I collagen genes contain "TATA" box and "CAT" box consensus sequences. An additional sequence required for transcription is similar to the consensus recognition sequence for nuclear factor-I. Mutations within this site prevents nuclear factor-I binding and also decreases transcription. A common feature of the fibrillar procollagen genes is the presence of enhancer sequences within their first intron, thought to determine tissue- and developmental-specific expression.[28]

mRNA for the cardiovascular collagens can be measured by Northern analysis in normal heart tissue and primary cultured cardiac cells, suggesting a continued synthesis of the proteins, or at least expression of the genes. Types I and III mRNA are expressed predominantly by cardiac and vascular fibroblasts, with little expression in the myocytes.[3] Type IV is expressed by both myocytes and fibroblasts. Increases in steady state mRNA levels of these collagens occur rapidly following the onset of hypertrophy in experimental animals due to pressure overload[24,29,30] and volume overload,[31] indicating that regulation of collagen deposition occurs, at least in part, at the transcription level. mRNA levels then fall to that of control animals, usually within 1 or 2 weeks of the initial rise. These early changes in gene expression demonstrate the rapidity with which the collagen producing cells respond to the stimulus.

Posttranslational Modifications

The pro α-chains are processed into triple helical procollagen, following extensive modifications that occur primarily in the cisternae of the endoplasmic reticulum. Prolyl hydroxylase catalyzes the hydroxylation of proline during polypeptide elongation and proceeds until virtually all Y-positioned prolines are hydroxylated. Hydroxyproline is essential for the stability of the triple helix. Under-hydroxylated procollagen cannot form triple helices and is therefore susceptible to degradation. Lysyl hydroxylase converts lysine to hydroxylysine (about seven residues per α-chain) and galactosyl and glucosyl transferases transfer carbohydrate moieties to the hydroxyl group of hydroxylysines in the helical regions. Mannose is also added to the carboxyl terminal of procollagen. Once translation is completed disulphide bridges are formed linking the pro α-chains at the C-terminal ends. The procollagen molecules are then packaged into vesicles in the Golgi complex and carried to the cellular membrane, where the procollagen is extruded from the cell by exocytosis.

Fiber Formation

Once released into the extracellular space, amino and carboxyl-peptidases remove the terminal extensions and collagen fiber formation occurs. However, immuno-electron microscopy studies have demonstrated that the thinner type I and III fibers appear to retain the N-terminal propeptide.[32] The N- and C-terminal propeptides may also exert a negative feedback effect on collagen synthesis.[33,34] These results suggest that propeptides may play critical roles both in fibrillogenesis and regulation of collagen synthesis. Fiber formation is a self-assembly process. The molecules align in quarter-stagger arrays, first forming microfibrils which are then linked to form larger fibers. The fibers are stabilized by the formation of intermolecular covalent crosslinks catalyzed by lysyl oxidase which readily binds to molecules arranged in fibers. Lysyl and hydroxylysyl residues, particularly in the nonhelical regions, undergo oxidative deamination to form allysine and hydroxyallysine. Intermolecular crosslinks form through the formation of a Schiff base between aldehyde-containing precursors and the side chains of a lysyl or hydroxylysyl residue in the helical region of an adjacent molecule (see ref. 35 for review). The nature of these crosslinks changes with age, from reducible crosslinks to a stable nonreducible form (through the formation of polyvalent crosslinks). There is some evidence that crosslinks may also form between type I and type III molecules supporting immunohistochemical evidence that type I and III molecules are present in the same fibrils.[36]

The Dynamic Nature of Cardiac Collagen Turnover

Early studies of collagen turnover suggested that collagen was virtually inert.[37] This is now recognized to be only partly true. Early techniques employed the "decay" method which involved measuring the decrease in the specific activity of proline in collagen following a single injection of a radio-labeled amino acid. This method did not allow for amino acid reutilization. Although hydroxyproline is not re-utilized, on collagen degradation, proline is recycled very efficiently (over 90%).[38] Continuous infusion methods for measuring

total protein synthesis rates reduced the problem of reutilization.[39,40] By adding the isotope continuously over several hours, the specific activity of the labeled amino acid rises to reach a plateau value which is maintained for several hours. Rates of protein synthesis are calculated in individual tissues from the specific activity of the free and protein-bound amino acids at the end of the infusion. A simpler approach is to inject a single flooding dose of unlabeled amino acid with the amino acid tracer, which rapidly floods all the tissue pools. This method, introduced by Henshaw et al.,[41] was adapted and validated by us for measuring collagen synthesis rates.[42] Using this method in rabbits the proline-specific activity in the tissue free pool reaches a plateau which is maintained for over 3 hours. The procollagen-specific activities (taken to represent the precursor pool) are between the plasma and the tissue free pool values, suggesting equilibration has been achieved between tissue compartments.

Despite the newly emergent techniques there have been few studies on the rates of collagen synthesis in the heart. We have shown collagen fractional synthesis rates of 3%/day and 6%/day in the right and left ventricles of 2-kg rabbits, respectively,[43] of which one third is degraded rapidly in both ventricles (see below). In comparison, values of 18%/day were found in both ventricles for noncollagen protein synthesis. In the rat fractional collagen synthesis rates of 9%/day were found at 6 months of age, this compares with 4%/day in the lung and <1%/day in skin.[44] Collagen synthesis rates decrease with increasing age in the rat heart (Figure 1).[44] This has also been demonstrated for other tissues such as lung.[44] There is no information on the rates of synthesis of the individual types in the heart. In the skin, it appears that collagen synthesis is more rapid for type I than type III. The half-life for processing type I procollagen in rabbit skin has been estimated at 26 minutes whereas the half-life for type III is 3.9 hours.[45]

The response of the collagen-producing cells to the stimulus for cardiac hypertrophy is very rapid and extensive. Only 2 days after pulmonary artery banding synthesis rates increase sixfold in the right ven-

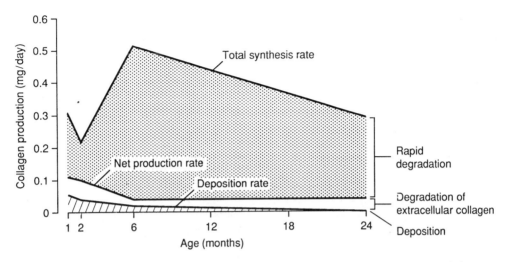

Figure 1. Age related changes in heart collagen metabolism. Collagen production and deposition (mg/day) were calculated in the hearts of rats from 1 to 24 months of age. Gross collagen synthesis (mg/day) represents the total amount of collagen synthesized in the heart calculated from measurements of collagen fractional synthesis rates and collagen content. The net production rate represents the total collagen synthesized minus the proportion that is degraded rapidly after synthesis (the shaded area). Deposition rates were based on the daily change in collagen content at the ages studied. Total collagen deposition is represented by the hatched area. The open area represents collagen degraded extracellularly, by metalloproteases. This figure was produced based on data obtained from the PhD thesis of Dr. Peter Mays.[107]

tricle, associated with an increase in the level of procollagen α_1(I) mRNA.[30] Bonnin et al. found an eightfold increase in collagen synthesis rates in the right ventricle 5 days after pulmonary artery banding in dogs.[46] A threefold increase in incorporation of ^{3}H-proline into hydroxyproline (measured in vitro) was observed 2 days after aortic constriction in the rat.[47] Right ventricular collagen synthesis rates increased threefold after 14 days in the bleomycin model in which the onset of pressure overload is more gradual.[43] Eleftheriades et al. saw no increase in collagen fractional synthesis rate until 16 weeks after the onset of moderate sustained hypertension in the young rat, demonstrating that the rapidity of the response may be dependent on the severity of the pressure overload.[48]

Fractional rates of collagen synthesis may be increased in the heart by an increase in synthesis per fibroblast and/or an increase in fibroblast number. An increase in collagen synthesis prior to an increase in DNA content, is evidence that an increase in synthesis by existing fibroblasts may occur prior to an increase in fibroblast number.[49] Increased levels of DNA during the development of cardiac hypertrophy are confined to fibroblasts and endothelial cells, since myocytes lose their mitotic activity during the early stages of development. Increased fibroblast and myofibroblast numbers have also been demonstrated morphometrically following the onset of pressure overload by pulmonary artery banding.[21] Taken together the data suggests that enhanced collagen production in the heart is increased by both mechanisms.

Degradation of Newly Synthesized Collagen

There are two principle pathways by which collagen is degraded; an intracellular pathway that degrades procollagen molecules rapidly after synthesis, and an extracellular pathway degrading fibrillar collagen. A significant proportion of the collagen synthesized in the heart is degraded rapidly. The proportion of collagen degraded by this pathway is about 60% of newly synthesized collagen in the 1-month-old rat heart[44] which is high compared to 28% and 6% in the lung and skin, respectively.[44] This value increases to over 90% by 6 months of age (see Figure 1).[44] In the adult rabbit values of 35%–50% are found in the ventricles.[30,43] These values are obtained by measuring the level of free labeled hydroxyproline in the tissue and comparing it to the total hydroxyproline radioactivity. Although this is susceptible to errors due to uptake from other tissues and losses into the circulation, the use of this method has been validated in vivo by McAnulty and Laurent.[50] It has been shown in vitro that free labeled hydroxyproline appears as early as 8 minutes after addition of radioisotope[51] suggesting that it is an intracellular process.

The intracellular pathway is thought to occur predominantly in lysosomes, although a small basal level of about 15% has been shown to be nonlysosomal.[52] It is unclear how the intracellular degradation processes are regulated or what determines the fate of the newly synthesized collagen molecule. No specific control mechanism has been identified. It may occur due to the activity of nonspecific proteases with other functions in the cell. It is clear that N-terminal motifs play key roles in the regulation of intracellular trafficking, particularly in directing proteins to lysosomes. Such a mechanism may be involved in determining the destination of the collagen molecule. Signal sequences have been identified that direct the collagen chains to the endoplasmic reticulum, for example.

Two functions have been proposed for this degradative pathway; first to prevent the secretion of defective molecules and second as a level of regulation of collagen production. The role of this degradative pathway as a regulator of collagen deposition has been demonstrated in several studies of hypertrophy or fibrotic disorders where enhanced collagen deposition is associated with a rise in the level of synthesis and a fall in the proportion of collagen degraded rapidly.[30,48,53]

Degradation of Extracellular Collagen

Collagens are degraded extracellularly due largely to the activity of matrix metalloproteases (see Chapter 13). Collagenolysis may be regulated at several sites including: biosynthesis and secretion of the latent enzyme procollagenase, predominantly by fibroblasts; activation of the latent enzyme by proteases; and inhibition of the active enzyme by protease inhibitors such as tissue inhibitor of metalloprotease (TIMP) and α_2-macroglobulin (for ref. 54). This degradative pathway plays a role in remodeling the collagen matrix during rapid tissue growth by degrading existing crosslinked collagen fibers. Collagenase cleaves the collagen molecules, in fibers, into a large fragment, TC_A (75% of the molecule's length) and a smaller TC_B fragment. The cleavage site is closer to the C-terminal and is specific for the peptide bond between glycine and leucine or glycine and isoleucine. Once the collagen molecule has been cleaved the triple helix unwinds and is degraded further by nonspecific proteases.

In the heart the extracellular pathway of degradation generally represents only a small proportion of the total collagen degraded (Figure 1), but may be important during the early stages of tissue remodeling. Six days after administration of bleomycin (which causes acute lung injury and the development of pulmonary hypertension), collagen concentration falls by almost 40%.[43] This occurs due to a fall in the total amount of collagen in the ventricle indicating a breakdown of part of the existing collagen matrix. This was supported by an increase in the proportion of free hydroxyproline found in this tissue. Scanning electron microscopy studies support this data.[18] These studies suggest that remodeling of the network occurs in order to accommodate the subsequent increase in muscle mass.

It is therefore clear that collagen composition can be increased by modulation at many sites in the metabolic pathways; with regulation at the level of transcription, translation, and also via altering the amount of collagen degraded, both intra- and extracellularly. Collagen deposition may also be increased by increasing the number of colla-

Regulation of sites in the pathway of collagen metabolism leading to an increased collagen deposition

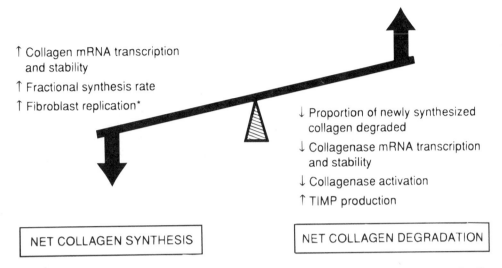

Figure 2. Regulation of sites in the pathway of collagen metabolism leading to an increased collagen deposition. Collagen deposition may be regulated at many sites in the synthetic and degradative pathways. This figure shows the processes that result in an increased deposition of collagen. *Collagen synthesis may be increased solely by increasing fibroblast number. This would result in an increase in collagen mRNA levels and collagen fractional synthesis rates in the tissue without increasing the rates of these two processes within each cell. If this scenario occurred the regulation of collagen deposition would be via completely different mechanisms, i.e. the regulation would be at the level of cell cycling rather than protein synthesis.

gen producing cells, by stimulating fibroblast replication or chemotaxis. The processes that may lead to increased collagen deposition are summarized in Figure 2. Cardiac fibroblasts are highly sensitive to external factors and rapidly respond to a change in their environment. Here we discuss the major stimuli currently under investigation that may be responsible for regulating fibroblast function in the heart during the development of hypertrophy and fibrosis.

The Regulation of Collagen Metabolism

The functional significance of collagen in the heart has now been established. That it turns over rapidly in the heart, even in the adult has shed light on the dynamic nature of the protein and the collagen-producing cells and has lead to a revised thinking

on how collagen deposition and remodeling can occur. These cells, predominantly fibroblasts in the heart, respond rapidly to physiological and pathological stimuli resulting in the production of new matrix which ultimately may lead to a compromise in heart function. We now need to identify the precise nature of the stimuli and the mechanisms by which collagen deposition is enhanced.

What Stimulates the Switch from a Compensatory Increase in Collagen to Fibrosis?

In addition to the stimuli for the compensatory increase in collagen deposition, there are further factors that result in the early, coordinate, increases in collagen and noncollagen proteins becoming a disproportionate increase in collagen deposition.

We hypothesize that during the compensatory phase of hypertrophy mechanical load stimulates both myocyte hypertrophy and collagen deposition—in a coordinate manner. Additional factors, in combination with, or produced or localized in response to, the mechanical load, further stimulate cardiac fibroblasts resulting in a disproportionate increase in collagen deposition (Figure 3). Such factors may include locally produced autocrine or paracrine agents, or factors that originate from the circulation and which are localized in the adventitia or interstitium, possibly due to increased permeability of the coronary vessels. Evidence implicating these processes are discussed below.

1. Mechanical Load

The view that biochemical signals regulate cell function has been challenged by evidence that mechanical load per se exerts important influences on cellular activity. Mechanical load appears critical not only for organ or tissue development but also to maintenance and functional adaptation in the adult. Abnormal mechanical forces may

Sources of fibroblast growth factors in the heart

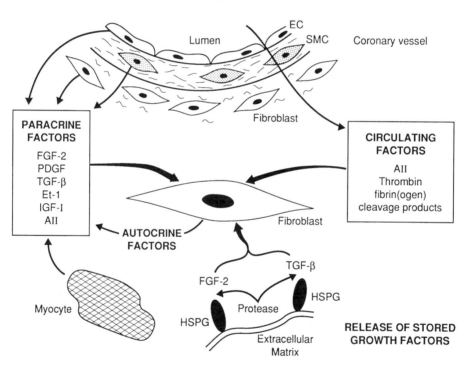

Figure 3. Sources of fibroblast growth factors in the heart. Many polypeptide growth factors that stimulate fibroblast activity have been identified as being produced by myocytes, endothelial cells, smooth muscle cells, and fibroblasts themselves. In the normal heart there may be a balance in the regulatory effects of these factors. Based on in vitro studies on endothelial cells, smooth muscle cells, and fibroblasts, mechanical load may increase the release of such factors thus stimulating increased fibroblast activity. In addition to autocrine and paracrine release, this figure also demonstrates that factors may arise from the circulation due to increased vascular permeability and through release from the extracellular matrix by proteases. The large fibroblast at the center of the figure may be an interstitial or adventitial fibroblast. This figure does not represent an exhaustive list of factors, but includes those in which significant evidence is available and which are discussed in the text. HSPG, heparan sulphate proteoglycans; Et, endothelin; IGF-1, insulin-like growth factor-1; IL-1, interleukin-1. See text for other abbreviations.

directly modulate gene expression leading to compensatory hypertrophic growth and ultimately to pathological conditions.

Mechanical forces are particularly important in the cardiovascular system where the tissues are constantly subjected to stresses and strains, with dramatic changes in these pressures occurring during development and disease. Cardiac growth due to pressure overload is associated with hypertrophy of cardiac myocytes and hyperplasia of fibroblasts and endothelial cells,[55] indicating that all cardiac cells may be influenced by mechanical load. Mechanical load may not be the sole influence, for example, following myocardial ischemia excess collagen deposition occurs as a wound healing response to hypoxia and tissue damage.

Cells respond to mechanical forces at three time-dependent levels. The first response occurs within milliseconds to seconds and includes activation of signal transduction pathways, such as opening of ion channels and activation of membrane-bound enzyme complexes, by which cells recognize changes in the mechanical environment and convert the mechanical event into chemical or electrical signals. In minutes to hours there are changes in gene transcription and morphology, such as cell orientation and cell shape. Finally after hours or days, there are changes in protein synthesis, the rate of cell division, and differentiation. Here we briefly discuss the processes involved, although it is important to note that little of the data described below has been obtained from cardiac fibroblasts.

Stimulation of Signal Transduction Pathways

Three events appear prominent in transducing a mechanical event into a cellular reaction: activation of ion channels; activation of membrane-bound enzyme complexes such as phospholipase C; and tension development transmitted via extracellular matrix receptors, such as integrins, linked through the cytoskeleton to the nucleus (Figure 4). These events may act independently or coordinately, and the nature of these responses is very cell dependent.

Stretch activated ion channels: One of the first responses to mechanical load, occurring within milliseconds, is the opening of selective stretch activated ion channels (SACs). The energy required to open these channels is provided by membrane strain rather than high energy phosphates. The channels are then kept open by energy derived from the flux of the ions. SACs have varying ion selectivities, although most are cation channels such as K^+, Na^+, or Ca^{2+}. SACs are transmembrane proteins linked in series to cytoskeletal strands[56] which, as described below, may participate actively in driving the load-induced response.

Activation of membrane-bound enzyme complexes: Stretch may alter the spacial arrangement, and thus activate, membrane-bound enzyme complexes. There is evidence that both adenylate cyclase and phospholipase C, generating cyclic AMP (CAMP) and inositol phosphates and diacylglycerol, respectively, are stimulated by mechanical load. The involvement of CAMP in the response to stretch appears complex and is dependent on cell type and the load applied. cAMP may be elevated following the application of mechanical load, but it may not be an important secondary messenger, in that it may not be necessary for stimulating a response.[57] Rosales and Sumpio demonstrated increased levels of inositol triphosphate and diacylglycerol in endothelial cells in response to cyclical strain.[58] This leads to increased levels of protein kinase C and the mobilization of internal calcium stores, thus stimulating cellular anabolic activity.

Cytoskeletal energy transfer: The cell is a tensile structure, with the cytoskeleton regulating cell shape due to the presence of contractile elements containing actin and myosin, and incompressible microtubules which hold the cell in its lowest energy state when the cell is in suspension.[59] When attached to an extracellular matrix the cytoskeleton is linked to matrix components, via integrin receptors, which 'pull' the cell into an elongated and flattened shape, creating tension within the cell. Many cells will only grow and replicate if attached to a substratum suggesting a requirement for this tensile state for cell function. Additional mechanical load may alter the arrangement of the underlying extracellular matrix leading

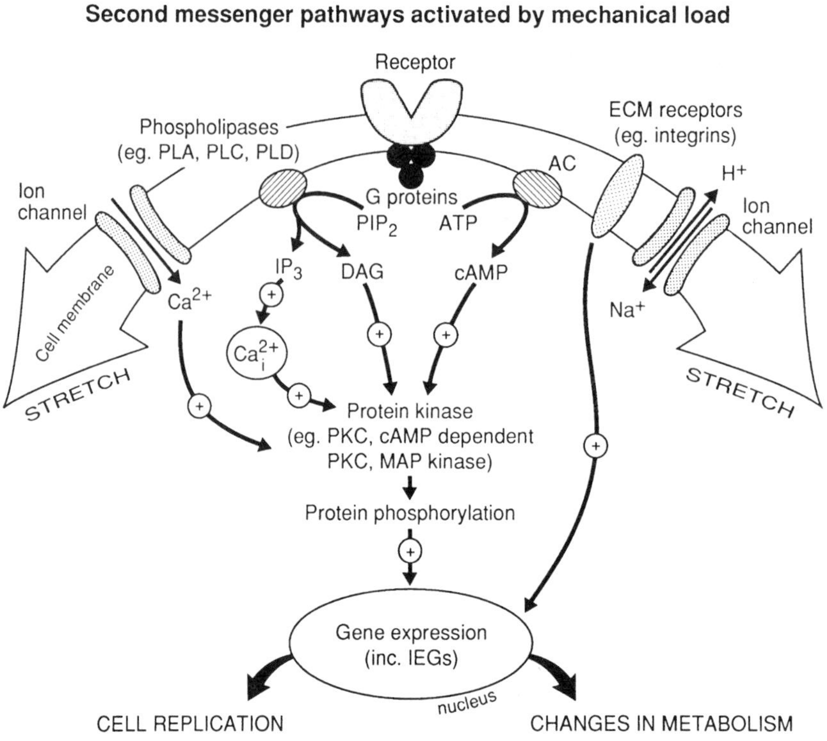

Second messenger pathways activated by mechanical load

Figure 4. Second messenger pathways activated by mechanical load. Mechanical load, represented by the arrows implying stretching of the cell membrane, leads to activation of many membrane-bound enzymes. Such activation results in a cascade of second messenger pathways resulting in increased gene expression, protein metabolism, and cell replication.

to changes in tension within the cell. The cytoskeleton is intimately linked to many cellular components such as ribosomes and the Golgi apparatus and also the nucleus. Tension created within the cytoskeleton may generate energy to drive metabolic processes associated with these organelles and regulate gene expression (reviewed by Bissel and Barcellos-Hoff).[60]

Stimulation of Gene Expression

The first response in terms of gene expression, is the stimulation of the immediate early genes. Increased expression of c-fos occurs 15 minutes after application of mechanical load to cardiac myocytes with the peak in mRNA levels at 30 minutes.[61] c-fos expression is also stimulated in the non-myocyte cells (predominantly fibroblasts).[62] c-myc, c-jun, JE, and Erg-1 are also increased in cardiac myocytes exposed to mechanical

load. Increased immediate early gene expression also occurs in vivo following application of pressure overload.[63] Komuro et al. determined that the signaling pathway for enhanced c-fos mRNA involved protein kinase C activity, possibly via activation of phospholipase C.[64]

Matrix protein gene expression increases upon mechanical stimulation, although this occurs later than the increase in oncogenic expression. mRNA levels for collagen type III were shown to increase 12 hours after application of cyclical stretch to neonatal cardiac fibroblasts[65] with no change in type I mRNA. This may reflect the extent of mechanical load applied and the time after which the measurements were made.

Cell Proliferation

Pressure overload leads to fibroblast and endothelial cell proliferation in the heart in vivo, suggesting that mechanical load influences cell replication.[21,49] In the vasculature, increased pressure stimulates an increase in the number of endothelial cells, medial smooth muscle cells, and fibroblasts in the adventitia. Cell replication also occurs in response to mechanical load in vitro, although this response is dependent on the cell type examined. Increased cell number is observed 1 to 2 days following the onset of mechanical load. Enhanced replication occurs for endothelial cells,[66] fibroblasts,[67] and smooth muscle cells.[68] We have shown that fibroblasts need only a trigger of 24-hour mechanical load in order for replication to occur to the same degree as that of 5 days of stretch.[67]

Protein Synthesis

Total protein synthesis increases in smooth muscle cells in response to mechanical load in vitro,[69] skeletal myoblasts,[70] and cardiac myocytes.[71] This protein accumulation is associated with cellular hypertrophy. Cyclic strain causes an increase in actin and myosin in airway smooth muscle cells[72] and fibroblasts.[73] Collagen synthesis is increased in aortic smooth muscle cells,[74] and pulmonary artery,[75] and cardiac[65,76] fibroblasts. Collagen synthesis is decreased, however, in response to mechanical strain in endothelial cells.[77] Elastin synthesis is increased in smooth muscle cell cultures in response to mechanical load.[78] An increase in fibronectin deposition occurs when mechanical load is applied to endothelial cells.[79] Thus mechanical load stimulates the synthesis of a diverse range of proteins, most notably the extracellular matrix proteins.

2. Polypeptide Growth Factors

Polypeptide growth factors such as platelet-derived growth factor (PDGF), basic fibroblast growth factor (FGF-2), and transforming growth factor-β (TGF-β) have been identified in the heart and are known to stimulate fibroblast function in vitro. PDGF is a fibroblast mitogen produced by a number of cell types including fibroblasts.[80] It has been implicated in develop-

ment,[81] atherosclerosis,[82] and wound healing.[83] We have demonstrated that it also stimulates cardiac fibroblast collagen synthesis and replication.[84] However Sarzani et al.[85] found no change in PDGF α- or β-receptor MRNA or PDGF B chain mRNA in hypertension induced cardiac hypertrophy. Thus a role for PDGF in cardiac hypertrophy in vivo has not yet been elucidated.

FGF-2 also stimulates cardiac fibroblast collagen synthesis and replication,[84] and is found in heart tissue associated with myocytes.[86] As a powerful angiogenic factor it may play a role in stimulating capillary growth during the hypertrophic process. Insulin-like growth factor-I stimulates myocyte protein synthesis[87] and stimulates cardiac fibroblast synthesis but not replication.[84] TGF-β is a most potent stimulator of fibroblast collagen synthesis in culture[84,88] and decreases the proportion of collagen degraded rapidly in lung[89] but not cardiac[84] fibroblasts.

Examination of growth factor production in response to mechanical load in cell culture has produced conflicting results. Vandenburgh found no production by myotubes exposed to increased mechanical load.[90] However, we found that human fetal lung fibroblasts produce autocrine factors, including PDGF, that stimulate fibroblast replication.[67,91] Wilson et al. also showed that smooth muscle replication was enhanced by mechanical stimulation through autocrine production of PDGF.[68] PDGF B chain mRNA levels in endothelial cells are affected by shear stress, although the data is conflicting as to whether mRNA levels are increased[92] or decreased.[93] Shear stress also increases FGF-2 mRNA levels.[93] Thus the response to mechanical load in terms of growth factor production appears highly cell specific. No data is available to date on cardiac fibroblast growth factor production.

Some cells require growth factors in the medium in order to respond to mechanical load. This has been demonstrated for replication by smooth muscle cells,[66] and collagen synthesis by cardiovascular fibroblasts.[76] Banes et al. demonstrated that vascular smooth muscle cells only replicate in response to mechanical load in the presence of growth factors such as PDGF and IGF-1.[66] However Wilson et al.[68] demonstrated enhanced vascular smooth muscle cells proliferation in the absence of growth factors in the media. This response may be due to the fact that these particular smooth muscle cells produce PDGF in an autocrine manner in response to mechanical load,[68] as we have shown for human fetal lung fibroblasts.[67] We have shown that cardiac fibroblasts require high serum levels in order to increase collagen production in response to mechanical load.[76] Thus autocrine growth factors may be produced in response to mechanical load, or be required, from a paracrine sources for example, to act synergistically with mechanical load to enhance fibroblast activity.

It is therefore clear that polypeptide growth factors are potent stimulators of fibroblast function, stimulating both replication and collagen metabolism. Evidence is emerging to indicate the presence of these factors in the normal and hypertrophying heart (Figure 3). Increased growth factor activity in hypertrophying hearts has been demonstrated in several models of pressure overload although the precise nature of these factors are not yet known.[94–96] More specifically, TGF-β mRNA is elevated in the early stages of cardiac hypertrophy induced by pressure overload.[29] Thus the combined evidence of their presence in heart tissue and their potent effects on fibroblasts in vitro suggests that growth factors may play a critical role in regulating cardiac collagen deposition in the normal and pressure overloaded heart.

3. Vasoactive Substances

An interesting hypothesis has emerged based on observations of vascular remodelling. Vasoconstrictor agents such as endothelin-1 and angiotensin II have been shown to stimulate cell activity in the pulmonary vessels whereas vasodilators such as prostacyclin appear to inhibit tissue growth. Thus a dual role has been suggested for these agents.[97]

Angiotensin II

The cardiac fibroblast may be exposed to increased levels of angiotensin II through an increased local production, possibly directly in response to the pressure overload, or due to increased permeability of the coronary vessels leading to an influx of the circulating substance. Considerable attention has focused on the role of the renin-angiotensin-aldosterone system, and more recently local tissue production of the hormones, in the development of cardiac fibrosis and is discussed in detail elsewhere in this book. Here we consider in vitro evidence that angiotensin II may be involved in regulating collagen deposition. Angiotensin II acts synergistically with mechanical load to stimulate smooth muscle cell replication, possibly due to the ability of angiotensin II to stimulate PDGF release.[98] It may act as a growth factor in its own right, with autocrine production being an initial mediator of stretch-induced hypertrophy of cardiac myocytes.[99] It does not stimulate replication of adult cardiac fibroblasts but has been shown to stimulate collagen synthesis at high concentrations.[100]

Endothelin

Mechanical force has a differential influence on the release of the vasoconstrictor, endothelin-1; mechanical load stimulates release,[101] while high shear stresses reduce release and mRNA levels.[102,103] The effect of shear on endothelin production is dependent on the level and duration of the stimulation, with sustained low levels causing an increase in endothelin production.[104] Suppression of this mesenchymal cell mitogen in areas of high shear forces may help prevent wall thickening in these areas. Sites of atherosclerosis are associated with areas of low (or turbulent) flow—with little evidence of the disease in regions of high flow. High flow, in addition to inhibiting endothelin production also stimulates the production of the antithrombotic agent, prostacyclin, and the fibrinolytic agent, tissue plasminogen activator, thus producing an appropriate environment for a nonthrombotic artery. Atherosclerosis develops particularly at bifurcations which in addition to low flow are regions in which the endothelium is subjected to great mechanical stresses and strains, thus providing an optimum mechanical environment for increased endothelin production.

Endothelin has differential effects on fibroblast function which are highly dependent on the tissue source of the cells. Endothelin-1 increases pulmonary artery fibroblast replication[105] and collagen synthesis (Keith Dawes, personal communication). It stimulates collagen synthesis and decreases degradation of newly synthesized collagen in human fetal lung fibroblasts, however it decreases synthesis and increases degradation in whole fetal rat fibroblasts.[106] Endothelin has no effect on cardiac fibroblast replication or collagen synthesis.[76]

It is becoming increasingly apparent that a particular cell phenotype is not regulated by one factor alone and that synergy and feedback mechanisms between many factors, including growth factors, extracellular matrix components, and the mechanical environment, are required for normal cell function. The regulation of collagen metabolism in the heart is no exception. One cannot consider a particular factor in isolation. However changes in the levels or composition of particular factors may tip the balance during disease processes, for example during the development of cardiac fibrosis. In these cases we may be able to dissect specific functions for particular factors. During the development of cardiac hypertrophy and fibrosis growth factors may play specific roles but it is likely that there are important interactions with other substances such as circulating hormones and that mechanical load per se will influence the cells responses.

In summary, collagen is turned over rapidly in the heart and, during the development of cardiac hypertrophy, enhanced collagen deposition may be achieved by an increase in collagen gene expression and synthesis and a decrease in the proportion of collagen degraded rapidly. Enhanced collagen production may also be accompanied by a change in the relative amounts of the fibrillar collagens types I and III. The mechanisms involved in stimulating collagen turnover are currently under investigation. Evidence suggests that mechanical load alone or acting synergistically with fibroblast growth factors may be a key modulator of cardiac fibroblast function and may

therefore play a role in the regulation of collagen deposition in the normal, hypertrophying, and fibrotic heart.

References

1. Van der Rest M, Garrone R. Collagen family of proteins. FASEB J, 1991;5:2814.
2. Kivirikko KI. Collagens and their abnormalities in a wide spectrum of diseases. Annals Med 1993;25:113.
3. Eghbali M, Czaja MJ, Zeydel M, et al. Collagen chain mRNAs in isolated heart cells from young and adult rats. J Mol Cell Cardiol 1988;20:267.
4. Borg TK, Caulfield JB. The collagen matrix of the heart. Fed Proc 1981;40:2037.
5. Turner JE, Laurent GJ. Increased type I collagen compared to type III during right ventricular hypertrophy in rabbits. Biochem Soc Trans 1986;14:1079.
6. Mays PK, Bishop JE, Laurent GJ. Age-related changes in the proportion of types I and III collagen. Mech Ageing Dev 988;45:203.
7. Schwartz D, Chin-Quee T, Veis A. Characterization of bovine anterior-lens-capsule basement-membrane collagen. Eur J Biochem 1980;103:21.
8. Paulsson M. Basement membrane proteins: structure, assembly, and cellular interactions. Crit Rev in Biochem and Mol Biol 1992;27:93.
9. Amenta PS, Gay S, Vaheri A, et al. The extracellular matrix is an integrated unit: ultrastructural localization of collagen types I, III, IV, V, VI, fibronectin and laminin in human term placenta. Collagen Relat Res 1986;6:125.
10. Birk DE, Fitch JM, Babiarz JP, et al. Collagen fibrillogenesis in vitro: interaction of types I and V collagen regulates fibril diameter. J Cell Sci 990;95:649.
11. Cole WG, Chan D, Hickey AJ, et al. Collagen composition of normal and myxomatous human mitral heart valves. Biochem J 1984;214:451.
12. Gay S, Rhodes RK, Gay RE, et al. Collagen molecules comprised of α_1(V)-chains (B-chains): an apparent localization in the exocytoskeleton. Collagen Relat Res 1981;1:53.
13. Kietly CM, Whittaker SP, Grant ME, et al. Type VI collagen microfibrils: evidence for a structural association with hyaluronan. J Cell Biol 1992;118:979.
14. Shimizu M, Umeda K, Sugihara N, et al. Collagen remodeling in myocardia of pa-

tients with diabetes. J Clin Pathol 1993;46: 32.

15. Rooney P, Wang M, Kumar P, et al. Angiogenic oligosaccharides of hyaluronan enhance the production of collagens by endothelial cells. J Cell Sci 1993;105:213.

16. Iruela-Arispe ML, Sage EH. Expression of type VIII collagen during morphogenesis of the chicken and mouse heart. Dev Biol 1991; 144:107.

17. Sawada H, Konomi H. The α1 chain of type VIII collagen is associated with many but not all microfibrils of elastic fibre system. Cell Structure and Function 1991;16:455.

18. Doering CW, Jalil JE, Janicki JS, et al. Collagen network remodelling and diastolic stiffness of the rat left ventricle with pressure overload hypertrophy. Cardiovasc Res 1988;22:686.

19. Low RB, Stirewalt WS, Hultgren P, et al. Changes in collagen and elastin in rabbit right-ventricular pressure overload. Biochem J 1989;263:709.

20. Weber KT, Janicki JS, Shroff SG, et al. Collagen remodeling of the pressure-overloaded, hypertrophied nonhuman primate myocardium. Circ Res 1988;62:757.

21. Leslie KO, Taatjes DJ, Schwarz J, et al. Cardiac myofibroblasts express alpha smooth muscle actin during right ventricular pressure overload in the rabbit. Am J Pathol 1991;139:207.

22. Fuster V, Danielson MA, Robb RA, et al. Quantitation of left ventricular myocardial fibre hypertrophy and interstitial tissue in human hearts with chronically increased volume and pressure overload. Circulation 1977;55:504.

23. Bishop JE, Greenbaum R, Gibson DG, et al. Enhanced deposition of predominantly type I collagen in myocardial disease. J Mol Cell Cardiol 1990;22:1157.

24. Chapman D, Weber KT, Eghbali M. Regulation of fibrillar collagen types I and III and basement membrane type IV collagen gene expression in pressure overloaded rat myocardium. Circ Res 1990;67:787.

25. Medugorac I, Jacob R. Characterization of left ventricular collagen in the rat. Cardiovasc Res 1983;17:15.

26. Mukherjee D, Sen S. Collagen phenotypes during development and regression of myocardial hypertrophy in spontaneously hypertensive rats. Circ Res 1990;67:1474.

27. Morioka S, Honda M, Ishikawa S, et al. Changes in contractile and non-contractile proteins, intracellular Ca^{2+} and ultrastructures during the development of right ven-

tricular hypertrophy and failure in rats. Jpn Circ J 992;56:469.

28. Bornstein P, Sage H. Regulation of collagen gene expression. Prog Nucl Acid Res Mol Biol 1989;37:67.

29. Villarreal FJ, Dillmann WH. Cardiac hypertrophy-induced changes in mRNA levels of TGF-beta 1, fibronectin and collagen. Am J Physiol 1992;262:H1861.

30. Bishop JE, Rhodes S, Laurent GJ, et al. Increased collagen synthesis and decreased collagen degradation in right ventricular hypertrophy induced by pressure overload. Cardiovasc Res 1994;28:1581–1585.

31. Penney DG, Bugaisky LB. Non-coordinate expression of collagen mRNAs during carbon monoxide-induced cardiac hypertrophy. Mol Cell Biochem 1992;109:37.

32. Fleischmajer R, Timpl R, Tuderman L, et al. Ultrastructural identification of extension aminopropeptides of type I and III collagens in human skin. Proc Natl Acad Sci, USA 1981;78:7360.

33. Weistner M, Krieg T, Horlein D, et al. Inhibiting effect of procollagen peptides on collagen biosynthesis in fibroblast cultures. J Biol Chem 1979;254:7016.

34. Aycock RS, Raghow R, Stricklin GP, et al. Post-transcriptional inhibition of collagen and fibronectin synthesis by a synthetic homolog of a portion of the carboxy-terminal propeptide of human type I collagen. J Biol Chem 1986;261:14355.

35. Yamauchi M, Mechanic GL. Cross-linking of collagen. In: Nimni ME, ed. Collagen. I. Biochemistry. Boca Raton, Fla: CRC Press 1988:157–172.

36. Henkel W, Glanville RW. Covalent crosslinking between molecules of type I and type III collagen. Eur J Biochem 1982;122: 205.

37. Neuberger A, Perrone JC, Slack HGB. The relative metabolic inertia of tendon collagen in the rat. Biochem J 1951;49:199.

38. Jackson SH, Heininger JA. Proline recycling during collagen metabolism as determined by concurrent $^{18}O_2$ and ^3H-labelling. Biochim Biophys Acta 1975;381:359.

39. Waterlow JC, Stephen JML. The measurement of total lysine turnover in the rat by intravenous infusion of L-[U-14C]lysine. Cell Signalling 1967;33:489.

40. Garlick PJ, Millward DJ, James WPT. The diurnal response of muscle and liver protein synthesis in vivo in meal-fed rats. Biochem J 1973;136:935.

41. Henshaw EC, Hirsch CA, Morton BE, et al. Control of protein synthesis in mammalian

tissues through changes in ribosome activity. J Biol Chem 1971;246:436.

42. Laurent GJ. Rates of collagen synthesis in lung, skin and muscle obtained in vivo by a simplified method using [3H] proline. Biochem J 1982;206:535.

43. Turner JE, Oliver MH, Guerreiro D, et al. Collagen metabolism during right ventricular hypertrophy following induced lung injury. Am J Physiol 1986;251:H915.

44. Mays PK, McAnulty RJ, Campa JS, et al. Age-related changes in collagen synthesis and degradation in rat tissues. Biochem J 1991;276:307.

45. Robins SP. Metabolism of rabbit skin collagen. Biochem J 1979;181:75.

46. Bonnin CM, Sparrow MP, Taylor RR. Collagen synthesis and content in right ventricular hypertrophy in the dog. Am J Physiol 1981;241:H708.

47. Turto H. Collagen metabolism in experimental cardiac hypertrophy in the rat and the effect of digitoxin treatment. Cardiovasc Res 1977;11:358.

48. Eleftheriades EG, Durand J, Ferguson AG, et al. Regulation of procollagen metabolism in the pressure-overloaded rat heart. J Clin Invest 1992;91:1113.

49. Skosey JL, Zak R, Martin AF. Biochemical correlates of cardiac hypertrophy. V. Labelling collagen, myosin and nuclear DNA during experimental myocardial hypertrophy in the rat. Circ Res 1972;31:145.

50. McAnulty RJ, Laurent GJ. Collagen synthesis and degradation in vivo. Evidence for rapid rates of collagen turnover with extensive degradation of newly synthesized collagen in tissues of the adult rat. Collagen Relat Res 1987;70:93.

51. Bienkowski RS, Cowan MJ, McDonald JA, et al. Degradation of newly synthesized collagen. J Biol Chem 1978;253:4356.

52. Bienkowski RS. Collagen degradation in human lung fibroblasts: extent of degradation, role of lysosomal proteases, and evaluation of an alternative hypothesis. J Cell Physiol 1984;121:152.

53. Laurent GJ, McAnulty RJ. Protein metabolism during bleomycin-induced pulmonary fibrosis in rabbits. Am Rev Respir Dis 1983; 128:82.

54. Stricklin GP, Hibbs MS. Biochemistry and physiology of mammalian collagenases. In Nimni ME, ed. Collagen. I. Biochemistry. Boca Raton, Fla: CRC Press, 1988:187–205.

55. Grove D, Nair KG, Zak R. Biochemical correlates of cardiac hypertrophy. III. Changes in DNA content; the relative contributions of polyploidy and mitotic activity. Circ Res 1969;25:463.

56. Sachs F. Ion channels as mechanical transducers. In: Stein WD, & Bronner F, eds. Cell Shape: Determinants, Regulation, and Regulatory role. New York, NY Academic Press, 1989:63–92.

57. Keeley FW, Bartoscewicz LA, Leenen FHH. The effect of wall stress on vascular connective tissue accumulation. Eur Respir Rev 3, 1993;16:623.

58. Rosales OR, Sumpio BE. Changes in cyclic strain increase inositol triphosphate and diacylglycerol in endothelial cells. Am J Physiol 1992;262:C956.

59. Ingber DE, Folkman J. Tension and compression as basic determinants of cell form and function: utilization of a cellular tensegrity mechanism. In: Stein WD, & Bronner F, ed, Cell Shape, Determinants, Regulation, and Regulatory Role. New York, NY: Academic Press, 1989;3–31

60. Bissel MJ, Barcellos-Hoff MH. The influence of extracellular matrix on gene expression: is structure the message? J Cell Sci 1987;327 8(Suppl.).

61. Komuro I, Kaida T, Shibazaki Y, et al. Stretching cardiac myocytes stimulates protooncogene expression. J Biol Chem 1990; 265:3595.

62. Sadoshima J, Jahn L, Takahashi T, et al. Molecular characterization of the stretch-induced adaptation of cultured cardiac cells. J Biol Chem 1992;267:10551.

63. Schneider MD, Roberts R, Parker TG. Modulation of cardiac genes by mechanical stress. The oncogene signalling hypothesis. Mol Biol Med 1991;8:167.

64. Komuro I, Katoh Y, Kaida T, et al. Mechanical loading stimulates cell hypertrophy and specific gene expression in cultured rat cardiac myocytes. J Biol Chem 1991;266:1265.

65. Carver W, Nagpal ML, Nachtigal M, et al. Collagen expression in mechanically stimulated cardiac fibroblasts. Circ Res 1991;69: 116.

66. Banes AJ, Baird CW, Dorofi D, et al. Cyclic mechanical load and growth factors stimulate endothelial and smooth muscle cell DNA synthesis. Eur Respir Rev 1993;3:16,: 618.

67. Bishop JE, Mitchell JJ, Absher PM, et al. Cyclic mechanical deformation stimulates human lung fibroblast proliferation and autocrine growth factor activity. Am J Respir Cell Mol Biol 1993;9:126.

68. Wilson E, Mai Q, Sudhir K, et al. Mechanical strain induces growth of vascular smooth

muscle cells via autocrine action of PDGF. J Cell Biol 1993;123:741.

69. Kollros PR, Bates SR, Mathews MB, et al. Cyclic AMP inhibits increased collagen production by cyclically stretched smooth muscle cells. Lab Invest 1987;56:410.

70. Vandenburgh H, Hatfaludy S, Karlisch P, et al. Skeletal muscle growth is stimulated by intermittent stretch-relaxation in tissue culture. Am J Physiol 1989;256:C674.

71. Terracio L, Peters W, Durig B, et al. Cellular hypertrophy can be induced by cyclical mechanical stretch in vitro. In: Skalak R, Fox CF, eds. Tissue Engineering. Alan R. Liss Inc, NY 1988;51–56.

72. Smith PG, Janiga KE, Ikebe M. Physical stress increases content of contractile proteins in airway smooth muscle (ASM) cells. Am Rev Respir Dis 1993;147:A253.

73. Pender N, McCulloch CAG. Quantitation of actin polymerization in two human fibroblast sub-types responding to mechanical stretching. J Cell Sci 1991;100:187.

74. Leung DYM, Glagov S, Mathews MB. Cyclic stretching stimulates synthesis of matrix components by arterial smooth muscle cells in vitro. Science 1976;191:475.

75. Butt RP, Laurent GJ, Bishop JE. Mechanical strain stimulates collagen synthesis by pulmonary artery fibroblasts. Eur Respir Rev 3, 1993;16:661.

76. Butt RP, Laurent GJ, Bishop JE. Mechanical load and polypeptide growth factors stimulate cardiac fibroblast activity. Annals NY Acad Sci. 1995;752:387–395.

77. Sumpio BE, Banes AJ, Link GW, et al. Modulation of endothelial cell phenotype by cyclic stretch: inhibition of collagen production. J Surg Res 1990;48:415.

78. Sutcliffe MC, Davidson JM. Effect of static stretching on elastin production by porcine aortic smooth muscle cells. Matrix 1990;10:148.

79. Gorfien SF, Winston FK, Thibault LE, et al. Effects of biaxial deformation on pulmonary artery endothelial cells. J Cell Physiol 1989;139:492.

80. Fabisiak JP, Absher M, Evans JN, et al. Spontaneous production of PDGF A-chain homodimer by rat lung fibroblasts in vitro. Am J Physiol 1992;263:L185.

81. Seifert RA, Schwartz SM, Bowen-Pope DF. Developmentally regulated production of platelet-derived growth factor-like molecules. Nature 1984;311:669.

82. Barret TB, Benditt EP. Platelet-derived growth factor gene expression in human atherosclerotic plaques and normal artery wall. Proc Natl Acad Sci USA 1988;85:2810.

83. Lynch SE, Nixon JC, Colvin RB, et al. Role of platelet-derived growth factor in wound healing: synergistic effects with other growth factors. Proc Natl Acad Sci USA 1987;84:7696.

84. Butt RP, Laurent GJ, Bishop JE. Enhanced collagen production and replication by cardiac fibroblasts in response to several classes of growth factors. Eut. J. Cell Biol. In Press.

85. Sarzani R, Arnaldi G, Chobanian V. Hypertension-induced changes of platelet-derived growth factor receptor expression in rat aorta and heart. Hypertension 1991;17:888.

86. Casscells W, Speir E, Sasse J, et al. Isolation, characterization, and localization of heparin-binding growth factors in the heart. J Clin Invest 1990;85:433.

87. Fuller SJ, Mynett JR, Sugden PH. Stimulation of cardiac protein synthesis by insulin-like growth factors. Biochem J 1992;282:85.

88. Varga J, Jiminez SA. Stimulation of normal fibroblast collagen production and processing by transforming growth factor-β. Biochem Biophys Res Commun 1986;138:974.

89. McAnulty RJ, Campa JS, Cambrey AD, et al. The effect of transforming growth factor-β on rates of procollagen synthesis and degradation in vitro. Biochim Biophys Acta 1991;1091:231.

90. Vandenburgh HH. Cell shape and growth regulation in skeletal muscle: exogenous versus endogenous factors. J Cell Physiol 1983;116:363.

91. Bishop JE, Butt RP, Laurent GJ. Mechanical force stimulates PDGF release by fibroblasts. J Endocrinol (Suppl.) 1992;132:276.

92. Hseih HJ, Li ND, Frangos JA. Shear-induced platelet-derived growth factor gene expression in human endothelial cells is mediated by protein kinase C. J Cell Physiol 1992;150:552.

93. Malek AM, Gibbons GH, Dzau VJ, et al. Fluid shear stress differentially modulates expression of genes encoding basic fibroblast growth factor and platelet-derived growth factor B chain in vascular endothelium. J Clin Invest 1993;92:2013.

94. Hammond GL, Wieben E, Markert CL. Molecular signals for initiating protein synthesis in organ hypertrophy. Proc Natl Acad Sci USA 1979;76:2455.

95. Sen S. Factors regulating myocardial hypertrophy in hypertension. Circulation 1987;75(Suppl. I):I81.

96. Bishop JE, Laurent GJ. Mediators affecting fibroblast function are present in hypertrophied rabbit right ventricles following the

development of pulmonary hypertension. Am Rev Respir Dis 1989;139(Suppl.):A171.

97. Peacock AJ, Dawes KE, Laurent GJ. Endothelial cell derived growth factors in pulmonary vascular hypertension. Eur Respir Rev 1993;3:16,:638.

98. Sudhir K, Wilson E, Chatterlee K, et al. Mechanical strain and collagen potentiate mitogenic activity of angiotensin II in rat vascular smooth muscle cells. J Clin Invest 1993;92:3003.

99. Sadoshima J, Xu Y, Slayter HS, et al. Autocrine release of angiotensin II mediates stretch-induced hypertrophy of cardiac myocytes in vitro. Cell 1993;75:977.

100. Brilla CG, Zhou G, Weber KT. Effects of angiotensin II and PGE2 on collagen synthesis in cardiac fibroblasts. Circulation 1993; 88(Suppl.):I-294.

101. Carosi JA, Eskin SG, McIntire LV. Cyclical strain effects on production of vasoactive materials in cultured endothelial cells. J Cell Physiol 1992;151:29.

102. Malek A, Izumo S. Physiological fluid shear stress causes down regulation of endothelin-1 mRNA in bovine aortic endothelium. Am J Physiol 1992;263:C389.

103. Sharefkin JB, Diamond SL, Eskin SG, et al. Fluid flow decreases preproendothelin-1 peptide release in cultured human endothelial cells. J Vasc Surg 1991;14:1.

104. Kuchan MJ, Frangos JA. Shear stress regulates endothelin-1 release via protein kinase C and cGMP in cultured endothelial cells. Am J Physiol 1993;264:H150.

105. Peacock AJ, Dawes KE, Shock A, et al. Endothelin-1 and endothelin-3 induce chemotaxis and replication of pulmonary artery fibroblasts. Am J Respir Cell Mol Biol 1992; 7:492.

106. Dawes KE, Cambrey AD, Campa JS, et al. Changes in collagen metabolism in response to endothelin-1: evidence for fibroblast heterogeneity. Submitted for publication 1994.

107. Mays PK. Age-related changes in collagen metabolism. PhD Thesis: University of London, 1990.

Chapter 13

Collagen Degradation After Myocardial Infarction

Jack P.M. Cleutjens, Ph.D.
Karl T. Weber, M.D.

Overview

The myocardium contains a cellular and extracellular compartment. Thirty to fourty percent of the cellular compartment consists of cardiac myocytes while 60%–70% are noncardiomyocytes.* Because of their dimensions cardiac myocytes occupy 66% of total myocardial volume, whereas the nonmyocytes, predominantly fibroblasts, endothelial cells, and to a lesser extent smooth muscle cells and mast cells together with the extracellular matrix, comprise the remainder of the tissue. The extracellular matrix consists of a structural protein network composed largely of type I and III fibrillar collagens.[1] These fibrous proteins are the major structural proteins in the tissue because of their rigidity and resistance to proteolytic digestion.[2]

The collagenous network consists of struts which connect cardiomyocytes to each other, cardiomyocytes to capillaries, cardiomyocytes to large collagen fibers, and of fine connections between large collagen fibers, which function as tethers and possibly as springs between myocytes.[3] A collagen weave surrounds groups of myocytes and has been associated with the elasticity of the heart.[3] The collagen network also contains coiled perimysial fibers, a fibrillar network that surrounds blood vessels and a complex network in the subendocardium and subepicardium.[4] The fibrillar collagen network has multiple functions,[5] e.g., alignment of cardiac myocytes and myocytes to capillaries,[4] prevention of excess myocyte and sarcomere stretch,[6] transmission of myocyte generated force to the ventricular chamber,[7] and imparting tensile strength and stiffness to tissue.[8] Disruption of the fibrillar collagen, which can occur with increased collagenolytic activity, can have multiple adverse consequences on the architecture and function of the myocardium.[1,5,9] In various studies only a moderate increase in the amount of collagen resulted in increased systolic and diastolic stiffness, whereas decreased levels of collagen can lead to myocardial dilatation or even rupture.

Besides the fibrillar collagen network the extracellular compartment consists of basement membranes, which envelope individual cardiomyocytes and smooth muscle cells, and which forms a layer to which endothelial cells are attached.[10] Basement membrane contains a structural backbone of type IV collagen to which other components like laminin, heparan sulphate proteoglycan, fibronectin, and other extracellular matrix components can attach.[11,12]

The enzymes involved in degradation of extracellular matrix components can be divided into four different classes: matrix metalloproteinases (MMPs) and serine pro-

* This work was supported in part by NIH grant R01-HL-31701, Netherlands Organization for Scientific Research (NWO) (Grant S 93.221.92) and Netherlands Heart Foundation (Grant 90.282).

teinases which react at neutral or slightly alkaline pH; and cysteine and aspartic proteinases which have optimal activity at acidic pH.[13]

Collagenolytic Activity

Matrix MMPs

Degradation of extracellular matrix is a normal process associated with morphogenesis, growth, angiogenesis, development, and wound healing under normal and pathological conditions.[13] Many of the matrix degrading enzymes are involved in diseases such as cancer. In tumor invasion, primary tumor cells escape their natural boundaries and intra- and extravasate before they come to reside at sites of metastasis. Many extracellular matrix components (e.g., basement membranes and fibrillar collagens in the interstitium) have to be degraded before tumor cells escape to form a metastatic lesion.

This chapter focuses principally on fibrillar collagen degradation, given the structural role of the interstitial fibrillar collagens in governing tissue architecture and function. Fibrillar collagens (types I, II [cartilage], and III collagen) are extremely resistant to cleavage by most proteinases, because collagen fibrils are tightly apposed, highly crosslinked and resistant to most extracellular matrix degrading enzymes.[2,13,14] The presence of covalently bound carbohydrate and fibril interaction with glycoproteins of the surrounding extracellular matrix components make it difficult to degrade interstitial collagens.[15] The only proteinases able to cleave native fibrillar collagen helices are interstitial collagenase also called collagenase (MMP-1, EC 3.4.24.7) and neutrophil collagenase (MMP-8). These enzymes cleave interstitial collagens at unique Gly-Leu or Gly-Ile sites in the native triple helix at $\frac{3}{4}$ from the N-terminal end, generating $\frac{3}{4}$ (TC^A) and $\frac{1}{4}$ (TC^B) collagen fragments also called gelatins.[13,16] The gelatins quickly unfold their triple helix conformation due to thermal degradation and can be further degraded into amino acids and oligopeptides by a number of less specific protein-

ases, such as gelatinases (MMP-2, a 72-kDa type collagenase; and MMP-9, a 92-kDa gelatinase), stromelysin (MMP-3), and serine proteases such as elastase and cathepsin G (Figure 1).[14,16] Another pathway of collagen degradation is endocytosis and intracellular degradation of larger collagen fragments by lysosomal enzymes at acidic pH. Predominantly cysteine proteinases produced by connective tissue and inflammatory cells, such as fibroblasts and macrophages, are involved in the intracellular degradation pathway.[17,18] Whether intracellular degradation plays a major role in the total degradation of collagen in the heart is still unknown.

The family of matrix MMPs are metal binding proteinases which are secreted as a latent proenzyme that requires subsequent extracellular activation. All MMPs have a putative Zn^{2+} binding site (HEXGH) as other zinc-containing proteases and MMPs require Ca^{2+} for stability and exhibit a preferred cleavage specificity for the N-terminal side of hydrophobic residues.[13,14,16]

Not only mature crosslinked fibrillar collagen can be degraded but also newly synthesized collagen. About 30% of newly synthesized collagen is degraded intracellularly within minutes of its synthesis.[19] This process can play a role in the deposition and fine tuning of an orderly and balanced collagen network.[2]

Tissue Inhibitors of Metalloproteinases (TIMPs)

Most of the matrix metalloproteinases (collagenases, gelatinases, and stromelysins) can be inhibited by a member of the family of tissue inhibitors of metalloproteinases (TIMPs).[13] Until now three members of this family have been described (TIMP-1, TIMP-2, and TIMP-3). These TIMPs bind only to the active site of the metalloproteinases and block access to substrate. This binding is very tight and is thought to be noncovalent with a very high K_d (10^{-9} to 10^{-10}). TIMP binds to metalloproteinases in a 1:1 molar ratio. Therefore small concentration changes of either components can result in marked changes in collagenolytic ac-

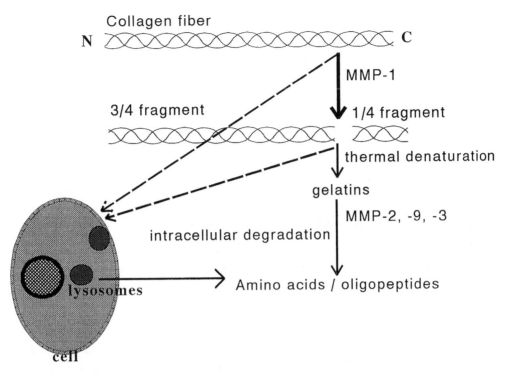

Figure 1. Schematic representation of interstitial collagen degradation pathways. MMP-1 collagenase; MMP-2, 72-kDa gelatinase; MMP-9, 92 kDa gelatinase; MMP-3 stromelysin.

tivity. Furthermore TIMP-1 forms a complex preferentially with MMP-9 (92-kDa type IV procollagenase), whereas TIMP-2 selectively complexes MMP-2 (72-kDa type IV procollagenase). TIMP-3 also called

SYNTHESIS

Collagen mRNA

Collagen fibril

$=$ *INHIBITION (TIMP)*

DEGRADATION Active MMP-1

ACTIVATION

Inactive proMMP-1

Collagenase mRNA

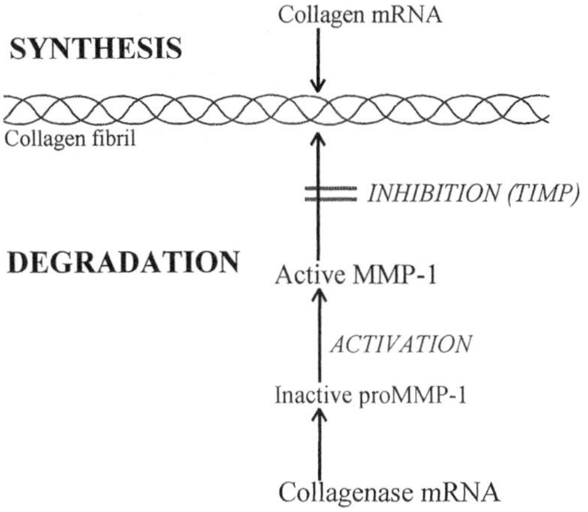

Figure 2. Schematic representation of the interstitial collagen turnover.

Chimp-3 is only described in chickens and only localized in the "insoluble" extracellular matrix.[20]

TIMPs reduce the activity of metalloproteinases and therefore limit the degradative activity of these enzymes (Figure 2). In addition to this function, a growth promoting effect of TIMP has been described and is known as erythroid potentiating activity (EPA). Besides cells of the erythroid system epithelial and mesenchymal cell growth may also be stimulated.[20]

Serum components, such as α2-macroglobuline, α1-macroglobuline, and α1-inhibitor-3 are also potent inhibitors of collagenase.[16] These macroglobulines serve as substrate for collagenase. After cleavage these macroglobulines bind to collagenase and disable the enzyme's matrix degrading capacity.[16,20]

Activation of MMPs

MMPs are synthesized as a pre-proenzyme and secreted as a latent proenzyme.

Cleavage of a region of approximately 10 to 80 amino acids from the N-terminus activates the proenzyme. The precise mechanism for the in vivo activation of latent MMPs is not fully understood. Plasmin derived from plasminogen by the action of plasminogen activators is one of the factors involved in MMP-1 and stromelysin activation in vivo.[14,16] Furthermore stromelysin (MMP-3) but also other peptidases are able to activate latent collagenase. In vitro mercurial compounds, plasmin and trypsin, can be used to artificially activate the latent proenzyme.[14,16] It has been suggested that a relative inaccessible sulfhydryl group is involved.[16] Upon activation the cysteine residue to which the sulfhydryl group is coupled is modified, exposed, or released by proteolysis and replaced by water, with the concomitant exposure of the active site. This is followed by an autolytic cleavage of the cysteine containing fragment.[21]

Collagenases present in an inactive form can be either inactive proenzymes as described above or an inactivated complex of active collagenase with its inhibitor which cannot be dissociated by gel filtration or ion exchange chromatography.[22] Whether in the latter case MMP can still be dissociated from its inhibitor and retain its activated state again is still unknown.

Collagenase Activity in the Heart After Myocardial Infarction

Collagenase was first localized in the heart by Montfort and Pérez-Tamayo.[23] Using immunohistochemistry with an antibody to rat uterus collagenase they showed that collagenase was present in the myocardium in interstitial spaces between myocardial fiber bundles and in the pericardium. Staining intensity was irregular and staining was only found in connective tissue areas bound to collagen fibers, reticulum fibers, and basement membranes. In short, collagenase was found in close contact to its substrate, fibrillar collagen. It is unknown whether this antibody could discriminate between active or latent collagenase and it is therefore unsure whether the observed immunostaining indicates that these collagen fibers are continuously remodeled by the collagenase present. The potential for rapid collagen turnover, however, is present in the heart. Tyagi et al.[24] found that most of the collagenolytic/gelatinolytic capacity in the normal rat heart is present in a latent form. When high collagenolytic activity is needed latent or inactivated collagenases can be easily activated.

Caulfield and Wolkowicz[25] demonstrated that disulfide reagents are capable of inducing a collagenolytic reaction in the isolated perfused heart. All components of the collagen matrix of the heart were degraded as demonstrated by scanning electron microscopy. Out of these results can be concluded that an inducible and active collagenolytic system exists in cardiac tissue and that this system may be expressed under conditions of oxidative stress.

What happens to the collagen network in the heart after ischemia? In early ischemia of the pig heart after left anterior descending coronary artery (LAD) occlusion the collagen network was studied with scanning and transmission microscopy.[26] Sato et al.[26] showed that at 40 minutes after coronary occlusion the collagen network became irregular in arrangement. At 2 hours after occlusion collagen fibrils and microfibrils in between cardiomyocytes became separated from the basement membrane, the banded pattern of collagen disappeared, and collagen fibrils, elastic fibers, and microfilaments were broken down and decreased in content. These results indicate that collagen and elastin breakdown may be related to observed cell injury.

Takahashi et al.[27] demonstrated that 1, 2, and 3 hours after LAD ligation in rats total collagen content was decreased in the infarct zone due to an increased breakdown of insoluble collagen. Also collagenase, neutral proteinase, and lysosomal serine protease activities were increased two to threefold, suggesting that an increase in these degradative enzymes may be responsible for the rapid degradation of extracellular matrix collagen after myocardial infarction. Loss of structural scaffold and mechanical coupling could account for abnormal wall motion (e.g., stunned myocardium).

Cardiomyocyte necrosis is not a major key factor in enhancing collagenase activity.

In stunned myocardium after repeated occlusion and reperfusion in dogs no cellular damage was observed by scanning and transmission electron microscopy.[28] The extracellular collagen matrix, however, was changed. The collagen weave surrounding myocytes disappeared completely and collagen struts, the interconnection between myocytes or myocytes and capillaries, became sparse or completely absent. This led to greater myocardial compliance and less effective contraction of the stunned myocardium. The mechanism responsible for increased collagenolysis was that more of the latent pool became activated, whereas the total (activated + latent) collagenolytic pool remained unchanged.[29] No changes in hydroxyproline concentration was found in the endocardium after myocardial stunning. This contrasts to the stunned midwall and epicardium where this amino acid marker of collagen was decreased, which could be due to the increased collagenolytic activity.

In a rat infarction model induced by ligation of the left coronary artery the temporal relationships between transcription of collagenase and TIMP mRNAs and activation of latent collagenase was studied. Furthermore, cells responsible for production of collagenase and TIMP mRNA were phenotyped.[30] Collagenolytic activity was determined by zymography.[31] Zymography has an advantage above biochemical collagen degradation assays because not only total collagenolytic activity is determined but also the different MMP subtypes involved can be measured (e.g., 72- and 92-kDa type collagenases/gelatinases, called MMP-2 and MMP9, and collagenase (MMP-1), a 54-kDa matrix MMP). After coronary ligation, a transient increase in collagenolytic activity was found only in the infarcted left ventricle and not in noninfarcted tissue or sham operated controls. Collagenolytic activity (MMP-1) was transiently increased from day 2 until day 7 following coronary ligation declining thereafter but only in the infarcted left ventricle. In contrast to the studies of Sato et al.[26] and Takahashi et al.[27] no increase in MMP-1 activity could be determined before day 2 after infarction. This suggests that MMP-1 is not the enzyme which breaks down the collagenous struts

and fibers early after ischemia. From these findings it is uncertain whether progressive dilatation and wall thinning which is frequently observed during heart failure is due to persistent activation of collagenase.

MMP-2 and MMP-9 (type IV collagenases/gelatinases) activity have also been found to be increased postinfarction. The activation pattern followed a similar time course as MMP-1. MMP-2 and MMP-9 activity were seen as the unreduced 62 and 58-kDa (MMP-2) and 92-kDa (MMP-9) lytic bands of these type IV collagenases/gelatinases.[32,33] Gelatinases can degrade the one and three quarter fragments of fibrillar collagen generated after cleavage with MMP-1,[13,14] which could account for the concomitant increase of collagenolytic activity of these MMPs.

Other collagenolytic enzymes, such as serine proteases (e.g., plasmin, cathepsin G) or lysosomal cysteine proteinases (e.g., cathepsin B) are probably involved in the early degradation of collagen following infarction. MMP-1 alone is not able to completely degrade insoluble collagen; a multienzyme system is therefore needed and must be active to fully degrade collagen.[34]

In contrast to the early activation of latent collagenases stored extracellularly, MMP-1 mRNA expression was detected only at day 7 following coronary ligation in the infarcted region of the left ventricle. It was not observed at other time points in the infarcted left ventricle and was not detected at all in either the noninfarcted interventricular septum or right ventricle or in either ventricle of sham operated rats. Posttranslational activation of stored extracellular latent collagenases seems to play a more important role in the regulation of myocardial collagenase activity following infarction than the synthesis of MMP-1 mRNA. It would appear that after infarcted tissue has been depleted of its latent pool of extracellular collagenase, through activation and utilization, MMP-1 mRNA is synthesized to replenish the latent procollagenase pool. The heart may therefore recognize and regulate its own store of collagenase through signals that remain to be elucidated.

TIMP mRNA expression accompanied

the activation of MMP-1, MMP-2, and MMP-9. Six hours after infarction TIMP mRNA was found to be increased in infarcted tissue reaching a peak on day 2. This peak overlapped the pattern of MMP activation, which began to rise 2 days after infarction. TIMP inhibits only the activated form of collagenases and gelatinases.[13,35] These findings suggest a direct regulation of TIMP transcription by activation of latent collagenases. A net balance in collagen degradation is therefore established by the equilibrium that exists between collagenase production and activation, on the one hand, and TIMP production on the other. Following infarction, the heart appears to regulate this balance and therefore the extent of collagen degradation.

Cells Involved in Production of MMPS and TIMPs

Many different cell types are capable of producing MMPs and TIMPs, but the main cell types involved are fibroblasts, macrophages, and polymorphonuclear leukocytes.[13]

After myocardial infarction, inflammatory cells invade infarcted tissue and contribute to collagen degradation. Collagen content could be preserved within 24 hours of infarction by making rats leukopenic by irradiation, which suggests that proteases produced by inflammatory cells, including polymorphonuclear leukocytes and monocytes,[36,37] are involved in the early degradation of collagen following infarction.[38]

In stunned myocardium, where ultrastructural evidence of collagen degradation was present in the absence of myocyte necrosis or inflammatory cells, an activation of latent collagenase, stored in the interstitial space, is likely operative.[28,29] A second route of increased collagenolytic activity could be that new synthesis of collagenase by cells present in the myocardium account for the degradation of the collagen matrix.

In our rat myocardial infarction model MMP-1 and TIMP mRNA producing cells within the myocardium were phenotyped by in situ hybridization, using probes for MMP-1 and TIMP in combination with immunohistochemistry on parallel tissue sec-

tions. TIMP mRNA producing cells were seen as early as day 2 after myocardial infarction, whereas the first MMP-1 mRNA producing cells were found mainly at day 7 postinfarction. MMP-1 and TIMP mRNA producing cells were predominantly localized in the area surrounding necrotic cardiomyocytes. In this area collagen mRNA and protein deposition also takes place.[39] The MMP-1 and TIMP mRNA producing cells were identified as fibroblasts or fibroblast-like cells and not endothelial cells or macrophages. Inflammatory cells were excluded, because of their size and because their proteases would be expected to be participatory earlier (e.g., day 1) in the wound healing response that follows coronary ligation.[38] From these results we concluded that collagenase and its inhibitor (TIMP) in the rat myocardial infarction model are most likely involved in the remodeling process in the infarcted left ventricle rather that in the early degradation of collagen struts between cardiomyocytes and capillaries which is related to proteolytic digestion induced by invading leukocytes.

Regulation of Collagenase Activity

Collagenolytic activity of tissue can be increased by activation of the latent pool of collagenases stored in the extracellular compartment. Collagenase activation has been demonstrated in the remodeling process found during wound healing in various tissues. Furthermore collagenolytic activity can be increased by a decrease in the concentration of inhibitor. Decreased TIMP levels were found in aortic aneurysms suggesting that increased collagenolytic activity was due to an imbalance in the collagenase inhibitor levels resulting in extracellular matrix degradation and subsequent aneurysms.[40] Decreased TIMP can lead to an increase in collagenase activity in metastatic cells. This enables tumor cells to penetrate their extracellular matrix rich environment and migrate to neighboring tissue.[41] Khokha et al.[42] demonstrated that an upregulation of TIMP suppresses metastatic capacity of cells. A fine tuned balance between collagenase and its inhibitors is necessary for normal tissue remodeling and function.[2,13] Small changes in this balance can have dramatic effects and form a potential danger for normal tissue function. Regulation of collagenolytic activity is related to secretion of collagenase when the enzyme is needed, a multistep activation of latent enzyme, and/or several tissue and blood inhibitors.

Therapeutic Use of TIMPs

Control of collagen deposition, when increased fibrosis is undesirable, could be achieved by intervention with collagen synthesis. Inhibition of collagen synthesis could be achieved by controlling intracellular hydroxylation using proline analogs, ascorbic acid deficiency, or iron chelators. Another approach is interference in collagen secretion or controlling maturation of collagen fibrils by β-aminopropionitrille or D-penicillamine which leads to poorly crosslinked collagen fibrils which therefore have less influence on tissue stiffness. Another route could be degradation of collagen by topical application of collagenase or scavenging TIMP which could lead to increased collagenolytic activity.[5] Because collagen turnover in a pathological lesion is generally much higher than found under normal circumstances and mostly a transient phenomenon, drugs which can selectively inhibit collagen synthesis or accelerate collagen degradation in a pathological lesion could be used.[5] Increased collagenolytic activity can have various adverse consequences on tissue function (e.g., cardiac dilatation or rupture or metastasis of tumor cells). It could be of great therapeutic use to control this disequilibrium between proteinase and its inhibitors.

Using metal chelators like EDTA and 1,10-phenanthroline or compounds with reactive sulfhydryl groups like cysteine, dithiothreitol, and D-penicillamine can reduce the collagenolytic activity directly. Another approach would be the use of inhibitors of MMPs. Recombinant TIMP,[43] isolated TIMP, or tetracyclines[20] can be used to regulate the collagenolytic activity by inhibiting the activated collagenases and/or forming a complex with the proteinases. Much re-

search will need to be done to determine the safety and efficacy of these drugs.

References

1. Weber KT. Cardiac interstitium in health and disease. J Am Coll Cardiol 1989;13: 1637–1652.
2. Werb Z. Degradation of collagen. In: Weiss JB, Jayson MI, eds. Collagen in Heart and Disease. Edinburgh: Churchill Livingstone, 1982:121–134.
3. Robinson TF, Factor SM, Capasso JM, et al. Morphology, composition, and function of struts between cardiac myocytes of rat and hamster. Cell Tissue Res 1987;249:247–255.
4. Caulfield JB, Borg TK. The collagen network of the heart. Lab Invest 1979;40:364–372.
5. Chvapil M. Experimental modification of collagen synthesis and degradation and their therapeutic applications. In: Weiss JB, Jayson MI, eds. Collagen in Heart and Disease. Edinburgh: Churchill Livingstone, 1982: 206–217.
6. Robinson TF, Cohen-Gould L, Factor SM. Skeletal framework of mammalian heart muscle. Arrangement of inter- and pericellular connective tissue structures. Lab Invest 1983;49:482–498.
7. Caulfield JB, Wolkowicz PE. Mechanisms for cardiac dilatation. Heart Failure 1990;6: 138–150.
8. Weber KT, Brilla CG, Janicki JS. Myocardial fibrosis: functional significance and regulatory factors. Cardiovasc Res 1993;27: 341–348.
9. Weber KT, Sun Y, Tyagi SC, et al. Collagen network of the myocardium: function, structural remodeling and regulatory mechanisms. (Review) J Mol Cell Cardiol 1994;26: 279–292.
10. Vracko R, Cunningham D, Frederickson RG, et al. Basal lamina of rat myocardium. Its fate after death of cardiac myocytes. Lab Invest 1988;58:77–87.
11. Bosman FT, Havenith MG, Visser R, et al. Basement membranes in neoplasia. Progress in Histochemistry and Cytochemistry 1992; 24:1–92.
12. Bosman FT, Havenith M, Cleutjens JPM. Basement membranes in cancer. Ultrastr Pathol 1985;8:291–304.
13. Murphy G, Reynolds JJ. Extracellular matrix degradation. In: Royce PM, Steinmann B, eds. Connective Tissue and its Heritable Disorders. Molecular, Genetic, and Medical Aspects. New York, NY: Wiley-Liss, 1993: 287–316.

14. Docherty AJ, Murphy G. The tissue metallo-proteinase family and the inhibitor TIMP: a study using cDNAs and recombinant proteins. Ann Rheum Dis 1990;49:469–479.
15. Kielty CM, Hopkinson I, Grant ME. Collagen: the collagen family: structure, assembly, and organization in the extracellular matrix. In: Royce PM, Steinmann B, eds. Connective Tissue and its Heritable disorders. Molecular, Genetics, and Medical Aspects. New York, NY: Wiley-Liss, 1993:103–147.
16. Woessner JF. Matrix metalloproteinases and their inhibitors in connective tissue remodeling. Faseb J 1991;5:2145–2154.
17. Everts V, Beertsen W, Tigchelaar-Gutter W. The digestion of phagocytosed collagen is inhibited by the proteinase inhibitors leupetin and E-64. Coll Rel Res 1985;5:315–336.
18. Beertsen W. Collagen phagocytosis by fibroblasts in the periodontal ligament of the mouse molar during the initial phase of hypofunction. J Dental Res 1987;66:1708–1712.
19. Bienkowski RS, Baum BJ, Crystal RG. Fibroblasts degrade newly synthesized collagen within the cell before secretion. Nature 1978; 276:413–416.
20. Denhardt DT, Feng B, Edwards DR, et al. Tissue inhibitor of metalloproteinases (TIMP, aka EPA): structure, control of expression and biological functions. Pharmacol Ther 1993;59:329–341.
21. Springman EB, Angleton EL, Birkedal-Hansen H, et al. Multiple modes of activation of latent human fibroblast collagenase: evidence for the role of a Cys73 active-site zinc complex in latency and a "cysteine switch" mechanism for activation. Proc Natl Acad Sci USA 1990;87:364–368.
22. Cawston TE, Galloway WA, Mercer E, et al. Purification of rabbit bone inhibitor of collagenase. Biochem J 1981;195:159–165.
23. Montfort I, Pérez-Tamayo R. The distribution of collagenase in normal rat tissues. J Histochem Cytochem 1975;23:910–920.
24. Tyagi SC, Matsubara L, Weber KT. Extraction and estimation of collagenase(s) activity by zymography in microquantities of rat myocardium. Clin Biochem 1993;26:191–198.
25. Caulfield JB, Wolkowicz P. Inducible collagenolytic activity in isolated perfused rat hearts. Am J Pathol 1988;131:199–205.
26. Sato S, Ashraf M, Millard RW, et al. Connective tissue changes in early ischemia of porcine myocardium: an ultrastructural study. J Mol Cell Cardiol 1983;15:261–275.
27. Takahashi S, Barry AC, Factor SM. Collagen degradation in ischaemic rat hearts. Biochem J 1990;265:233–241.
28. Zhao M, Zhang H, Robinson TF, et al. Pro-found structural alterations of the extracellular collagen matrix in postischemic dysfunctional ("stunned") but viable myocardium. J Am Coll Cardiol 1987;10:1322–1334.
29. Charney RH, Takahashi S, Zhao M, et al. Collagen loss in the stunned myocardium. Circulation 1992;85:1483–1490.
30. Cleutjens JPM, Kandala JC, Guarda E, et al. Regulation of collagen degradation in the rat myocardium after infarction. J Mol Cell Cardiol. (In press)
31. Heussen C, Dowdle EB. Electrophoretic analysis of plasminogen activators in polyacrylamide gels containing sodium dodecyl sulfate and copolymerized substrates. Anal Biochem 1980;102:196–202.
32. Overall CM, Wrana JL, Sodek J. Independent regulation of collagenase, 72-kDa progelatinase, and metalloendoproteinase inhibitor expression in human fibroblasts by transforming growth factor-beta. J Biol Chem 1989;264:1860–1869.
33. Brown PD, Levy AT, Margulies IMK, et al. Independent expression and cellular processing of Mr 72,000 type IV collagenase and interstitial collagenase in human tumorigenic cell lines. Cancer Res 1990;50: 6184–6191.
34. Leibovich SJ, Weiss JB. Failure of human rheumatoid collagenase to degrade either normal or rheumotoid arthritic polymeric collagen. Biochim Biophys Acta 1971;251: 109–118.
35. Emonard H, Grimaud JA. Matrix metalloproteinases. A review. Cell Mol Biol 1990;36: 131–153.
36. Pyke C, Ralfkiaer E, Tryggvason K, et al. Messenger RNA for two type IV collagenases is located in stromal cells in human colon cancer. Am J Pathol 1993;142:359–365.
37. Welgus HG, Campbell EJ, Cury JD, et al. Neutral metalloproteinases produced by human mononuclear phagocytes. Enzyme profile, regulation, and expression during cellular development. J Clin Invest 1990;86: 1496–1502.
38. Cannon RO, Butany JW, McManus BM, et al. Early degradation of collagen after acute myocardial infarction in the rat. Am J Cardiol 1983;52:390–395.
39. Cleutjens JPM, Van Krimpen C, Smits JFM, et al. Increase of type I and III collagen mRNA and protein in the infarcted and noninfarcted rat heart after myocardial infarction. (Abstract) J Mol Cell Cardiol 1991; 23(Suppl. V):S60.
40. Brophy CM, Marks WH, Reilly JM, et al. Decreased tissue inhibitor of metalloprotei-

nases (TIMP) in abdominal aortic aneurysm tissue: a preliminary report. J Surg Res 1991; 50:653–657.

41. Ponton A, Coulombe B, Skup D. Decreased expression of tissue inhibitor of metalloproteinases in metastatic tumor cells leading to increased levels of collagenase activity. Cancer Res 1991;51:2138–2143.

42. Khokha R, Zimmer MJ, Wilson SM, et al. Up-regulation of TIMP-1 expression in F16-F10 melanoma cells suppresses their metastatic ability in chick embryo. Clin Exp Metastasis 1992;10:365–370.

43. DeClerck YA, Yean T-D, Chan D, et al. Inhibition of tumor invasion of smooth muscle layers by recombinant human metalloproteinase inhibitor. Cancer Res 1991;51:2151–2157.

Chapter 14

The Pathogenesis of Atherosclerosis

Shogo Katsuda, M.D., Isao Nakanishi, M.D.

Introduction

Atherosclerosis is an arterial disease that is recognized to be the major cause of death in the United States, Europe, and Japan.[1] Because atherosclerosis progresses insidiously for many years before symptoms develop, its cause and pathogenesis have been difficult to elucidate. Yet in the past decade or two, cellular and molecular approaches to the study of the cells of the arterial wall and lipid metabolism have provided numerous insights into the pathogenesis of the disease. Today we have advanced the understanding that ultimate lesions of atherosclerosis represent the culmination of a series of cellular and molecular events in which there is proliferation of both smooth muscle cells and macrophages which had previously entered the arterial intima. The interactions among these cells and the endothelial cells and T lymphocytes that had also entered the lesion lead to a massive fibroproliferative response, in which the smooth muscle cells produce connective tissue matrix. Thus, the interaction between different cell types is the fundamental event in the disease. This is reminiscent of the cell-cell interaction observed in the healing of wounded or inflamed tissues, where monocytes/macrophages and lymphocytes migrate into the lesion and modulate the functions of fibroblasts such as cell proliferation and synthesis of extracellular matrix.[2,3] From these viewpoints, it is possible to consider that the progression of atherosclerosis also involves processes similar to wound healing where destruction and remodeling of extracellular matrix is one of the key events.

This chapter will review current knowledge on the pathogenesis of atherosclerosis, and the role of the extracellular matrix in the pathogenesis of atherosclerosis will be considered.

The Lesions of Atherosclerosis

Of the three layers of the artery, the intima is the cell layer principally involved in atherosclerosis, although secondary changes are often found in the media. Three classic types of lesion are recognized: the fatty streak; the fibrous plaque or atheromatous plaque; and the so-called "complicated plaque."[4] Fatty streaks, commonly occurring early in life, are yellowish, relatively flat lesions that extend in the direction of blood flow. They are likely, but yet unproven, precursors of more advanced lesions. The lesion is characterized by an intimal aggregation of lipid-rich smooth muscle cells and macrophages (foam cells) and some T lymphocytes (Figure 1). Most of the lipid is in the form of cholesterol and cholesteryl esters. Although there are few fibrous elements in the area where foam cells aggregated densely, there are various amounts of extracellular matrix components in the areas where cells are sparsely distributed. Fibrous plaques, the most characteristic lesions of advancing atherosclerosis, are whitish in gross appearance and are elevated so that they protrude into the lumen. Plaques exhibit histologic variabil-

From Weber KT, MD *Wound Healing in Cardiovascular Disease*, Armonk, NY, Futura Publishing Company Inc., © 1995.

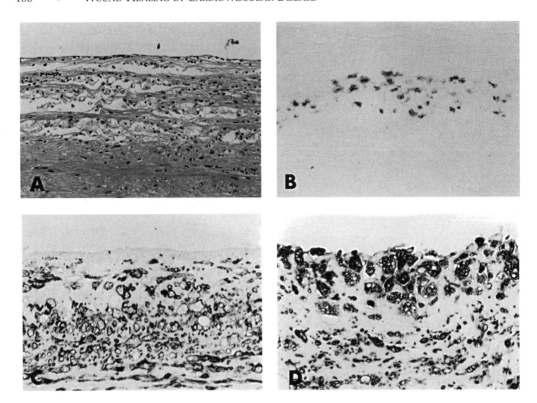

Figure 1. Fatty streak of the aorta. A: Hematoxylin and eosin stain, demonstrating an accumulation of subendothelial foam cells. B: Anti-T lymphocyte antibody OPD 4 immunocytochemical preparation, demonstrating T cell composition of the lesion. C: Antimuscle actins antibody HHF35, demonstrating smooth muscle cell-derived foam cells near base of the lesion. D: antimacrophage antibody HAM56, demonstrating significant numbers of macrophage-derived foam cells confined largely to the more superficial aspects of the lesion. (A, original magnification ×200; B-D, original magnification ×400).

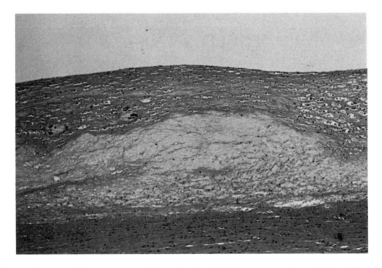

Figure 2. Fibrous plaque of the aorta consists of a basal atheroma and overlying fibrous cap. Hematoxylin and eosin stain (×64).

ity, but a typical cellular plaque consists of a fibrous cap and a deeper necrotic core (atheroma) (Figure 2). Fibrous caps are composed mostly of smooth muscle cells and dense connective tissue containing collagen, elastic fibers, proteoglycans, and glycoproteins. Macrophages and smooth muscle cells with variable amounts of lipid and T lymphocytes are beneath and to the side of fibrous cap. Atheromas contain cellular debris, extracellular lipid, cholesterol crystals, and occasional calcium deposits. The complicated plaques appear to be fibrous plaques that have been altered by hemorrhage, ulceration, calcification, and superimposed thrombosis.

In summary, the lesions of atherosclerosis are characterized by three fundamental phenomena: proliferation of smooth muscle cells; accumulation of extracellular matrix components including collagen, elastic fibers and proteoglycans; and deposition of intracellular and extracellular lipid. Therefore, any hypothesis that attempts to explain the pathogenesis of atherosclerosis must account for these phenomena, and ultimately explain the role of major risk factors, particularly hyperlipidemia, hypertension, and smoking in the development of the disease.

Response-to-Injury Hypothesis of Atherosclerosis

Although several theories explaining the pathogenesis of atherosclerosis based on analyses of animal models and human atherosclerotic lesions have been proposed, the current trend is to consider atherosclerosis as a response of the arterial wall to a variety of injurious agents, and that multiple pathogenetic mechanisms contribute to the formation of the lesions. Favored today and receiving the greatest attention is the response-to-injury hypothesis proposed by Ross and Glomset.[5–7] We will now review this attractive hypothesis of atherosclerosis.

Sequence of Events in Atherosclerosis

Chronic Endothelial Injury and Endothelial Dysfunction

Chronic or repeated injury to the endothelial cells is the keystone of the response-to-injury hypothesis. As a result of exposure to injurious agents such as oxidized low density lipoprotein (ox LDL), hypertension, hemodynamic disturbances (shear stress, turbulent flow), circulating endotoxins, carbon monoxide, viruses, and homocysteine, subtle changes occur in the endothelial cells of the artery as well as in the circulating leukocytes. Such subtle forms of injury to the endothelial cells lead to dysfunctional changes in these cells and induce increased permeability and formation of specific adhesive glycoproteins, such as vascular cell adhesion molecule-1 (VCAM-1),[8] on the surface of the endothelial cells.

Increased permeability of endothelial cells results in increased accumulation of plasma proteins, particularly low density lipoprotein (LDL) in hypercholesterolemia, beneath the endothelial cells. This is rapidly followed by attachment, adhesion, and spreading of peripheral blood monocytes and T lymphocytes at sites where endothelial dysfunction have occurred, notably at branches and bifurcations of the arteries. These cells adhere due to the formation of a series of adhesive cell surface glycoproteins by the endothelial cells and leukocytes, which interact in a ligand-receptor manner. Thus, the earliest changes induced by injurious agents appear to be altered endothelial permeability together with the adherence of leukocytes representing the first phase of an inflammatory response.

Intimal Aggregation of Macrophages, T Lymphocytes, and Smooth Muscle Cells

Following adhesion to endothelial cells, monocytes and T lymphocytes migrate across the surface of the endothelial cells, probe between the junctions of the endothelial cells, and are chemotactically attracted into the subendothelial space where they begin to accumulate within the intima, resulting in an early, highly specialized form of chronic inflammation. This process of chemotaxis can be generated by a number of molecules that are expressed by endothelial cells and/or smooth muscle cells, including monocyte chemotactic protein-1 (MCP-1)[9] and ox LDL. Platelets may become involved at these sites due to separations that occur between retracted endothelial cells, exposing the underlying cells or connective tissue matrix. Monocytes become transformed into macrophages in the intima and avidly engulf lipoproteins, largely ox LDL by the so-called scavenger pathway,[10] to become foam cells. In addition, early in the evolution of the lesion, medial smooth muscle cells migrate into the intima where they proliferate and some take up lipoprotein particles to also be transformed into foam cells. The formation of the foam cells and their continued aggregates in the intima, together with the accompanying T lymphocytes, lead to the first ubiquitous lesion of atherosclerosis, the fatty streak.

Fibrous Plaque Formation and Further Lesion Progression

If the injurious agents, whether hypercholesterolemia or factors associated with hypertension, cigarette smoking, etc., continue to be exposed to the arterial wall, the inflammatory response also continues. With time, foam cell– and T lymphocyte-rich lesions become converted to lesions enriched in smooth muscle cells. The smooth muscle cells in the lesions can synthesize the bulk of the connective tissue matrix including collagen, elastic fibers, and proteoglycans. A number of growth factors have been implicated in the migration and proliferation of smooth muscle cells, most importantly "platelet-derived growth factor" (PDGF),[11] released from platelets adherent to the focus of endothelial injury but also produced by macrophages, endothelial cells, and smooth muscle cells in response to the release of cytokines such as tumor necrosis factor (TNF),[12] interleukin-1 (IL-1),[13] and interferon (INF)-γ[14] generated by macrophage–T lymphocyte interactions as described below. If the conditions that induce the response continue for a long enough period of time, the cellular fatty lesion is modified by the further deposition of collagen, elastic fibers, and proteoglycans, and ultimately become fibrous plaques. The advanced lesion, or fibrous plaque, then can intrude into the arterial wall. Figure 3 summarizes the sequential events of atherogenesis in the response-to-injury hypothesis.

The "response-to-injury hypothesis" suggests that the entire process of lesion for-

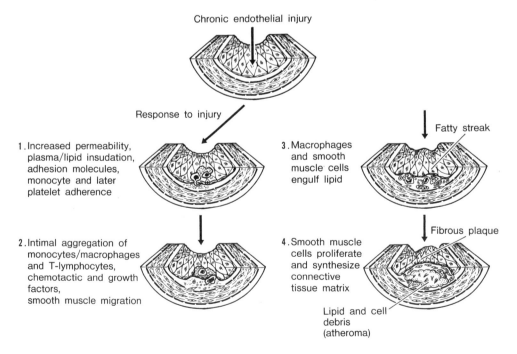

Figure 3. Hypothetical sequence of events in atherosclerosis.

mation begins as a protective, inflammatory response, which in time and with continuing injury become excessive. In its excess, both the inflammation and the fibrous, connective tissue proliferation become the disease entity.

Cellular Interactions and Growth Regulatory Molecules

It has now become apparent that a complex network of cellular interactions among endothelial cells, monocyte/macrophages, platelets, T lymphocytes, and smooth muscle cells determine the direction in which the lesions will go and that growth factors and cytokines induce and regulate numerous critical cell functions.

Although many growth regulatory molecules and cytokines may be formed within the lesions of atherosclerosis, several of the molecules such as PDGF, basic fibroblast growth factor (bFGF),[15] heparin-binding epidermal growth factor-like growth

factor (HB-EGF),[16] insulin-like growth factor-1 (IGF-1),[17] IL-1, TNFα, colony-stimulating factor (CSF)[18] and transforming growth factor-β (TGF-β)[19] are potentially important in cell proliferation. Among them, PDGF, bFGF, and IGF-1 may be critical to the proliferation of smooth muscle cells and possibly endothelial cells.[20] Macrophage replication can potentially occur through the action of CSFs formed by endothelial cells, smooth muscle cells, or the macrophages themselves. Although IL-1, TNFα, and TGF-β have numerous effects upon smooth muscle cells, they can also induce secondary gene expression in smooth muscle cells for PDGF-AA, thus inducing the cells to make growth-stimulatory molecules in which they can potentially stimulate themselves in an autocrine fashion.[20] In a similar fashion, these three molecules can stimulate endothelial cells in vitro by inducing PDGF-BB formation. Macrophages, a source of all three of these molecules, can provide direct paracrine stimulation by secreting both chains of PDGF. PDGF-B chain protein has

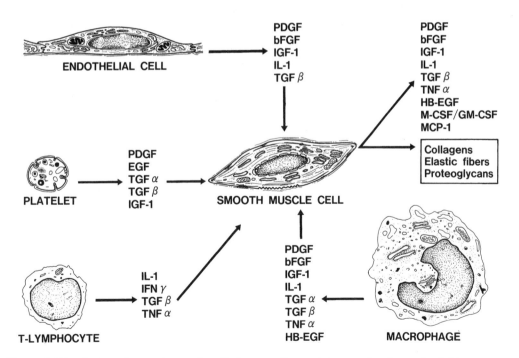

Figure 4. Stimulation of smooth muscle cells by growth regulatory molecules and cytokines generated from endothelial cells, platelets, T lymphocytes, and macrophages. Smooth muscle cells responded to these molecules synthesize extracellular matrix proteins as well as growth factors and cytokines.

been observed in macrophages in all phases of atherogenesis.[21] Thus, PDGF could be a principal mediator of smooth muscle cell proliferation in vivo by paracrine stimulation of macrophages or endothelial cells, or by autocrine stimulation of the smooth muscle cells. HB-EGF is as potent a mitogen in vitro for smooth muscle cells as PDGF, and it can be synthesized by both macrophages and smooth muscle cells.[16,22] However, little is known of the role that it may play in vivo.

As a potential balance to these mitogens, several factors are also potent inhibitors of the replication of smooth muscle cells or endothelial cells. These include TGF-β, IL-1, and INFγ. When each of these is present in high concentrations, it can inhibit the proliferative effect of the secreted PDGF-AA that it has induced by downregulating the relevant PDGF receptor molecules.[23]

A number of the mitogenic molecules that can be formed by activated macrophages, endothelial cells or smooth muscle cells can also act as chemoattractants for some of the other cells. PDGF,[24] IGF-1[20] and bFGF[25] are potent chemoattractants for smooth muscle cells, FGF for endothelial cells,[20] and M-CSF for monocyte-derived macrophages.[20] Macrophages and smooth muscle cells can also generate additional chemoattractants for monocytes such as MCP-1 and ox LDL.

Although many growth regulatory molecules have been characterized, none of them works alone in the process of atherogenesis. Through a network of cellular interactions, one molecule impinging on a target cell can modulate the expression of a second molecule from the target cell that can then either stimulate its neighbors in a paracrine way, or itself in an autocrine way. Figure 4 shows the stimulation of smooth muscle cells, which appear to sit in a pivotal position in the coordination of fibroproliferative events, by the growth regulatory molecules and cytokines formed by endothelial cells, platelets, macrophages, and T-lymphocytes.

Extracellular Matrix and Atherosclerosis

As described above, the entire process of atherogenesis is a specialized type of chronic inflammatory response.[7,20] In this sense, the most fundamental change in atherosclerosis is a remodeling of the original structure of the intima induced by an increase in extracellular matrix, in other words a kind of fibrosis developing in the intima. This intimal fibrosis has several characteristic features that differ from those of fibrosis developing in other tissues including the production of extracellular matrix by smooth muscle cells and the deposition of large amounts of intracellular and extracellular lipid. Such differences lead to the formation of fibrofatty lesions peculiar to atherosclerosis.

In this section, we will first consider the intimal and medial extracellular matrix, which is deeply involved in atherosclerosis, and next discuss the development and progression of atherosclerosis from the aspect of extracellular matrix.

Extracellular Matrix Components of the Arterial Wall

Of the various components of the extracellular matrix present in the intima and media, we will describe here collagen, elastic fibers, and hyaluronic acid and proteoglycans.

Collagen

Collagen is the main structural component of the extracellular matrix. It is formed by three polypeptide chains, referred to as alpha chains, and is a protein group having triple helical and globular domains. At the present time, 30 gene families of alpha chain have been identified, with the types of collagen formed by them differentiated as types I to XVI.[26,27] The distribution of each type of collagen shows cell or tissue specificity. In human arterial wall five types of collagen (I, III, IV, V, and VI) are distributed, accounting for 20% of the dry weight of the aorta and 40% of medium and small-sized arteries.[28] In tissue, types I, III, and V are distributed as collagen fibers. Studies using the double immunoelectron microscopic method have revealed that the collagen fibers of the corium dermis form hybrid fibers consisting of types I and III collagen.[29]

Hybrids of types I and V collagen have also been reported,[30] and it seems likely that in the arterial wall as well heterotypic fibrils containing molecules of type III collagen and type V collagen in addition to type I collagen molecules may predominate. Types I and III collagen possess resilience and elasticity, respectively.[28] Also, type V collagen when present in large amounts forms thin fibers,[31] and thus collagen fibers, with type I collagen as the base, by altering the proportion of types III and V can meet various functional demands.

By electron microscopy, type VI collagen is observed as a branching network of filaments (Figure 5). Type VI collagen binds with the core protein of chondroitin sulfate proteoglycan on the cell surface,[32] and can also bind with type I collagen[33] and hyaluronic acid.[34] Accordingly, this collagen is involved in the binding of the cell and other extracellular matrix components, and is thought to play an important role in preserving the three-dimensional structure of tissue and directing tissue remodeling.

Type IV collagen is found only in basement membrane, along with other unique proteins such as laminin, heparin sulfate proteoglycan, and nidogen/entactin.[26] Principal among the biological activities of basement membrane are cell support, selective molecular sieving, and the ability to bind to cells and regulate their migration, growth, and differentiation.

Elastic Fibers

Elastic fibers as observed under the electron microscope consist of two morphologically completely different components: a central amorphous region; and microfibrils with a diameter of 10 to 12 nm located around the periphery of the amorphous component. This central amorphous region composing upward of 90% of the mature elastic fiber is made up of elastin, an extremely hydrophobic, insoluble protein,[35] while the microfibrils are made up of a number of components including glycopro-

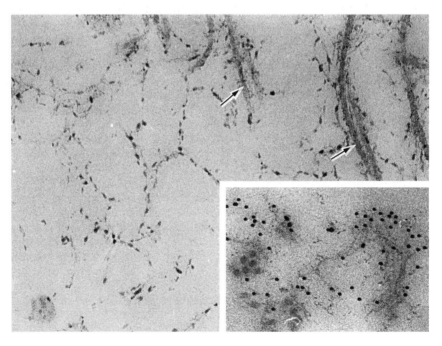

Figure 5. Transmission electron photomicrograph showing a branching network of filaments present around and between cross-banded collagen fibers (arrows) (×45,000). Inset shows immunoelectron photomicroscopic localization of type VI collagen. Filamentous structure is labeled with antitype VI collagen antibody (×45,000). (From Katsuda et al, Arterioscler Thromb 1992 :494–502, with permission of the American Heart Association.)

teins such as fibrillin.[36] Elastin accounts for 50% of the dry weight of the aorta and 20% of medium and small-sized arteries.[28] Extracellular elastin, which is resilient, and contraction filament bundles within the smooth muscle cells work in tandem to provide resilience and contractility to the arteries.[37]

Morphological evidence suggests that microfibrils may serve as a nidus for the deposition of elastin and serve to determine the shape and direction of elastic fibers. However, functional significance of the relationship between the amorphous component and the microfibrils remains an important unsolved question.

Hyaluronic Acid and Proteoglycans

Glycosaminoglycan is the major structural component of the matrix filling the space between the fiber components (Figure 6B), and hyaluronic acid, chondroitin sulfate, heparan sulfate, and dermatan sulfate, each with a specific function, are present in the arterial wall.[38] Heparan sulfate, chondroitin sulfate, and dermatan sulfate covalently bind to core proteins and exist as proteoglycans. These proteoglycans are each produced from endothelial and smooth muscle cells, with the former producing mainly heparan sulfate proteoglycans, and the latter mainly chondroitin sulfate and dermatan sulfate proteoglycans.

Heparan sulfate proteoglycans are present mainly in basement membrane, and have important functions in mediating interactions between cells and matrix and control of plasma protein permeation. In addition, by binding with antithrombin III they exert an anticoagulation effect. Chondroitin sulfate proteoglycans together with hyaluronic acid fill up the interfiber space and thereby maintain the viscoelasticity of the artery. Dermatan sulfate proteoglycans are closely associated with the surface of collagen fibers at regular intervals and play a role in fiber formation.

Destruction of Intimal Matrix and Development of Atherosclerosis

Increased endothelial permeability and subsequent intimal edema is generally ac-

cepted as evidence of vascular injury.[39] As shown in Figure 6A, one of the first observable events in atherosclerosis is the accumulation of edema fluid associated with swelling and partial loss of the endothelial cell basement membrane, disappearance of the reticular structure made up of hyaluronic acid and proteoglycans, and disruption of collagen fibers. Thus, destruction of the normal structure of the intima occurs. At the site of injury, endothelial cells, platelets, and monocytes/macrophages release chemotactic factors to smooth muscle cells such as PDGF,[24] IGF-1,[20] and bFGF.[25] Some components of edema fluid including fibrinogen and fibrin are also chemotactic for smooth muscle cells.[40] Smooth muscle cells in the media recognize these chemotactic factors, and migrate into the intima in which these factors are present at high concentrations (Figure 6A).

Contractile activity of medial smooth muscle cells is vital for normal functioning of the artery. This activity is achieved through attachment of the cells to each other and to extracellular matrix components around them. For smooth muscle cells to migrate, therefore, the cells have to degrade their own basement membranes, their intercellular attachments, and release themselves from their restricted environment and then destroy the adjacent extracellular matrix which acts as a barrier to cell motility by various matrix-degrading enzymes. We have reported that matrix metalloproteinase-1 (MMP-1, interstitial collagenase), MMP-2 (72-kDa gelatinase/type IV collagenase), and MMP-9 (92-kDa gelatinase/type IV collagenase) produced by smooth muscle cells might play an important role in the process of the migration.[41] Jackson et al.[42] have also suggested that plasmin, a serine proteinase, is potentially involved in the migration of smooth muscle cells.

During the migration into the intima and/or within the intima, smooth muscle cells change the phenotype from "contractile" to "synthetic" state[43,44] and proliferate in response to growth factors and cytokines released by macrophages, T lymphocytes, endothelial cells, and by themselves as described above. The synthetic state smooth muscle cells actively produce components of the extracellular matrix such as collagen,

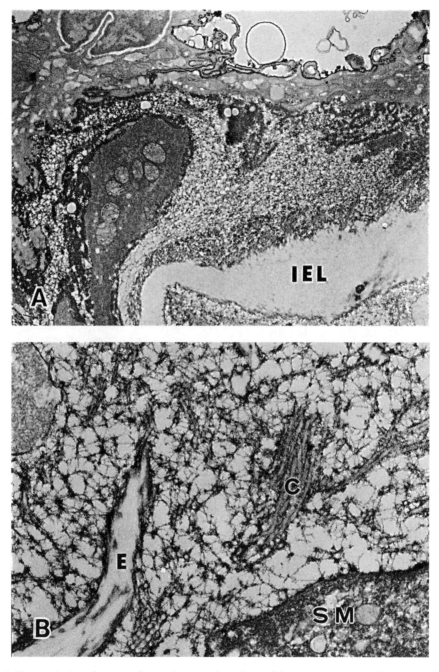

Figure 6. Transmission electron photomicrographs taken of the common carotid arteries of rabbits that were partially constricted with silver cuff. A: The intima 3 days after constriction, showing subendothelial edema. The intima is widened and occupied by flocculent materials of edema fluid associated with destruction of the normal structure. A smooth muscle cell is migrating from the media into the intima through the gap of the internal elastic lamina (IEL). Ruthenium red stain (×10,800). B: The intima 7 days after constriction, showing repair of the destroyed structure. The intimal matrix is reconstructed by newly synthesized collagen fibers (C), elastic fiber (E), and hyaluronic acid and proteoglycans which are filling the space between the fibers. SM-smooth muscle cell. Ruthenium red stain (×26,000).

elastic fibers, hyaluronic acid, and proteo-glycans, and repair the destroyed intimal structure (Figure 6B). Thus, the destruction of intimal matrix is a key step in develop-ment of the disease. As shown in Figure 6B, initial matrix is a loosely connected tissue rich in hyaluronic acid and proteoglycans, which provides a good support for further cell migration. Smooth muscle cells con-tinue to migrate into the injured intima and elaborate a new, more structurally sound extracellular matrix.

Matrix Remodeling and Progression of Atherosclerosis

Over long periods intimal injury and the reparative response elicited by this in-jury are repeated, during the course of which destruction of the intimal matrix is also added resulting from the release of var-ious matrix-degrading enzymes released by macrophages which have a biophylactic function and other cells present in the le-sions. As part of the reparative response to various types of injuries, fibrosis proceeds while the structure of the intima is being remodeled.

Collagen

Collagen increases in parallel with inti-mal thickening, reaching levels 5 to 20-fold of normal.[45] In normal arteries, types I and III collagen account for 30% and 70%, re-spectively, while in atherosclerosis this pro-portion is reversed with type I making up 65% and type III 35%.[46] Immunohistochem-ical analysis of the distribution of each colla-gen type in atherosclerotic lesions reveals several interesting findings.[47] Types I and III collagen are distributed together in all thickened intima while, notably, the stain-ing of type V collagen is enhanced as the lesion evolves (Figure 7A). Biochemical studies as well have documented increased type V collagen in atherosclerotic lesions,[48] with type V collagen deposition and lesion progression showing an intimate connec-tion. Because type V collagen is known to increase in atherosclerotic lesions but also in such fibrosing lesions as scar tissue[49] and scirrhous carcinoma,[50] this type of collagen

appears to be involved in progressive fibro-sis. The increase in type V collagen holds in check the thickness of fibers and may repre-sent a reaction of the organism to maintain the flexibility of the arterial wall.

Type IV collagen also increases with progression of the lesion.[51] Medial smooth muscle cells and those in early atheroscle-rotic lesions are surrounded by relatively thin type IV collagen, while cells in ad-vanced lesions are surrounded by thick type IV collagen with, in particular, elongated cells around atheroma surrounded by mul-tilayered type IV collagen (Figure 7B). These findings correspond to the multilayered structure of the basement membrane as ob-served with the electron microscope, with this thickening and formation of multiple layers in the basement membrane possibly acting as a cushion to protect the cell from the vascular hemodynamic forces exerted by the protruding lesion.[52] In addition, thickening of the basement membrane is a marker of decreased proliferative ability and of cell senescence,[52] with the basement membrane becoming a site of calcium pre-cipitation as well.

Type VI collagen is invariably present in areas of intimal thickening (Figure 7C). This collagen, although degraded by human neutrophil elastase,[53] is resistant to various matrix-degrading enzymes re-leased by smooth muscle cells and macro-phages, and so plays a vital role in protect-ing the intima from enzymatic degradation and providing structural unity to the inti-mal connective tissue. In addition, type VI collagen can bind to von Willebrand factor, and by forming a complex in vascular sub-endothelium plays a role in platelet aggre-gation.[54]

In this way, each collagen increases in parallel with evolution of the lesion, while in the atheroma extensive degradation of collagens occur (Figure 7D). These findings suggest that collagens preserve the patho-physiological and functional integrity of the arterial wall by providing mechanical sup-port as well as assuring the proper interac-tion of cells during the formation of athero-sclerotic lesions.

TGF-β promotes synthesis of collagens I, III, IV, and V by cultured arterial smooth muscle cells,[55,56] whereas IL-1 conversely

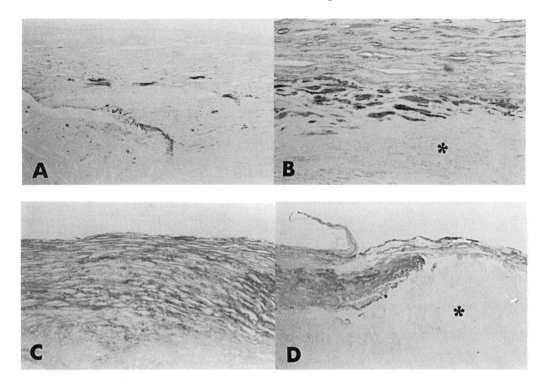

Figure 7. Photomicrographs showing fibrous plaques immunostained for collagens. A: Localization of type V collagen, showing irregular distribution and concentration in the fibrous cap. B: localization of type IV collagen. Note increased deposition of collagen near the atheroma (*). C: Localization of type VI collagen, showing diffuse distribution throughout the thickened intima. D: Localization of type III collagen in a large fibrous plaque with impending ulceration. Collagen is not present in the atheroma (*). (A-D, original magnification ×109. From Katsuda et al., Arterioscler Thromb 1992 : 494–502, with permission of the American Heart Association.)

suppresses it.[56] PDGF suppresses the synthesis of type IV collagen[56] while enhancing that of types I, III,[55] and V.[57] INFγ, a product of activated T lymphocytes, decreases the collagen synthesis by cultured smooth muscle cells and inhibits the augmentation in collagen synthesis produced by PDGF and TGF-β.[55] Jaeger et al.[58] demonstrated that expression of mRNAs of types I and III collagen in cells occurs in the vicinity of macrophages, whereas no mRNA-containing cells could be detected in the intima and media of the normal artery as well as in fibrous plaques free of macrophages. These results strongly suggest that a variety of growth regulatory molecules and cytokines regulate collagen synthesis by smooth muscle cells in the lesions, and macrophages and T lymphocytes play an important role in this process.

Collagen degradation as well as collagen synthesis are equally critical to matrix remodeling, in which the resorption is tightly regulated by a complex interplay of cell-cell and cell-matrix interactions involving the production of enzymes, inhibitors, and regulatory molecules such as growth factors and cytokines. Matrix metalloproteinases (MMPs) are thought to be major enzymes in extracellular matrix degradation in normal and pathological states.[59,60] Actually, MMPs such as MMP-1, MMP-2, MMP-3 (stromelysin-1), and MMP-9, that cleave collagen types I, III, IV, and V, denatured collagens (gelatins) and other matrix proteins, and their inhibitors, the tissue inhibitors of matrix metalloproteinases (TIMPs)[59] have been demonstrated in macrophages and smooth muscle cells in atherosclerotic lesions (Katsuda et al., unpublished observations). In addition, plasminogen activator and plasmin are deeply involved in atherogenesis.[61] Plasmin has been shown to initiate the autoactivation of many MMPs by cleavage of the peptide.[59] Finally, of particular interest is the extensive degradation of collagen in the atheroma. An excess of collagenolytic enzymes over inhibitors together with decreased synthesis of collagen by injured smooth muscle cells in the atheroma might contribute significantly to tissue destruction.

Elastic Fibers

Remodeling of elastic fibers is also a closely related process in the disease. In areas of intimal thickening in the neonatal aorta, elastic fibers show an arrangement in which they stick out facing the lumen, while as the lesion progresses with increasing age the elastic fibers develop a dense sponge-like structure. However, as the lesion becomes even more advanced destruction of the elastic fibers becomes striking. Elastic fibers are markedly decreased and disappear, particularly within the atheroma.[62] By electron microscopy, excessive accumulation of microfibrils in elastin degraded sites is seen, and when the elastic fibers are partially ruptured, bundles of microfibrils seem to join the ends of the ruptured portions as noted in Figure 8. These findings may also be interpreted as reflecting the destruction and repair of elastic fibers in atherosclerosis. Growth regulatory molecules and cytokines play an important role in the remodeling and turnover of elastin. TGF-β[63] and IGF-1[64] enhance the synthesis of elastin in arterial smooth muscle cells, and EGF[65] inhibits elastin synthesis. We have demonstrated that MMP-2 and MMP-9 produced by smooth muscle cells and macrophages can degrade elastin,[66,67] and that the production of MMP-9 by macrophages was remarkably stimulated by TNFα and IL-1.[68]

Biochemical analysis has demonstrated that the elastic fibers in atherosclerotic lesions are characterized by increases in polar amino acid and cholesterol content,[69] with associated calcium deposition.

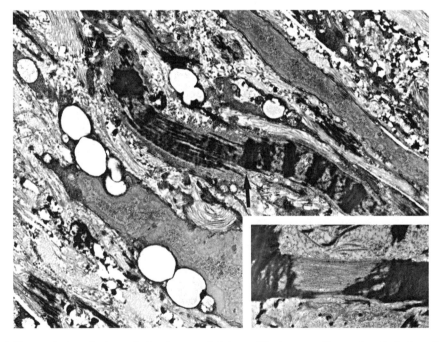

Figure 8. Transmission electron photomicrograph taken of the human atherosclerotic lesion, showing degraded elastic fiber (arrow). Tannic acid stain ($\times$9,000). Inset shows the bundle of microfibrils bridging the gap between the interrupted elastic fiber. Tannic acid stain ($\times$10,000).

Hyaluronic Acid and Proteoglycans

In the early stage of atherosclerosis, first hyaluronic acid and then chondroitin sulfate proteoglycans increase, while in the later stage the proportion of dermatan sulfate proteoglycans increase.[70] Since hyaluronic acid holds large amounts of water,[70] the increase in hyaluronic acid in the early stage is involved in the development of intimal edema, while the increase in dermatan sulfate proteoglycans in the later stage is thought to play an important role in collagen fiber formation.[38] TGF-β binds strongly to the small chondroitin-4-sulfate proteoglycan core protein in the matrix, whereas bFGF and related growth factors have high affinity for heparan sulfate proteoglycans such as basement membrane heparan sulfate proteoglycan,[71] and they can be released from sequestered form by matrix degradation.[2] Thus, proteoglycans are important storage site for growth regulatory molecules. Plasma lipoproteins infiltrating the intima bind to collagen, elastin, proteoglycans, and other components of the extracellular matrix and are taken up within the cell, preventing their diffusion and leading to their deposition in the intima. For lipoproteins to be taken up by macrophages they must undergo some kind of modification or degeneration. Binding to proteoglycans is also thought to be involved in their modification.[38] A recent study using the double immunoelectron microscopic method has demonstrated the colocalization of apoprotein B, which is the main apoprotein of LDL, and chondroitin sulfate in the extracellular matrix and foam cells of atherosclerotic lesions,[72] confirming the importance of proteoglycans in lipid deposition.

Summary and Conclusions

We have reviewed current concepts of the pathogenesis of atherosclerosis, and discussed the development and progression of this disease, emphasizing the role of extracellular matrix in response to injury. We now recognize the major roles that changes in synthesis and degradation of extracellular matrix play not only in inflammation and wound healing but also in atherosclerosis. It is the integrated interplay between cell-cell and cell-extracellular matrix, mediated by growth regulatory molecules and cytokines that determines whether or not a lesion will progress, remain static, or undergo regression. If the injury is subtle and/or transient, repair is successful in restoring normal intimal structure and function. If the injury continues chronically over a sufficiently long period of time, lesions continue to undergo intense remodeling and progress to a point at which clinical sequelae develop. Elucidation of integrated interplay controlling tissue repair and remodeling should provide insights for understanding why an outcome of injury leads to either normal tissue repair or progression to disease.

Acknowledgment: We are very grateful to Professor Russell Ross, of the Department of Pathology, University of Washington, Seattle, for reviewing this manuscript.

References

1. World Health Organization. Classification of atherosclerotic lesions. WHO Tech Rep Serv 1985;143:1.
2. Davidson JM. Wound repair. In: Gallin JI, Goldstein IM, Snyderman R, eds. Inflammation: Basic Principles and Clinical Correlates. New York, NY: Raven Press, 1992:809.
3. Kumar V, Cotran RS, Robbins SL. Basic Pathology. Philadelphia, Pa: W.B. Saunders Company, 1992:47.
4. Schoen FJ. Blood vessels. In: Cotran Rs, Kumar V, Robbins SL, eds. Pathological basis of disease. Philadelphia: W.B. Saunders Company. 1994:467
5. Ross R, Glomset JA. The pathogenesis of atherosclerosis. N Engl J Med 1976;295:369,420.
6. Ross R. The pathogenesis of atherosclerosis—an update. N Engl J Med 1986;314:488.
7. Ross R. The pathogenesis of atherosclerosis: a perspective for the 1990s. Nature 1993;362:801.
8. Cybulsky MI, Gimbrone MA Jr. Endothelial expression of a mononuclear leukocyte adhesion molecule during atherogenesis. Science 1991;251:788.
9. Takeya M, Yoshimura T, Leonard EJ, et al. Detection of monocyte chemoattractant protein-1 in human atherosclerotic lesions by an antimonocyte chemoattractant protein-1

monoclonal antibody. Hum Pathol 1993;24: 534.

10. Brown MS, Goldstein JL. Lipoprotein metabolism in the macrophage: implications for cholesterol deposition in atherosclerosis. Ann Rev Biochem 1983;52:223.

11. Ross R, Raines EW, Bowen-Pope DF. The biology of platelet-derived growth factor. Cell 1986;46:155.

12. Old LJ. Tumor necrosis factor (TNF). Science 1985;230:630.

13. Raines EW, Dower SK, Ross R. IL-1 mitogenic activity for fibroblasts and smooth muscle cells is due to PDGF-AA. Science 1989;243:393.

14. Hansson GK, Jonasson L, Holm J, et al. γ-interferon regulates vascular smooth muscle proliferation and Ia antigen expression in vivo and in vitro. Circ Res 1988;63:712.

15. Klagsbrun M, Edelman ER. Biological and biochemical properties of fibroblast growth factors: implications for the pathogenesis of atherosclerosis. Arteriosclerosis 1989;9:269.

16. Higashiyama S, Abraham JA, Miller J, et al. A heparin-binding growth factor secreted by macrophage-like cells that is related to EGF. Science 1991;251:936.

17. Cercek B, Fishbein C, Forrester JS, et al. Induction of insulin-like growth factor 1 mRNA in rat aorta after balloon denudation. Circ Res 1990;66:1755.

18. Clinton SK, Underwood R, Hayes L, et al. Macrophage colony stimulating factor gene expression in vascular cells and in experimental and human atherosclerosis. 1992;140: 301.

19. Moses HL, Yang EY, Pietenpol JA. TGF-β stimulation and inhibition of cell proliferation: new mechanistic insights. Cell 1990;63: 245.

20. Ross R. Atherosclerosis: a defense mechanism gone awry. Am J Pathol 1993;143:987.

21. Ross R, Masuda J, Raines EW, et al. Localization of PDGF-B protein in macrophages in all phases of atherogenesis. Science 1990;248: 1009.

22. Besner G, Higashiyama S, Klagsbrun M. Isolation and characterization of a macrophage-derived heparin-binding growth factor. Cell Regul 1990;1:811.

23. Battegay EJ, Raines EW, Seifert RA, et al. TGF-β induces bimodal proliferation of connective tissue cells via complex control of an autocrine PDGF loop. Cell 1990;63:515.

24. Grotendorst GR, Seppa HEJ, Kleinman HK, et al. Attachment of smooth muscle cells to collagen and their migration toward platelet derived growth factor. Proc Natl Acad Sci USA 1981;78:3669.

25. Jackson CL, Reidy MA. Basic fibroblast growth factor: its role in the control of smooth muscle cell migration. Am J Pathol 1993;143:1024.

26. Kielty CM, Hopkinson I, Grant ME. Collagen: the collagen family: structure, assembly, and organization in the extracellular matrix. In: Royce PM, Steinmann B, eds. Connective Tissue and its Heritable Disorders. Molecular, Genetic, and Medical Aspects. New York, NY: Wiley Liss, 1993:103.

27. van der Rest M, Garrone R. Collagen family of proteins. FASEB J 1991;5:2814.

28. Barnes MJ. Collagens in atherosclerosis. Collagen Rel Res 1985;5:65.

29. Fleischmajer R, MacDonald ED, Perlish JS, et al. Dermal collagen fibrils are hybrids of type I and type III collagen molecules. J Struct Biol 1990;105:162.

30. Birk DE, Fitch JM, Babiarz JP, et al. Collagen type I and type V are present in the same fibril in the avian corneal stroma. J Cell Biol 1988;106:999.

31. Linsenmayer TF, Bibney E, Igoe F, et al. Type V collagen: molecular structure and fibrillar organization of the chicken al(v) NH2-terminal domain, a putative regulator of corneal fibrillogenesis. J Cell Biol 1993;121:118.

32. Stallcup WB, Dahlin K, Shuttleworth CA. Interaction of the NG 2 chondroitin sulfate proteoglycan with type VI collagen. J Cell Biol 1990;111:3177.

33. Bonaldo P, Russo V, Bucciotti F, et al. Structural and functional features of the α3 chain indicate a bridging role for chicken collagen VI in connective tissues. Biochemistry 1990; 29:1245.

34. Kielty CM, Whittaker SP, Grant ME, et al. Type VI collagen microfibrils: evidence for a structural association with hyaluronan. Journal 1992;118:979.

35. Rosenbloom J. Elastin: an overview. Methods Enzymol 1987;144:172.

36. Sakai LY, Keene DR, Engvall E. Fibrillin, a new 350-kD glycoprotein, is a component of extracellular microfibrils. J Cell Biol 1986; 103:2499.

37. Davis EC. Smooth muscle cell to elastic lamina connections in developing mouse aorta. Role in aortic medial organization. Lab Invest 1993;68:89.

38. Wight TN. Cell biology of arterial proteoglycans. Arteriosclerosis 1989;9:1.

39. Yoshida Y, Sue Y, Okano M, et al. The effects of augmented hemodynamic forces on the progression and topography of atherosclerotic plaques. Ann N Y Acad Sci 1990;598: 256.

40. Naito M, Hayashi T, Kuzuya N, et al. Effects

of fibrinogen and fibrin on the migration of vascular smooth muscle cells in vitro. Atherosclerosis 1990;83:9.

41. Katsuda S, Okada Y, Okada Y, et al. In vitro analysis of arterial smooth muscle cell migration: relationship between cells and extracellular matrix. (Abstract) Circulation 1992; 86(Suppl.)68.

42. Jackson CL, Raines EW, Ross R, et al. Role of endogenous platelet derived growth factor in arterial smooth muscle cell migration after balloon catheter injury. Arterioscler Thromb 1993;13:1218.

43. Campbell GR, Campbell JH. Recent advances in molecular pathology: smooth muscle phenotypic changes in arterial wall homeostasis: implications for the pathogenesis of atherosclerosis. Exp Mol Pathol 1985;42: 139.

44. Thyberg J, Hedin U, Sjolund M, et al. Regulation of differentiated properties and proliferation of arterial smooth muscle cells. Arteriosclerosis 1990;1:96.

45. McCullagh KC, Ehrhast LA. Increased arterial collagen synthesis in experimental canine atherosclerosis. Atherosclerosis 1974; 19:13.

46. McCullagh KA, Balian G. Collagen characterization and cell transformation in human atherosclerosis. Nature 1975;258:73.

47. Katsuda S, Okada Y, Minamoto T, et al. Collagens in human atherosclerosis. Immunohistochemical analysis using collagen type specific antibodies. Arterioscler Thromb 1992;12:494.

48. Ooshima A. Collagen αB chain: increased proportion in human atherosclerosis. Science 1981;213:666.

49. Ehrlich HP, White BS. The identification of αA and αB collagen chains in hypertrophic scar. Exp Mol Pathol 1981;34:1.

50. Minamoto T, Ooi A, Okada Y, et al. Desmoplastic reaction of gastric carcinoma: a light- and electron-microscopic immunohistochemical analysis using collagen type-specific antibodies. Human Pathol 1988;19:815.

51. Murata K, Motoyama T, Kotake C: Collagen types in various layers of the human aorta and their changes with the atherosclerotic process. Atherosclerosis 1986;60:251.

52. Ross R, Wight TN, Strandness E, et al. Human atherosclerosis I. Cell constitution and characteristics of advanced lesion of the superficial femoral artery. Am J Pathol 1984; 144:79.

53. Kielty CM, Lees M, Shuttleworth A, et al. Catabolism of intact type VI collagen microfibrils: susceptibility to degradation by serine proteinases. Biochem Biophys Res Commun 1993;191:1230.

54. Rand JH, Patel ND, Schwarz E, et al. 150-kD von Willebrand factor binding protein extracted from human vascular subendothelium is type VI collagen. J Clin Invest 1991; 88:253.

55. Amento EP, Ehsani N, Palmer H, et al. Cytokines and growth factors positively and negatively regulate interstitial collagen gene expression in human vascular smooth muscle cells. Arterioscler Thromb 1991;11:1223.

56. Okada Y, Katsuda S, Watanabe H, et al. Collagen synthesis of human arterial smooth muscle cells: effects of platelet-derived growth factor, transforming growth factor-β1 and interleukin-1. Acta Pathol Jpn 1993; 43:160.

57. Okada Y, Katsuda S, Matsui Y, et al. The modulation of collagen synthesis in cultured arterial smooth muscle cells by platelet-derived growth factor. Cell Biol Int Rep 1992; 16:1015.

58. Jaeger E, Rust S, Roessner A, et al. Joint occurrence of collagen mRNA containing cells and macrophages in human atherosclerotic vessels. Atherosclerosis 1991;31:55.

59. Murphy G, Reynolds JJ. Extracellular matrix degradation. In: Royce PM, Steinmann B, eds. Connective Tissue and its Heritable Disorders. Molecular, Genetic and Medical Aspects. New York, NY: Wiley Liss, 1993:287.

60. Woessner JF. Matrix metalloproteinases and their inhibitors in connective tissue remodeling. FASEB J 1991;5:2145.

61. Tanaka K, Sueshi K. Biology of disease. The coagulation and fibrinolysis systems and atherosclerosis. Lab Invest 1993;69:5.

62. Katsuda S, Okada Y, Nakanishi I. Abnormal accumulation of elastin associated microfibrils during elastolysis in the arterial wall. Exp Mol Pathol 1990;52:13.

63. Liu J, Davidson JM. The elastogenic effect of recombinant transforming growth factor-beta on porcine aortic smooth muscle cells. Biochem Biophys Res Commun 1988;154: 895.

64. Badesch DB, Lee PDK, Parks WC, et al. Insulin-like growth factor 1 stimulates elastin synthesis by bovine pulmonary arterial smooth muscle cells. Biochem Biophys Res Commun 1989;160:382.

65. Tokimitsu I, Tajima S, Nishikawa T. Preferential inhibition of elastin synthesis by epidermal growth factor in chick aortic smooth muscle cells. Biochem Biophys Res Commun 1990;168:850.

66. Okada Y, Katsuda S, Okada Y, et al. An elas-

tinolytic enzyme detected in the culture medium of human arterial smooth muscle cells. Cell Biol International 1993;17:863.

67. Katsuda S, Okada Y, Okada Y, et al. 92-kDa gelatinase/type IV collagenase can degrade elastin of arterial wall. (Abstract) Circulation 1993;88:I-620.

68. Watanabe H, Nakanishi I, Yamashita K, et al. Matrix metalloproteinase-9 (92-kDa gelatinase/type IV collagenase) from U937 monoblastoid cells: correlation with cellular invasion. J Cell Sci 1993;104:991.

69. Kramsch DM, Franzblau C, Hollander W. The protein and lipid composition of arterial elastin and its relationship to lipid accumulation in the atherosclerotic plaque. J Clin Invest 1971;50:1666.

70. Helin P, Lorenzen I, Garbarsch C, et al. Repair in arterial tissue: morphological and biochemical changes in rabbit aorta after a single dilatation injury. Circ Res 1971;29:542.

71. Ruoslahti E, Yamaguchi Y. Proteoglycans as modulators of growth factor activities. Cell 1991;64:867.

72. Galis ZS, Alavi MZ, Moore S. Co-localization of aortic apoprotein B and chondroitin sulfate in an injury model of atherosclerosis. Am J Pathol 1993;142:1432.

Chapter 15

Proteinases and Inhibitors
in Aortic Aneurysms

G. Scott Herron, Ph.D., M.D., Elaine N. Unemori, Ph.D.,
Ronald J. Stoney, M.D.

Abdominal Aortic Aneurysms

A Multifactorial Disease

Abdominal aortic aneurysms (AAA) occur when mechanical and hemodynamic forces deform and irreversibly dilate a structurally altered infrarenal aortic wall. A unifying hypothesis linking these processes to the pathogenesis of AAA, however, remains unsettled.

The atherosclerotic process,[1,2] age-related degenerative and adaptive changes of the aortic wall,[3–5] smoking,[6,7] inflammatory reactions[8,9] and heritable connective tissue metabolic defects[10–12] all may contribute to "acquired" or "nonspecific" AAA disease. However, one factor that is central to all these processes involves the control of aortic connective tissue degradation, particularly during the initial pathogenic insult but also in the mid and end-stage repair response.

AAA disease is characterized by destruction of the aortic wall microarchitecture. The regularly arranged lamellar and fibromuscular units comprising aortic media are fragmented and reduced to a thin sclerotic shell.[13] This layer, nearly devoid of smooth muscle, separates a thrombosed, atherosclerotic lumen from an invariably inflammatory, fibrotic adventitia containing a vigorous neovascular component. These histologic changes represent the end point of a multifactorial disease process that be-

lies complex cellular and molecular events in AAA disease.

It is the active remodeling process of the aortic wall and ongoing inflammation that implicate matrix-degrading proteinases as paramount in AAA disease. The purpose of this chapter is to review the current state of knowledge concerning extracellular matrix degradation in AAA and present evidence that both normal repair or "adaptive" mechanisms in combination with immune-mediated tissue destruction appear to play important roles in AAA disease.

Matrix Metabolism in AAA

The strength and elasticity of the aortic wall are provided for by the two most abundant structural proteins of the aorta, the interstitial collagens and elastin. Together with vascular smooth muscle cells these components are arranged in lamellar units that define the major structural support of the aortic wall.[14] Destruction of these units has focused attention on hydrolytic enzymes and changes in the biochemical composition of normal and diseased aortic wall. Little is known, however, about repair responses in the adult human aorta and whether it has the capacity to reform lamellar units. Furthermore, it is unknown whether the mechanism(s) of AAA rupture represents an end-stage outcome AAA dilation or if a specific pathological process precipitates this grave event.[15]

From Weber KT, MD *Wound Healing in Cardiovascular Disease*, Armonk, NY, Futura Publishing Company Inc., © 1995.

Loss of collagen and elastin was originally described by Sumner, et al. who showed AAA tissues contain marked decreases in the concentrations of both collagen and elastin.[16] It is now clear, however, that simple "loss" of these proteins does not explain the complexity of aortic matrix metabolism in AAA disease. There is ample evidence for compensatory synthesis and accumulation of both collagen and elastin during AAA expansion.[17] The concept of a balance between matrix synthesis and degradation favoring the latter, therefore, includes the notion that provisional and replacement matrix components do not maintain the tensile strength of the aorta in the proteolytic environment of AAA tissue.

Elastic Tissue

It is now generally agreed that elastic tissue failure is the primary event that results in aortic wall dilation seen in AAA.[13,18–22] Exactly what elastic tissue "failure" means at the molecular level in AAA disease remains to be shown, as controversy exists regarding the initial site of elastin degradation within the aortic wall, the initial enzyme species responsible, the cell type(s) involved in this elastolysis, the effects of microfibrillar protein metabolism, and the role of compensatory elastin synthesis in the process of continued dilation.

Turnover of elastin within the uninjured adult aorta is negligible, however, AAA disease is characterized by a tenfold decrease in insoluble elastin concentration (normalized to total protein) relative to undiseased aorta.[23] This apparent depletion is caused by "dilution" of elastin with other matrix proteins synthesized within the aneurysm wall.[16] Although collagen synthesis increases, its deposition is not enough to explain this dilution effect and the identity of the majority of these other matrix proteins is currently unknown (see below).[17]

Minor components of aortic elastic tissue have received increasing attention in aneurysmal disease, particularly with respect to arteriomegaly and multiple aneurysms. Marked increases in elastic microfibrillar proteins were found in AAA tissues and this finding has been observed in other wounded vascular tissues.[23,24] These proteins may constitute the "other" category of matrix components responsible for apparent depletion of elastin seen in AAA tissue.[17]

Abnormalities in a specific microfibrillar protein, fibrillin, have been found in Marfan syndrome patients and it is now known that the FBN1 gene on chromosome 15q21.1 is the locus for mutations that result in a spectrum of connective tissue diseases.[25,26] Aneurysmal dilations of the aorta are characteristic of Marfans, however, it is unknown to what extent "familial" AAAs involve the FBN1 gene[10] or the collagen genes (see below).

Collagens

Experimentally, loss of aortic interstitial collagen results in rapid vessel dilation and rupture[19] and most would agree that ultimately, collagen must fail for an aneurysm to rupture. However, considerable variability in the amount of collagen has been found in AAA tissues.[27–29] Such variability may reflect vascular repair processes at different stages of AAA development,[30] the intensity of inflammation,[31] the subtype of AAA disease examined,[32] aortic tissue sampling, or the reporting of collagen concentration versus content.[17]

Fibrosis of both the neointima/atherosclerotic plaque and the adventitia appears to be responsible for the direct positive correlation that is observed between aneurysm size and collagen content.[17] Changes in the ratio of type I and III collagen have been excluded as a factor in AAA disease.[28,32]

Heritable defects in types I and III collagen resulting in abnormal fibril formation have been found in some families with aortic aneurysms,[12] however, >80% of AAA patients have no familial history of aneurysmal disease.[33] It is possible that mutations will be found in minor collagen genes, particularly those which provide solid state template information for interstitial collagen fibril assembly in different subsets of AAA patients.

To date, little specific information is available on the role of proteoglycan core proteins syndecan, aggrecan, versican, decirin, or their polysaccharide components in AAA disease. Adhesive glycoproteins, such as, tenacin and fibronectin or basement membrane components, particularly laminin isoforms, have not been analyzed in AAA tissues.

Posttranslational Modification

Abnormalities in connective tissue crosslinks, extracellular processing, and fibrillogenesis have been implicated in AAA since the early work of Sandberg, et al.[34] Several animal models have demonstrated the reproducibility of aneurysmal dilation when elastin crosslinking is deficient.[35,36] More recent work has documented, however, that elastin crosslinks are not deficient in human AAA tissue.[23] Other posttranslational modification defects may contribute to the susceptibility of newly secreted collagen and elastin to degradation in AAA tissue,[37–39] although no biochemical proof of this has been reported in the human.

It thus appears that many common pathways of altered aortic matrix deposition and dissolution ultimately result in irreversible dilations of the aorta. The next section details this latter process in infrarenal AAA disease.

AAA Matrix Degradation

Coordinate disassembly of extracellular matrix involves manifold, redundant enzymatic and inhibitor systems.[40,41] In physiological remodeling, matrix degradation is precisely controlled through a combination of proteinase cascade systems,[42] tissue compartmentalization,[43] cell surface, and pericellular localization.[44–46] However, pathological states of matrix degradation, including AAA disease, appear to result from tissue "self destruction," in which cytokines stimulate proteinase synthesis and activation without compartmentalization or physiological dampening by ubiquitous inhibitors.

As detailed below, much is now known about the different types of proteinases and inhibitors present in the walls of both normal and diseased aortas. What remains to be shown in the case of AAA disease is the specific contributions from each cell type present in aortic tissue during the evolution of a normal vessel to an AAA.

Serine Proteinases

Certain connective tissues can be degraded very effectively by two serine proteinase systems, the plasminogen-dependent pathway[44] and the neutrophil serine proteinase pathway.[47] The former appears to mediate degradation of provisional and rapidly remodeling matrices but leaves interstitial collagens intact, while the latter is capable of degrading mature interstitial collagenous tissue, elastic tissue, and basement membrane components.[40,42] Currently, many of the enzymes and inhibitors comprising these two systems have been found in AAA tissues, however, their specific roles are unclear. Table 1 shows these two serine proteinase systems, their cellular sources and identification in AAA tissue.

Historically, Loeven speculated that increased elastase activity may be associated with aging of the vasculature and arterial disease.[48] Experimental evidence for this elastolytic activity was first reported in aortic tissue[49] and serum[50,51] from AAA patients using synthetic peptides as substrates. These "elastase-like" activities were attributed to leukocyte elastase, a 29-kDa serine proteinase present in the azurophilic granules of polymorphonuclear leukocytes.[52] Campa et al.[20] subsequently identified leukocyte elastase as one of the elastolytic activities in both atherosclerotic and aneurysmal aortic wall. The neutrophil serine proteinase, cathepsin G, has not been identified in AAA disease, however, examination for its presence has not been reported.

Plasminogen-dependent serine proteinase have great potential for aortic wall destruction and most of these have been identified in AAA tissue. Substrate gel zymography on casein has identified a major proteinase in AAA tissues at approximately 80-kDa (Figure 1) that is partially blocked by serine proteinase inhibitors, however, most of the activity is not.[53] Tilson and Newman[54] identified plasmin as one of the proteinases contributing to this activity on casein zymograms, with the remaining activity due to activated gelatinase-B/MMP-9.

"Plasminogen activators, u-PA and t-PA, have also been identified in AAA tis-

Table 1

Matrix-Degrading Serine Proteinases		
Name	*Source*	*Found in AAA**
Plasminogen system:		
Plasmin	Serum	Yes; Immunological
Plasminogen Activators		
u-PA	Mesenchymal Cells	Yes; Zymography
	Macrophage, PMN	
t-PA	Mesenchymal Cells	Yes; Zymography
PMN System		
Elastase	PMN	Yes; Immunological
Cathepsin G	PMN	No
Others		
Elastase	Smooth Muscle Cell	Yes; Immunological
Elastase	Pancreas	Yes; Immunological
Tissue Kallikrien	Endothelial Cell	No

* 'Yes' indicates that the protein has been positively identified in AAA tissue either by immunological reactivity and/or by zymography. 'No' indicates that the protein either has not been
specifically tested for in AAA tissue or that it has not been found.

sues.[121] t-PA synthesized by cells of the vascular wall represented the vast majority of both activity and enzyme species present, however, u-PA was also found and interestingly, it was associated with a specific mononuclear cell infiltrate."

Other serine proteinases have been implicated in AAA disease, including pancreatic elastase[55] and smooth muscle elastase.[56] Tissue kallikrien, a very efficient activator of the gelatinase-B/MMP-9, is present in the intima of aortic wall[57] but has not been reported in AAA tissue.

Serine Proteinases Inhibitors

Table 2 shows the major members of serine proteinase inhibitor super family, the Serpins.[58] Cohen and coworkers[59] suggested that AAA disease, like emphysema, involves elastic tissue destruction and therefore is likely to manifest abnormalities in the control of aortic wall elastase activity. Decreases in the levels of α_1 proteinase inhibitor (α_1 PI) have been reported in the serum and in tissue extracts of AAA patients[60] and alterations in the ratio of elastase activity to α_1 PI favoring net elastase activity have been found in ruptured AAAs and in patients with multiple aneurysms.[61]

Although serine elastases have been shown to comprise only a minor component of the total elastase activity of AAA tissue,[20] Mitchell et al. presented the case of a ruptured mesenteric arterial aneurysm in a patient who was homozygous for mutant α_1 PI.[62] Increased expression of type 1 plasminogen activator inhibitor mRNA was observed in severely atherosclerotic aortas, including AAA.[122] The presence of α_2 plasmin inhibitor and the three other plasminogen activator inhibitors have not been reported in AAA tissue. The presence of α_2 plasmin inhibitor and the four plaminogen activator inhibitors have not been reported in AAA tissue.

Metalloproteinases

The matrixins or matrix metalloproteinase (MMP) gene family comprise nine or more zinc-dependent, neutral endopeptidases exhibiting hydrolytic activity against all connective tissue substrates tested. The proteins share structural and sequence homology, as well as, zymogen activation features.[63] They differ, however, in their substrate specificities, inhibitor profiles, and cellular sources (Table 3).

Initial zymographic analysis revealed the presence of at least three of the matrixins in AAA tissues and these include MMP-2,

AORTIC PROTEINASES BY ZYMOGRAPHY

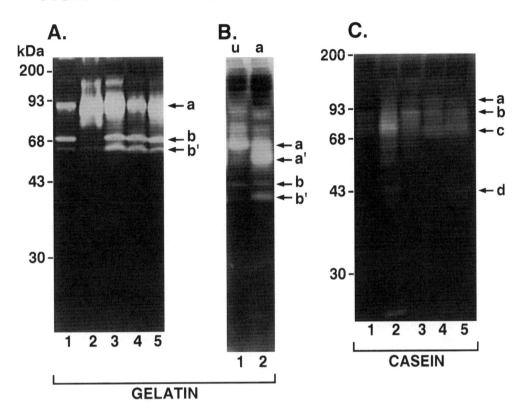

Figure 1. Distribution of proteinases in aortic tissue detergent extracts as revealed by zymography on gelatin (A and B) and casein (C) substrates. In A and C lane 1 represents a normal aortic sample from an accident victim (26-year old) and lanes 2 to 5 represent extracts from four different AAA patients. In B, lanes 1 and 2 represent a single AAA extract before (u, unactivated) and after (a, activated) activation with 10-mM aminophenylmecuric acetate. Molecular weight markers (in kilo-Daltons) are shown at the left of A and C. To the right of each gel are letters indicating the best candidate enzyme species as indicated below. On gelatin (A and B): a = Proenzyme form of gelatinase-B/MMP-9 at 92 kDa; a' = Activated form of gelatinase-B/MMP-9 at 84 kDa; b = Proenzyme form of gelatinase-A/MMP-2 at 72 kDa; b' = Activated form of gelatinase-A/MMP-2 at 66 kDa. On casein (C): a = Proenzyme form of gelatinase-B/MMP-9 at 92 kDa; b = Activated form of gelatinase-B/MMP-9 at 84 kDa; c = Multiplet representing plasmin at 80 kDa and t-PA at 75 kDa—several faint multiplets between 45 and 60 kDa represent various forms of stromelysin/MMP-3; and d = Multiplet representing the two forms of u-PA at 48 and 35 kDa and several other unidentified proteinases between 35 to 45 kDa. Reprinted with permission.[53]

MMP-3, and MMP-9 and their respective activation products (Figure 1). However, one MMP which could not be positively identified in earlier studies was fibroblast type collagenase/MMP-1.[53]

Different extraction conditions used by subsequent workers combined with immunoblotting unequivocally identified MMP 1 in AAA tissues.[64,65] This confirmed several previous reports, dating back to 1980, in which variably increased levels of collagenase activity were found in AAA tissue extracts.[27,39,66,67] Interestingly, degradation products of MMP-1 at 22, 25 and 27-kDa have been identified in AAA tissue extracts that are not found in control aortas.[65] The

Table 2

Serpin Family Serine Proteinase Inhibitors

Name	Activity	Found in AAA*
Alpha-1 Proteinase Inhibitor	Serine Elastases	Yes
Alpha-2 Anti-Plasmin	Plasmin	No
Plasminogen Activator Inhibitors		
PAI-1	u-PA and t-PA	No
PAI-2	u-PA and t-PA	No
PAI-3	Protein C	No
Protease Nexin	u-PA and t-PA	No

* Indicates major inhibitory activity.

† Indicates that the protein has been positively identified by immunologic reactivity in AAA issues.

activity of the 25-kDa species is not blocked by tissue inhibitors of metalloproteinase (TIMP).[68]

Stromelysin/MMP-3,[64] gelatinase-*B*/MMP-9,[53,54,64] and gelatinase-*A*/MMP-2[53] (J.T. Powell, personal communication) have all been identified in AAA tissues by a variety of methods. Gelatinase-A and -B appear to be responsible for most of the MMP activity seen on casein zymograms (Figure 1) and together represent the major metalloelastases of AAA extracts.

Evidence for differential regulation of the two gelatinases in AAA patients comes from our initial observations using aortic biopsies obtained during aneurysmectomy.[53] Aortic extract from the patient seen in lane 2 of Figure 1 shows the absence of gelatinase-*A*/MMP-2, whereas, all other AAA patients we examined and even con-

Table 3

Matrixin Family Metalloproteinases

Name	Abbreviation	MW‡	Substrates§	Found in AAA‖
Fibroblast-Type Collagenase	FIB-CL/MMP-1	57kDa/52kDa	Interstitial Collagens	Yes
PMN-Type Collagenase	PMN-CL/MMP-8	75kDa	same as MMP-1	No
Stromelysin-1	SL-1/MMP-3	60kDa/55kDa	PG Core, Elastin, BMZ/Matrix	Yes
Stromelysin-2	SL-2/MMP-10	60kDa/55kDa	same as MMP-3	No
Stromelysin-3	SL-3/MMP-11	?	?	No
72Kd Gelatinase*	Gel-A/MMP-2	75kDa	Gelatin, same as MMP-3	Yes
92Kd Gelatinase	Gel-B/MMP-9	92kDa	same as MMP-2	Yes
Matrilysin/PUMP-1†	PUMP-1/MMP-7	28kDa	same as MMP-3 and	No
Macrophage Metallo Elastase	MME	53kDa	Elastin	No
Membrane-Type MMP	MT-MMP	66kDa	MMP-2	No

* Other names inlcude Type IV collagenase.

† Other names include Putative Metalloproteinase-1.

‡ Indicates major proenzyme species and their respective glycosylated isoforms.

§ Substrate specificities listed are major categories and do not indicate individual proteins; for more detail please refer to recent reviews (40–42).

‖ Indicates that the protein has been positively identified in AAA tissue by either immunologic reactivity or by zymography.

trol aortic tissue contain this species. Furthermore, there appears to be a marked increase in caseinolytic activity from this same patient centered at approximately 75 to 80-kDa, where activated gelatinase-*B*/MMP-9, t-PA, and plasmin are located. Correlation of this phenomenon with clinical phenotype and inflammation, however, must be addressed in future studies (see below).

Another clue to the differential regulation of the gelatinases in AAA disease comes from our observation that there appears to be a reciprocal relationship between gelatinase-*A*/MMP-2 and gelatinase-*B*/MMP-9 secretion that is correlated with location of the aortic biopsy. We showed that an undilated region of the aorta secretes more gelatinase-*B*/MMP-9 and less gelatinase-*A*/MMP-2 relative to dilated aortic tissue taken from the same patient, using organ culture media and gelatin affinity chromotography.[53]

Perhaps related to the above phenomenon is the observation that the presence of gelatinase-*A*/MMP2 is negatively associated with aneurysm diameter and medial inflammation (J.T. Powell, personal communication). Powell and her colleagues also examined a polymorphic locus, microsatellite mfd24, close to the gelatinase-A/MMP-2 on chromosome 16 and found alterations in DNA sequence in thirty AAA patients relative to thirty controls. The authors hypothesize that early aneurysmal dilation may be mediated by this MMP in genetically susceptible patients and that an immune-mediated clearance of gelatinase-A may be partially responsible for its tissue levels (see below).

Using recombinant TIMP-1 affinity chromatography, Tilson and Newman have identified several cleavage products of gelatinase-*B*/MMP-9.[54] In addition, a 32-kDa caseinase with no crossreactivity to MMPs 1, 3, and 9 was also isolated by this technique but not further characterized. These authors suggest that gelatinase-B is the metalloelastase responsible for initial elastolysis seen in early aneurysmal dilation[69] and believe that a specific monocytic inflammatory cell is the source of this enzyme.[54]

Matrilysin/MMP-7, neutrophil collagenase/MMP-8 and the stromelysin isoforms, MMP-3 and MMP-10 have not been specifically identified in AAA tissues. However, their putative activities as visualized by zymography have been previously reported[53,64,70] and it is likely that many of these will be identified, in variable concentrations and perhaps at different stages of AAA development in diseased tissue from AAA patients.

Metalloproteinase Inhibitors

The tissue inhibitors of metalloproteinases (TIMPs) represent two structurally similar low molecular weight proteins which form essentially irreversible 1:1 complexes with all active MMPs.[71–73] The specificities for TIMP-1 and TIMP-2 differ significantly (Table 4), in that the former seems to inhibit MMP-1 and MMP-3 while the latter is more effective against the gelatinases. In addition, both species bind tightly to the zymogen state of the two gelatinases and modify activation pathways in a complex manner.[74–76] In fact, the control of gelatinase-A activation by TIMPs represent another level of MMP regulation that is just now being realized.[77]

TIMP-1 was originally identified in aortic tissue organ cultures where it was shown to represent over 50% of the total radiolabeled protein secreted by AAA tissue.[53] Increases in the activities several MMPs were noted in AAA tissue extracts after TIMPs were inactivated by reduction and alkylation.[64]

Initial attempts at quantifying the level of TIMP showed decreases in immunoreactive material in AAA extracts versus normal aortic controls.[78] However, this has not been

Table 4

Tissue Inhibitors of Metalloproteinases

Name	Activity	Found in AAA*
TIMP-1	CL/SL > GL	Yes
TIMP-2	GL > CL/SL	No
TIMP-3	?	No

* Indicates that protein has been positively identified by immunologic reactivity in AAA tissues.

repeated and a follow-up study in which TIMP-1 transcripts were evaluated by Northern blotting showed no differences between AAA and control TIMP-1 mRNA expression by fibroblasts under nonstimulated conditions.[79] In addition, these investigators screened six AAA patients for DNA sequence abnormalities and found no restriction site polymorphisms by Southern analysis using TIMP-1 as a probe. However, a C to T transition was detected at the same nucleotide position in 2 of the 6 patients TIMP mRNA. Although the latter point mutation was silent at the protein level, it may be used as an informative marker for linkage studies in the future.

The control of TIMP-1 or TIMP-2 synthesis, secretion, and activity in AAA tissues warrants investigation, however, no reports have addressed these parameters yet; in fact, TIMP-2 has not been identified in AAA tissue. Nolan et al.[80] examined TIMP-1 and TIMP-2 transcript levels in normal human arterial smooth muscle cells in response to various cytokines and found a decrease in TIMP-2 level in response to TNF-α. Interestingly, TIMP-1 can be inactivated by neutrophil elastase[81] which has been identified in AAA tissues.

Finally, the existence of a plasmin-independent, cell surface mechanism for the specific activation of the gelatinase-A/TIMP-2 complex has been shown by several recent studies.[82–84] Its significance in the control of gelatinase-A activity has profound implications for early events in angiogenesis, tumor cell invasion, and tissue remodeling as seen in diseases such as AAA.

α_2 Macroglobulin

This tetrameric serum proteinase inhibitor, synthesized by the liver, inactivates all classes of endopeptidases by a unique "bait and trap" mechanism.[85] It is thought to be confined to the vasculature because of its large size (780-kDa), however, both macrophages and mesenchymal cells have been shown to synthesize α_2M[86,87] and significant tissue penetration occurs during states of inflammation due to capillary leakage. α_2M concentrations in interstitial fluids of inflamed tissues are as much as 100- to 1000-fold greater than TIMP concentrations.[88,89] The fact that collagenase/MMP-1 preferentially binds to α_2M in a mixture of both TIMP and α_2M strongly suggests that α_2M is a key player in the regulation of MMP activity in AAA.[40]

Uptake of α_2M-proteinase complexes by inflammatory cells bearing the α_2M receptor/low density lipoprotein receptor-related protein (LRP) has been shown to have clinical significance in a variety of diseases characterized by connective tissue remodeling.[90] Powell and colleagues have identified α_2M activity in AAA tissue extracts and examined the relationship between gelatinase-A activity and inflammatory infiltrates using KSCN inactivation (J. T. Powell, personal communication). Their results show a negative correlation between the degree of inflammation and gelatinase-A/MMP-2 activity, suggesting that macrophages are clearing AAA tissue of α_2M-gelatinase-A via the α_2M-LRP receptor. This phenomenon may help explain why gelatinase-A activity was absent in one AAA sample as revealed by zymography (Figure 1).

The immunological implications of this receptor-mediated proteinase uptake system involving macrophages in AAA disease could lie in antigen presentation to T cells and immunoglobulin synthesis by B cells. Although no anti-extracellular matrix protein antibodies have been reported in AAA disease, it is conceivable that they are involved in immune-mediated tissue destruction observed in the aortic wall. Additionally, it is known that macrophages can be activated by this same "proteinase-activated" α_2M system, thus providing a local self-amplification cycle of connective tissue destruction.[90]

Localization of Proteinases and Inhibitors

Histochemical and ultrastructural studies have examined the loss of connective tissue within AAA tissue as an indirect means to localize proteolytic activity. While most authors agree that medial elastolysis is the primary event in AAA formation,[18–21] both adventitial elastolysis and collagenolysis appear to be important for continued dilation.[13,17] Medial degeneration is not unique to AAA; atherosclerotic plaques are associated with atrophy and thinning of the media with focal erosions evident beneath plaque debris.[30]

Most of the cells present within AAA tissue have been implicated either in the direct secretion of proteinases and inhibitors or in their mediation of proteinase induction via cytokine networks in AAA tissue. These cells include both large vessel and microvascular endothelial cells,[53] smooth muscle cells,[56] aortic mesenchymal cells,[91] macrophages,[8,54,92–94] leukocytes,[49–51] and T-lymphocytes and B-lymphocytes and plasma cells.[8,31,95]

Most studies directed at localizing proteinases and inhibitors within the aortic wall have utilized vascular "stripping" or anatomical dissection of medial from adventitial tissue. The separated tissues are then extracted and assayed for proteolytic/inhibitory activities either by incubation with various substrates or by zymography. Using a combination of both techniques, the majority of gelatinase-B/MMP-9 was concentrated in the luminal portion of the media, while collagenase/MMP-1 and stromelysin/MMP-3 were found in the adventitia.[64]

To date, only one report has localized proteinases and inhibitors within the aortic wall using immunohistochemical techniques on AAA tissues.[53] Marked staining of both gelatinase-B/MMP-9 and TIMP-1 was localized to vasa vasorum in both the adventitia and media of tissue taken during surgical repair of a 5-cm AAA. High power examination showed the staining associated with the vessels themselves and not inflammatory cells. These findings stand as the only direct evidence for localized secretion of proteinases and inhibitors from noninflammatory cells.

Chronic inflammatory infiltrates consisting of T-lymphocytes, macrophages, and plasma cells distinguish AAA from either normal aorta or atherosclerotic tissue.[8,94] Macrophages play a dominant role in wound repair and pathological tissue remodeling as sources of both hydrolases and cytokines[96,97] and are likely to be the source of several important elastolytic hydrolases

in AAA disease.[54] It is unknown whether truly "inflammatory AAAs"[98–100] and idiopathic retroperitoneal fibrosis are distinct clinical entities or represent the extreme end of the "aortitis" immunological spectrum.[101]

AAA Pathogenesis

Several leading hypotheses defining pathogenic steps in AAA formation include: (1) arterial remodeling in response to atherosclerotic plaque formation[30]; (2) a genetically determined imbalance in serine[56] and/or matrix MMP activities (J.T. Powell, personal communication)[11] and; (3) heritable mutations in specific matrix proteins.[10–12,102] That all three of these theories include shared elements argues in favor of a process that unifies them; inflammatory cell infiltration may be such a process. Hypertension, smoking, and age have been identified as risk factors for AAA development and are likely to exacerbate the fundamental pathogenic processes detailed above.

It should be noted that there are no reports of heritable connective tissue diseases in which mutations have been found in matrix-degrading hydrolases or their promoter elements. However, there are many examples of both dominant and recessively inherited mutations in collagens, elastic tissue associated proteins, adhesive glycoproteins, and their respective posttranslational processing enzymes.[103] More importantly, there is evidence that the "remodeling" or "degradative" phenotype of resident cells within damaged tissue of heritable connective tissue diseases is abnormally expressed, contributing to matrix degradation by highly upregulated proteinase gene transcription.[104] It is possible that this phenotypic response results from abnormal ECM-cell signaling mechanisms generated by mutant ECM.[119,120]

Inflammation is central to AAA pathogenesis and its contribution to matrix remodeling cannot be over emphasized. However, whether it represents a primary event[31,94,101] or is secondary to the chemotactic properties of matrix degradation products and/or local cytokines[56,64,93] remains to be shown.

Role of Medial Neovascularization in AAA

Like other tissues, the vasculature attempts to recapitulate itself in response to damage or wounding. However, unlike other encapsulated organs the cells comprising blood vessels are genetically programmed to "invade" other tissues through the process of angiogenesis.[105] This invasive phenotype manifests early in development, as seen in arterial remodeling in the placenta[106-108] and throughout life during wound healing.[109] Angiogenic disease processes in which new vessels interfere with tissue structure and/or function include diabetic retinopathy and nephropathy, tumor-induced neovascularization, and perhaps atherosclerosis. Connective tissue degrading enzymes secreted by both invading and resident cell types are characteristic of all these processes.[44,77]

New blood vessel growth is well documented in AAA disease, however, the causes and consequences of this process are unclear. Atherosclerotic plaque invariably stimulates an angiogenic response from the vasa vasorum.[110-112] Arterial remodeling in response to vascular wounding stimulates a similar response with intense proliferation of vasa[113,114] and is known to complicate balloon angioplasty. Macrophages, present in large numbers in AAA tissues, are potent inducers of angiogenesis[115] and are the major source of IL-8 and MCP-1 in AAA tissue.[31] Local tissue hypoxia generated by metabolism of inflammatory cells and possibly, ischemia of the vasa caused by increased tangential stress during dilation of the aorta, may stimulate new blood vessel growth.[116]

Medial invasion by capillaries may compromise the structural integrity of the infrarenal aorta, since this segment of the human aorta lacks medial vasa in the normal human adult.[30] Immunolocalization of gelatinase-B/MMP-9 to the vasa vasorum in AAA tissue[53] strongly suggests that secretion of this potent metalloelastase[117] by sprouting capillaries contributes to medial destruction seen in AAA.

Summary and Conclusions

The active remodeling processes observed in AAA disease derive from a complex series of events that cause destruction of aortic wall microarchitecture. The result of this process, irreversible vascular dilation, is a phenotypic response of the vasculature shared by various heritable connective tissue diseases, aging, and by compensatory arterial enlargement observed in response to atherosclerotic plaque or changes in hemodynamics. While the current status of AAA research cannot differentiate the exact contributions made by each of these processes it is nevertheless possible to identify major potential steps in the development of AAA disease. These steps include initial aortic wall elastolysis, inflammation, provisional matrix synthesis and local amplification of proteinase cascade cycles. Repetition of these steps in the infrarenal aortic wall likely results in failure of this tissue due to net matrix degradation.

The majority of basic investigations on AAA disease describe the composition and characteristics of end-stage pathological tissue and therefore, it is difficult to address the issue of primary events. By analogy with other pathological connective tissue processes, however, the combined action of both serine and metalloproteinases and lack of local control by their endogenous inhibitors appears to overwhelm the reparative capacity of the infrarenal aorta.

While considerable progress has been made during the past two decades on the pathogenesis of AAA disease, several important questions remain unanswered. Some of these questions include:

1. What are the sources, location, and types of proteinases responsible for the initial elastolysis observed in early dilation?
2. What is the contribution of the normal compensatory or wound repair mechanisms within the aortic wall to continued dilation?
3. What are the various control mechanisms which limit proteolytic activities within the aortic wall with respect to: (a) zymogen activation pathways; (b) local levels of TIMPs

and Serpins; (c) tissue clearance of activated proteinases by α_2M and its effect on antigen presentation; and (d) cytokine stimulation of proteinase gene expression?
4. What is the effect of medial neovascularization on the tensile strength of the infrarenal aorta? and
5. What is the role of heritable ECM defects in "acquired" or "nonspecific" AAA pathogenesis?

There are few animal models of AAA that duplicate all characteristics of the human disease. The aneurysm-prone mouse,[36] the elastase infusion rat model[18] and the monkey atherosclerotic regression model,[1] serve as excellent systems to test the validity of the steps mentioned above. In addition, the best candidates for either reversion or prevention of arterial enlargement observed in these models appear to be specific proteinase inhibitors. While surgical correction of AAA disease currently offers our only effective means of treatment, the near future holds promise for therapeutic trials of these agents. Specific MMP inhibitors are currently meeting with great success in other human diseases in which the balance of matrix metabolism favors net degradation.

References

1. Zarins CK, Xu C, Glagov S. Aneurysmal enlargement of the aorta during regression of experimental atherosclerosis. Vasc Surg 1992;15:90–101.
2. Reed D, Reed C, Stemmermann G, et al. Are aortic aneurysms caused by atherosclerosis. Circulation 1992;85:205–211.
3. Masuda H, Bassiouny HS, Glagov S, et al. Artery wall restructuring in response to increased flow. Surg Forum 1989;40:285–286.
4. Robert L, Jacob MP, Frances C. Interaction between elastin and elastases and its role in the ageing of the arterial wall, skin and other connective tissues. A review. Mech Aging Dev 1984;28:155–166.
5. Schlatmann TJM, Becker AE. Histologic changes in the normal aging aorta: implications for dissecting aortic aneurysm. Am J Cardiol 1977;39:13–20.
6. Cohen JR, Sarfati I, Wise L. The effect of cigarette smoking on rabbit aortic elastase activity. J Vasc Surg 1989;9:580–582.
7. Auerbach O, Garfinkel L. Atherosclerosis and aneurysm of the aorta in relation to smoking and age. Chest 1980;78:805–809.
8. Koch AE, Haines GR, Rizzo RJ, et al. Human abdominal aortic aneurysms: immunophenotypic analysis suggesting an immune-mediated response. Am J Pathol 1990;137:1199–1219.
9. Pearce WH, Koch A, Haines GR, et al. Cellular components and immune response in abdominal aortic aneurysms. Surg Forum 1991;42:328–330.
10. Berg MA, Tynan K, Aoyama T, et al. Aortic aneurysm in a family with a glycine-to-serine substitution in the FBN-1 gene. [Abstract] Am J Hum Genet 1993;53(Suppl.): 151.
11. Tilson MD, Newman K. Rationale for molecular approaches to the etiology of abdominal aortic aneurysm disease. J Vasc Surg 1992;15:924–925.
12. Kontusaari S, Tromp G, Kuivaniemi, et al. A mutation in the gene for type III procollagen (COL3A1) in a family with aortic aneurysms. J Clin Invest 1990;86:1465–1473.
13. White JV, Haas K, Phillips S, et al. Adventitial elastolysis is a primary event in aneurysm formation. J Vasc Surg 1993;17: 371–381.
14. Wolinsky H, Glagov S. A lamellar unit of aortic medial structure and function in mammals. Circ Res 1967;20:99–111.
15. Swanson RJ, Littooy FN, Hunt TK, et al. Laparotomy as a precipitating factor in the rupture of intra-abdominal aneurysms. Arch Surg 1980;115:299–304.
16. Sumner DS, Hokanson DE, Strandness DE. Stress-strain characteristics and collagen-elastin content of abdominal aortic aneurysms. Surg Gynecol Obstet 1970;130: 459–466.
17. Baxter BT, Halloran BG. Matrix protein metabolism in abdominal aortic aneurysms. In: Yao JST, Pearse WH, eds. Aneurysms: New Findings and Treatments. Norwalk, Conn: Appleton & Lange, 1994:25–34.
18. Anidjar S, Salzman JL, Gentric D. Elastase-induced experimental aneurysms in rats. Circulation 1990;82:973–981.
19. Dobrin PB, Baker WH, Gley WC. Elastolytic and collagenolytic studies of arteries. Arch Surg 1984;119:405–409.
20. Campa JS, Greenhalgh RM, Powell JT. Elastin degradation in abdominal aortic aneurysms. Atherosclerosis 1987;65:13–21.
21. Reilly JM, Brophy CM, Tilson MD. Characterization of an elastase from aneurysmal aorta which degrades intact aortic elastin. Ann Vasc Surg 1992;6:499–502.

22. Powell JT. Dilation through loss of elastin. In: Greenhalgh RM, Mannick JA, eds. The Cause and Management of Aneurysms. Philadelphia, Pa: Saunders, 1990:89–96.

23. Baxter BT, McGee GS, Shively VP, et al. Elastin content, cross-links, and mRNA in normal and aneurysmal human aorta. J Vasc Surg 1992;16:192–200.

24. Katsuda S, Yoshikatsu O, Nakanishi I. Abnormal accumulation of elastin-associated microfibrils during elastolysis in the arterial wall. Exp Mol Pathol 1990;52:13–24.

25. Dietz HC, McIntosh I, Sakai LY, et al. Four novel FBN-1 mutations: significance for mutant transcript level and EGF-like domain calcium binding in the pathogenesis of Marfan syndrome. Genomics 1993;17: 468–475.

26. Francke U, Furthmayr H. Genes and gene products involved in Marfan syndrome. Sem Thorac Cardiovasc Surg 1993;5:3–10.

27. Menashi S, Campa JS, Greenhalgh RM, et al. Collagen in abdominal aortic aneurysm: typing, content and degradation. J Vasc Surg 1987;6:578–582.

28. Rizzo RJ, McCarthy WJ, Dixit SN, et al. Collagen types and matrix protein content in human abdominal aortic aneurysms. J Vasc Surg 1989;10:365–373.

29. McGee GS, Baxter BT, Shively VP, et al. Aneurysm or occlusive disease: factors determining the clinical course of atherosclerosis of the infrarenal aorta. Surgery 1991;110: 370–376.

30. Zarins CK, Glagov S. Atherosclerotic process and aneurysm formation. In: Yao JST, Pearse WH, eds. Aneurysms: New Findings and Treatments. Norwalk, Conn: Appleton & Lange, 1994:35–48.

31. Koch AE, Kunkel SL, Pearse WH, et al. Enhanced production of the chemotactic cytokines interleukin-8 and monocyte chemoattractant protein-1 in human abdominal aortic aneurysms. Am J Pathol 1993;142: 1423–1431.

32. Powell J, Greenhalgh RM. Cellular, enzymatic, and genetic factors in the pathogenesis of abdominal aortic aneurysms. J Vasc Surg 1989;9:297.

33. Anidjar S, Kieffer E. Pathogenesis of acquired aneurysms of the abdominal aorta. Ann Vasc Surg 1992;6:298–305.

34. Sandberg LB, Hackett TN, Carnes WH. The solubilization of an elastin-like protein from copper-deficient porcine aorta. Biochim Biophys Acta 1969;181:201.

35. Boucek RJ, Gunja-Smith Z, Nobel NL, et al. Modulation by propanolol of the lysyl cross-links in aortic elastin and collagen of the aneurysm-prone, mottled mouse. Biochem Pharmacol 1983;32:275–280.

36. Rowe DW, McGoodwin EB, Martin GR, et al. Decreased lysyl oxidase activity in the aneurysm-prone, mottled mouse. J Biol Chem 1977;252:939–942.

37. Sakalihasan N, Heyers A, Nusgens BV, et al. Modifications of the extracellular matrix of aneurysmal abdominal aortas as a function of their size. Eur J Vasc Surg 1993;7: 633–637.

38. Tilson MD. Histochemistry of aortic elastin in patient with non-specific aortic aneurysmal disease. Arch Surg 1988;123:503–505.

39. Webster MW, McAuley CE, Steed DL, et al. Collagen stability and collagenolytic activity in the normal and aneurysmal human abdominal aorta. Am J Surg 1991;161: 635–638.

40. Birkedal-Hansen H, Moore WGI, Bodden MK, et al. Matrix metalloproteinases: a review. Crit Rev Oral Biol Med 1993;4: 197–250.

41. Matrisian LM. Metalloproteinases and their inhibitors in matrix remodeling. Trends Genet 1990;6:121.

42. Murphy G, Reynolds JJ. Extracellular matrix degradation. In: Royce PM, Steinmann B, eds. Connective Tissue and Its Heritable Disorders. New York, NY: Wiley-Liss, 1993: 287–316.

43. Unemori EN, Bouhana KS, Werb Z. Vectorial secretion of extracellular matrix proteins, matrix degrading proteinases, and tissue inhibitor of metalloproteinases by endothelial cells. J Biol Chem 1990;265: 445–451.

44. Moscatelli D, Rifkin DB. Membrane and matrix localization of proteinases: a common theme in tumor cell invasion and angiogenesis. Biochim Biophys Acta 1988;948: 67–85.

45. Monsky WL, Kelly T, Lin C, et al. Binding and localization of 72kDa matrix metalloproteinase at cell surface invadopodia. Cancer Res 1993;53:3159–3164.

46. Moser TL, Enghild JJ, Pizzo SV, et al. The extracellular matrix proteins laminin and fibronectin contain binding domains for human plasminogen and tissue plasminogen activator. J Biol Chem 1993;268: 18917–18923.

47. Weiss SJ. Tissue destruction by neutrophils. N Engl J Med 1989;320:365–376.

48. Loeven WA. Elastolytic enzymes in the arterial wall. J Atheroscl 1969;9:35–45.

49. Busuttil RW, Rinderbreicht H, Flesher A, et al. Elastase activity: the role of elastase in

aortic aneurysm formation. J Surg Res 1982; 32:214–217.

50. Cannon DJ, Read RC. Blood elastolytic activity in patients with aortic aneurysm. Ann Thorac Surg 1982;32:214–217.

51. Brown SL, Backstrom B, Busuttil FW. A new serum proteolytic enzyme in aneurysm pathogenesis. J Vasc Surg 1982;2: 393–399.

52. Travis J. Structure, function, and control of neutrophil proteinases. Am J Med 1988;84: 37–42.

53. Herron GS, Unemori E, Wong M, et al. Connective tissue proteinases and inhibitors in abdominal aortic aneurysms. Arterioscler Thromb 1991;11:1667–1677.

54. Tilson MD, Newman KA. Proteolytic mechanisms in the pathogenesis of aortic aneurysms. In: Yao JST, Pearse WH, eds. Aneurysms: New Findings and Treatments. Norwalk, Conn: Appleton & Lange, 1994:3–10.

55. Dubick MA, Hunter GC, Perez-Lizano E, et al. Assessment of the role of pancreatic proteases in human abdominal aortic aneurysms and occlusive disease. Clin Chem Acta 1988;177:1–10.

56. Cohen JR, Sarfati I, Danna D, et al. Smooth muscle cell elastase, atherosclerosis and abdominal aortic aneurysms. Ann Surg 1992; 216:327–330.

57. Menashi S, Desrivieres S. Activation of the 92kDa collagenase by tissue kallikrein. In: Inhibition of Matrix Metalloproteinases: Therapeutic Potential. Tampa, Fla: New York Academy of Sciences & Long Island Jewish Medical Center, 1994:40.

58. Carrell RW, Barwell DR. Serpins: the superfamily of plasma serine proteinase inhibitors. In: Barrett AJ, Salvesen G, eds. Proteinase Inhibitors. Amsterdam: Elsevier, 1986: 403–420.

59. Cohen JR, Mandell C, Margolis I, et al. Altered aortic protease and antiprotease activity in patients with ruptured abdominal aortic aneurysms. Surg Gynecol Obstet 1987;164:355–358.

60. Cohen JR, Mandell C, Chang JB, et al. Elastin metabolism of the infrarenal aorta. J Vasc Surg 1988;7:210–214.

61. Cohen JR, Sarfati I, Ratner L, et al. Alpha 1-antitrypsin phenotypes in patients with abdominal aortic aneurysms. J Surg Res 1990;49:319–321.

62. Mitchell MB, McAnena OJ, Rutherford RB. Ruptured mesenteric artery aneurysm in a patient with alpha 1-antitrypsin deficiency: etiologic implications. J Vasc Surg 1993;17: 420–424.

63. Woessner JF Jr. Matrix metalloproteinases and their inhibitors in connective tissue remodeling. FASEB J 1991;5:2145–2154.

64. Vine N, Powell JT. Metalloproteinases in degenerative aortic disease. Clin Sci 1991; 81:233–239.

65. Irizarry E, Newman RM, Gandhi RH, et al. Demonstration of interstitial collagenase in abdominal aortic aneurysm disease. J Surg Res 1993;54:571–574.

66. Busuttil RW, Abou-Zam-zam AM, Machleder HI. Collagenase activity of the human aorta: a comparison of patients without abdominal aortic aneurysms. Arch Surg 1980;115:1373–1378.

67. Zarins CK, Runyon-Hass A, Zatina MA, et al. Increased collagenase activity in early aneurysmal dilatation. J Vasc Surg 1986;3: 238–248.

68. Clark IM, Cawston TE. Fragments of human fibroblast collagenase: purification and characterization. Biochem J 1989;263: 201–206.

69. Nackman GB, Halpern V, Gandhi R, et al. Induction of endogenous proteinases and alterations of extracellular matrix in a rat model of aortic aneurysm formation. Surg Forum 1991;42:348–350.

70. Brophy CM, Sumpio B, Reilly JM, et al. Electrophoretic characterization of protease expression in aneurysmal aorta: report of a unique 80 kDa elastolytic activity. Surg Res Commun 1991;10:315–321.

71. Cawston TE. Proteinase inhibitors of metallo-proteinases. In: Barrett AJ, Salvesen G, eds. Proteinase Inhibitors. Amsterdam: Elsevier, 1986:589–610.

72. Stetler-Stevenson WG, Krutzch HC, Liotta LA. Tissue inhibitor of metalloproteinase (TIMP-2). A new member of the metalloproteinase inhibitor family. J Biol Chem 1989;264:17374–17378.

73. DeClerk YA, Yean T-D, Ratzkin BJ, et al. Purification and characterization of two related but distinct metalloproteinase inhibitors secreted by bovine aortic endothelial cells. J Biol Chem 1989;264:17445–17453.

74. Goldberg GI, Marmer BL, Grant GA, et al. Human 72-kDa type IV collagenase forms a complex with a tissue inhibitor of metalloproteinases designated TIMP-2. Proc Natl Acad Sci USA 1989;86:8207–8211.

75. Howard EL, Bullen EC, Banda MJ. Regulation of the autoactivation of human 72-kDa progelatinase by tissue inhibitor of metalloproteinase-2. J Biol Chem 1991;266: 13064–13069.

76. Kleiner DE, Tuuttila A, Tryggvason K, et al. Stability analysis of latent and active 72-kDa collagenase: the role of tissue inhibitor

of metalloproteinases-2 (TIMP-2). Biochemistry 1993;32:1583–1592.

77. Stetler-Stevenson WG, Aznavoorian S, Liotta L. Tumor cell interactions with the extracellular matrix during invasion and metastasis. Ann Rev Cell Biol 1993;9:541–573.

78. Brophy CM, Marks WH, Reilly JM, et al. Decreased tissue inhibitor of metalloproteinases (TIMP) in abdominal aortic aneurysm tissue: a preliminary report. J Surg Res 1991; 50:653–657.

79. Tilson MD, Reilly JM, Brophy CM, et al. Expression and sequence of the gene for tissue inhibitor of metalloproteinases in patients with abdominal aortic aneurysms. J Vasc Surg 1993;18:266–270.

80. Nolan KD, Mesh CL, Shively VP, et al. Cytokines modulate matrix metalloproteinase and TIMP gene expression. Surg Forum 1991;42:346–347.

81. Okada Y, Watanabe S, Nakanishi I, et al. Inactivation of tissue inhibitor of metalloproteinases by neutrophil elastase and other serine proteinases. FEBS Lett 1988; 229:157–160.

82. Murphy G, Ward R, Gavrilovic J, et al. The C-terminal domain of 72 kDa gelatinase A is not required for catalysis, but is essential for membrane activation and modulates interactions with tissue inhibitors of metalloproteinases. Biochem J 1992;283:637–641.

83. Strongin AY, Marmer BL, Grant GA, et al. Plasma membrane-dependent activation of the 72-kDa type IV collagenase is prevented by complex formation with TIMP-2. J Biol Chem 1993;268:14033–14039.

84. Brown PD, Kleiner DE, Unswerth EJ, Stetler-Stevenson WG. Cellular activation of the 72 kDa type IV procollagenase/TIMP-2 complex. Kidney Int 1993;43:163–170.

85. Sottrup-Jensen L. α-Macroglobulins: structure, shape, and mechanism of proteinase complex formation. J Biol Chem 1989;264:11539–11542.

86. Mosher DF, Wing DA. Synthesis and secretion of α-2 macroglobulin by cultured human fibroblasts. J Exp Med 1976;143:462–467.

87. Hovi T, Mosher D, Vaheri A. Cultured human monocytes synthesize and secrete α-2 macroglobulin. J Exp Med 1977;145:1580–1585.

88. Cawston TE, McLaughlin P, Hazleman BL. Paired serum and synovial fluid values of α-2 macroglobulin and TIMP in rheumatoid arthritis. Br J Rheumatol 1987;26:354–358.

89. Hayakawa T, Yamashita K, Kodama S, et al. Tissue inhibitor of metallo-proteinases and collagenase activity in synovial fluid of human rheumatoid arthritis. Biomed Res 1991;12:169–173.

90. Chu CT, Oury TD, Enghild JJ, et al. Adjuvant-free in vivo targeting. J Immunol 1994; 152:1538–1545.

91. Evans CH, Georgescu HI, Lin CW, et al. Inducible synthesis of collagenase by cells of aortic origin. J Surg Res 1991;51:399–404.

92. Davidson JM, Hill KE, Mason ML, et al. Longitudinal gradients of collagen and elastin gene expression in the porcine aorta. J Biol Chem 1985;260:1901–1908.

93. Brophy CM, Reilly JM, Smith GJW, Tilson ND. The role of inflammation in nonspecific abdominal aortic aneurysm disease. Ann Vasc Surg 1991;5:229–233.

94. Louwrens H, Pearse WH. Role of inflammatory cells in aortic aneurysms. In: Yao JST, Pearse WH, eds. Aneurysms: New Findings and Treatments. Norwalk, Conn: Appleton & Lange, 1994:11–24.

95. Beckman EN. Plasma cell infiltrates in abdominal aortic aneurysm. Am J Clin Pathol 1986;85:21–24.

96. Shapiro SD, Kobayashi DK, Pentland AP, et al. Induction of macrophage metalloproteinases by extracellular matrix. Evidence for enzyme- and substrate-specific responses involving prostaglandin-dependent mechanisms. J Biol Chem 1993;268:8170–8175.

97. Adams DO, Hamilton TA. Macrophages as destructive cells in host defense. In: Gallin JI, Goldstein IM, Snyderman R, eds. Inflammation: Basic Principles and Clinical Correlates. New York, NY: Raven Press, 1992:637–662.

98. Walker DI, Bloor K, Williams G, et al. Inflammatory aneurysms of the abdominal aorta. Br J Surg 1972;59:609–614.

99. Rose AG, Dent M. Inflammatory variant of abdominal atherosclerotic aneurysm. Arch Pathol 1981;105:409–413.

100. Goldstone J, Malone JM, Moore WS. Inflammatory aneurysms of the abdominal aorta. Surgery 1978;83:425–430.

101. Ramshaw AL, Parums DV. The distribution of adhesion molecules in chronic periaortitis. Histopathology 1994;24:23–34.

102. Francke U, Furthmayr H. Marfan's syndrome and other disorders of fibrillin. N Engl J Med 1994;330:1384–1385.

103. Beighton P. Molecular nosology of heritable disorders of connective tissue. In: Beighton P, ed. McKusick's Heritable Disorders of Connective Tissue. Fifth ed. St. Louis, Mo: Mosby, 1993:699–716.

104. Unemori EN, Mauch C, Hoeffler W, et al. Constitutive activation of the collagenase promoter in recessive dystrophic epidermolysis bullosa fibroblasts: role of endogenously activated AP-1. Exp Cell Res 1994; 211:212–218.

105. Folkman J, Shing Y. Angiogenesis. J Biol Chem 1992;267:10931–10934.

106. Fernandez PL, Merino MJ, Nogales FF, et al. Immunohistochemical profile of basement membrane proteins and 72 kDa type IV collagenase in the implantation placental site. Lab Invest 1992;66:572–579.

107. Strickland S, Richards WG. Invasion of the trophoblasts. Cell 1992;71:355–357.

108. Enders AC, King BF. Early stages of trophoblastic invasion of the maternal vascular system during implantation in the macaque and baboon. Am J Anat 1991;192:329–346.

109. Banda MJ, Howard EW, Herron GS, et al. Regulation of connective tissue turnover by metalloproteinase inhibitors. In: Janssen H, Rooman R, Robertson JIS, eds. Wound Healing. Petersfield: Wrightson, 1991: 61–70.

110. Heistad DD, Armstrong ML, Marcus ML. Hyperemia of the aortic wall in atherosclerotic monkeys. Circ Res 1981;48:669–675.

111. Kahlon R, Shapero J, Gotlieb AI. Angiogenesis in atherosclerosis. Can J Cardiol 1992; 8:60–64.

112. Bo WJ, Mercuri M, Tucker R, et al. The human carotid atherosclerotic plaque stimulates angiogenesis on the chick chorioallantoic membrane. Atherosclerosis 1992;94: 71–78.

113. Zollikofer CL, Redha FH, Bruhlmann WF, et al. Acute and long-term effects of massive balloon dilation on the aortic wall and vasa vasorum. Radiology 1987;164:145–149.

114. Edelman ER, Nugent MA, Smith LT, et al. Basic fibroblast growth factor enhances the coupling of intimal hyperplasia and proliferation of the vasa vasorum in injured rat arteries. J Clin Invest 1992;89:465–473.

115. Sunderkotter C, Steinbrink K, Goebeler M, et al. Macrophages and angiogenesis. J Leukoc Biol 1994;55:410–422.

116. Knighton DR, Hunt TK, Scheuenstuhl H, et al. Oxygen tension regulates the expression of angiogenesis factor by macrophages. Science 1983;221:1283–1285.

117. Senior RM, Griffin GL, Fliszar CJ, et al. Human 92 and 72 kDa type IV collagenases are elastases. J Biol Chem 1991;266: 7870–7875.

118. Greenwald RA, Golub LM. Closing remarks. In: Greenwald RA, Golub LM, eds. Inhibition of Matrix Metalloproteinases: Therapeutic Potential. Tampa, Fla: New York Academy of Sciences, 1994.

119. Hynes RO. Integrins: versatility, modulation, and signaling in cell adhesion. Cell 1992;69:11–25.

120. Damsky CH, Werb Z. Signal transduction by integrin receptors for extracellular matrix: cooperative processing of extracellular information. Curr Opin Cell Biol 1992;4: 772–781.

121. Reilly J, Sicard G, Lucore C. Abnormal expression of plasminogen activators in aortic aneurysmal and occlusive disease. J Vasc Surg 1994;19:865–872.

122. Schneiderman J, Sawdey MS, Keeton MR, et al. Increased type 1 plasminogen activator inhibitor gene expression in atherosclerotic human arteries. Proc. Natl. Acad. Sci. USA, 1992;89:6998–7002.

Chapter 16

Circulating Hormones of the Renin-Angiotensin-Aldosterone System and Myocardial Fibrosis in Left Ventricular Hypertrophy

Christian G. Brilla, M.D., Ph.D., Karl T. Weber, M.D.

Abstract Summary

Based on epidemiologic findings of the Framingham heart study, left ventricular hypertrophy (LVH) is the major risk factor associated with the appearance of symptomatic heart failure. However, it is not the growth of cardiac myocytes that appears to be responsible for an abnormal structural remodeling of the hypertrophied heart leading to pathological LVH. Instead, nonmyocyte cells, whose behavior and growth are under control of growth factors including circulating hormones of the renin-angiotensin-aldosterone system (RAAS), are important.

This has been demonstrated in in vivo studies of experimental hypertension, where an abnormal fibrous tissue response was found in states of an activated RAAS in both the hypertensive, hypertrophied left ventricle as well as the normotensive, non-hypertrophied right ventricle. In contrast, no myocardial fibrosis was found in either ventricle when the RAAS was not stimulated despite comparable degrees of arterial hypertension and LVH. These findings suggest that a circulating hormone of the RAAS, which gained access to the common coronary circulation of the ventricles, was involved in the regulation of the myocardial collagen matrix. This hypothesis has been confirmed in various animals models in which plasma concentrations of angiotensin II (AngII) and aldosterone (ALDO) were varied. Based on morphological and biochemical findings it can be concluded that arterial hypertension (i.e., an elevation in coronary perfusion pressure), together with elevated circulating AngII or ALDO, are associated with cardiac fibroblast activation and the resultant development of reactive interstitial and perivascular fibrosis that occurs within the normal connective tissue structures of the myocardium irrespective of cardiac myocyte necrosis and scarring. Subsequently, this hypothesis has been tested in in vitro studies using cultured, adult, rat cardiac fibroblasts where collagen synthesis normalized to total protein synthesis was increased by AngII or ALDO in a dose-dependent manner and under serum free conditions. In addition, matrix metalloproteinase 1 (MMP-1) activity, which is the key enzyme of collagen degradation, could be suppressed by AngII. In contrast, MMP-1 activity was not altered by ALDO. Thus, the net effect of either effector hormone of the RAAS on adult cardiac fibroblasts is collagen accumulation.

[1] This work was supported in part by NIH Grant #R01-HL-31701 and Deutsche Forschungsgemeinschaft Grant #Br1029–1.

From Weber KT, MD *Wound Healing in Cardiovascular Disease*, Armonk, NY, Futura Publishing Company Inc., © 1995.

In various forms of acquired and genetic arterial hypertension, where the circulating or tissue RAAS are respectively activated, these hormonal systems determine whether myocardial structure will be altered in that myocardial failure will develop due to progressive fibrosis. Accordingly, suppression of the RAAS by either chronic angiotensin-converting enzyme (ACE) inhibition or ALDO receptor antagonism has shown that myocardial fibrosis of the hypertensive heart can be prevented or even regressed.

Introduction

According to the longitudinal study, conducted over the past three decades in Framingham, Massachusetts, left ventricular hypertrophy (LVH) is the primary risk factor associated with the appearance of myocardial failure.[1,2] The hypertrophic growth of cardiac myocytes accounts for the increment in myocardial mass and, therefore, for the development of LVH. Why the growth of these muscle cells would prove either adaptive or pathological has been an enigma. One line of reasoning has suggested that it is not the hypertrophic growth of myocytes that is responsible for pathological LVH.[3,4] Instead, pathological LVH has been attributed to the growth and altered behavior of nonmyocyte cells. The subsequent remodeling of myocardial structure they create alters its mechanical behavior leading to diastolic and/or systolic failure and ultimately symptomatic heart failure. Nonmyocyte cells include cardiac fibroblasts, whose growth and enhanced collagen synthesis and/or suppressed collagen degradation are responsible for the accumulation of collagen within the cardiac interstitium, where type I collagen is the major fibrillar component of the extracellular matrix that accounts for myocardial stiffness.

The structural remodeling and accumulation of fibrillar collagen that occurs in different disease states, together with its functional consequences, have been examined in various species.[3-5] In particular, the mechanisms responsible for disproportionate collagen accumulation, or fibrosis, have been addressed[4,6] and the following identi-fied: (1) signals mediating fibroblast and cardiac myocyte growth are largely independent of one another; (2) fibrous tissue accumulation occurs as either a reactive or a reparative process, based on whether or not there is parenchymal cell loss (i.e., myocyte necrosis); and (3) activation of the renin-angiotensin-aldosterone system (RAAS) with elevations in circulating angiotensin II (AngII) and aldosterone (ALDO) is related to the abnormal fibrous tissue response in acquired or genetic arterial hypertension. In contrast, collagen concentration remains normal in the hypertrophied myocardium seen with low-renin states, e.g., in arteriovenous fistula or chronic anemia, as well as with thyroxine[6] or growth hormone administration. This is also the case for an atrial septal defect[7] and when arterial hypertension is created by banding the abdominal aorta below the renal arteries,[8] when renal perfusion is not impaired, and therefore the RAAS is not activated.

In examining the structure of the hypertrophied left ventricle in hypertension it will be difficult to identify the trophic factors responsible for myocyte and nonmyocyte cell growth. This problem is partially resolved by considering that the right and left ventricles are anatomically arranged *in series* and *in parallel* with respect to their common coronary circulation. In the absence of pulmonary venous hypertension due to left heart failure, the right ventricle represents a negative internal control relative to the role of hemodynamic factors, such as elevated ventricular systolic and/or diastolic pressures. Contrariwise, a circulating hormone that may be involved in mediating nonmyocyte cell growth, independent of ventricular pressure, would make the right ventricle a positive internal control in that it too would demonstrate a structural remodeling independent of hemodynamic factors. Furthermore, in vitro studies using cultured adult cardiac fibroblasts, where in addition to hemodynamics other growth factors can be excluded under serum free conditions, are helpful to examine the role of the RAAS effector hormones, AngII and ALDO, on fibroblast-mediated collagen synthesis and degradation and to determine the major role of these circulating hormones in mediating myocardial fibrosis and thereby pathological LVH.

Myocardial Growth and Circulating Hormones

Cell Population of the Myocardium

The myocardium is composed of different cells. Cardiac myocytes are the largest of these cells and occupy 75% of the structural space of the myocardium; these parenchymal cells, however, comprise only one third of all cardiac cells.[9,10] Two thirds of all myocardial cells are nonmyocyte cells: endothelial cells; vascular smooth muscle cells; cardiac fibroblasts, belonging to a family of fibroblast-like cells including pericytes, myofibroblasts and interstitial fibroblasts, which are responsible to both produce and degrade the structural components of the myocardial collagen matrix; and finally macrophages and mast cells, involved in inflammatory processes during a wound healing response to any injury, i.e., hypertension, myocardial infarction, or infective heart disease.

Cardiac fibroblasts are multipotential cells free to move within the cardiac interstitium. Fibroblasts contain the mRNA for type I and type III collagens, the major fibrillar collagens of the myocardium.[11,12] These collagens are involved in the interstitial and perivascular fibrosis of the myocardium[13] and the replacement scarring that follows cell death.[14]

Circulating Hormones and the Myocardium

Circulating hormones (e.g., growth hormone, thyroxine, and norepinephrine) are known to regulate cardiac myocyte growth.[15–17] In addition mechanical conditions (e.g., stretch) also contribute to the growth of cardiac myocytes while myocyte generated AngII may act as an autocrine growth factor released from myocytes in response to stretch or hemodynamic load.[18–20] Whether stretch would also promote the growth of cardiac fibroblasts or enhance their synthesis of collagen, in a manner

analogous to stress-mediated collagen deposition in bone, is uncertain. Mechanical factors would not appear to account for the disproportionate accumulation of collagen that occurs with LVH in some conditions and not others despite comparable elevations in wall stress due to ventricular pressure or volume overload. Myocardial fibrosis was present in renovascular hypertension (RHT) when the RAAS was activated, as measured by its circulating effector hormones, AngII and ALDO[8]; however, it was absent with infrarenal banding when the RAAS was not stimulated,[8] although systemic pressures and subsequent LVH were similar compared with RHT (Figure 1). Likewise, progressive interstitial and perivascular fibrosis occurred in either ventricle in RHT or with chronic exogeneous ALDO administration, i.e., it appeared in the pressure overloaded and hypertrophied left ventricle as well as in the nonoverloaded, nonhypertrophied right ventricle (vide infra). In addition, types I and III collagen gene expression and collagen synthesis are temporally dissociated from the onset of myocyte growth.[21,22] Therefore, trophic factors which mediate myocyte and nonmyocyte (i.e., cardiac fibroblast) cell growth in the myocardium can be independent of one another. Clearly, the increase in cardiac myocyte mass in the athlete's heart or the LVH known to occur with hyperthyroidism are independent of the development of myocardial fibrosis which does not occur in these entities.

Functional Significance of Myocardial Fibrosis

The stress-strain relationship of the myocardium has been used to determine the functional impact of collagen accumulation on systolic and diastolic myocardial stiffness.[23–26] Diastolic stiffness is increased at both 8 and 12 weeks of experimentally induced renovascular hypertension (2-kidney-1-clip model), while the force-generating capacity of the myocardium is enhanced thereby preserving systolic function (e.g., ejection fraction). At 32 weeks, in addition to diastolic dysfunction at rest with elevated left ventricular filling pressure systolic dys-

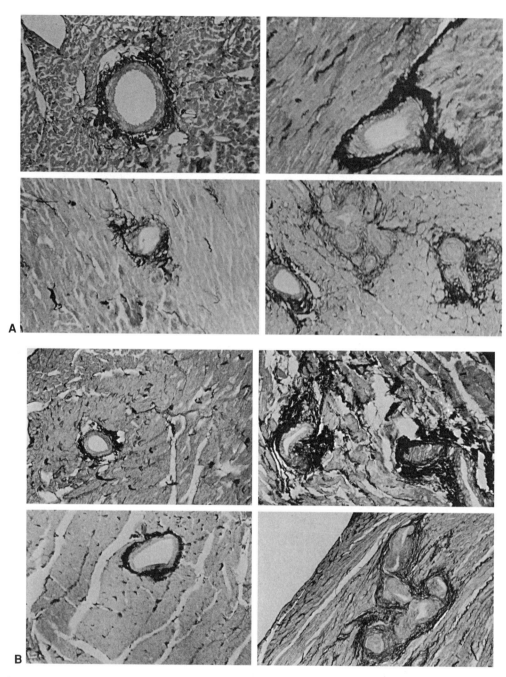

Figure 1. Photomicrographs of picrosirius red stained myocardium under direct light (×40, original magnification). A:) Left ventricle: unoperated control (upper left), renovascular hypertension (RHT, upper right), infrarenal banding (IRB, lower left), and aldosterone administration (ALDO, lower right). Collagen fibers appear black while the media of intramural coronary arteries and myocytes are gray. The normal interstitial collagen and meshwork of collagen surrounding an intramyocardial coronary artery are shown in the upper left panel. With RHT, interstitial and perivascular fibrosis is evident. Such a remodeling of the myocardium was not found with IRB. Following chronic ALDO administration, an interstitial and perivascular fibrosis was seen. B:) Right ventricle: unoperated control (upper left), RHT (upper right), IRB (lower left), and ALDO administration (lower right).

—legend continues on facing page

function with chamber dilatation and reduced ejection fraction appears.[27] Thus, the accumulation of fibrillar collagen is a major determinant of impaired myocardial stiffness and pump dysfunction and its progressive accumulation accounts for ventricular dysfunction that first appears during diastole and subsequently involves systole.

Myocardial Fibrosis and Plasma Angiotensin II

Cardiac Myocyte Necrosis and Reparative Fibrosis

The possibility that elevations in circulating AngII were responsible for cardiac myocyte necrosis[28] was investigated using in vivo antimyosin antibody labeling, a marker of abnormal sarcolemmal permeability and impending myocyte death. Intraperitoneal administration of subhypertensive doses of AngII was used together with this immunolabeling technique. Myocyte labeling was observed within 24 hours of AngII administration, but not thereafter. After continuous AngII administration for 2 weeks, microscopic scarring was seen in the left ventricle on day 14. The amount of scarring, however, involved only a small portion (<1%) of the myocardium and was not found in untreated control animals (unpublished observations).

In renovascular hypertension, where plasma AngII and ALDO are known to be significantly increased,[8] antimyosin labeling was found within 24 hours,[28] but not afterwards. This evidence of parenchymal cell injury was not seen when captopril, an angiotensin converting enzyme inhibitor, was given prior to inducing renal ischemia. Antimyosin labeling, as a marker of myocyte necrosis,[28] and microscopic scarring[29] were not observed when comparable arterial hypertension and LVH were induced by placing a constrictive band on the abdominal aorta below the renal arteries. In this model of nonrenovascular hypertension an elevation in plasma AngII or ALDO does not occur.[8]

Thus, available evidence suggests that elevations in plasma AngII, whether induced by exogenous administration or increased endogenously in response to renal ischemia, are associated with early cardiac myocyte necrosis and a subsequent reparative fibrosis. Initially, the degree of scarring, and by implication the extent of cell loss, however, is modest. After 8 weeks, a larger degree of scarring is evident and may be related to altered myocardial potassium balance. At 12 weeks, and beyond, a reparative fibrosis appears in the endomyocardium in rats with RHT.[30] This much later event may be related to the structural remodeling of intramyocardial coronary arteries with impaired blood flow that eventuate in additional myocyte necrosis.

Reactive Fibrosis

After 8 weeks of RHT,[8] a diffuse interstitial and perivascular fibrosis was seen in both the normotensive, nonhypertrophied right ventricle and the hypertensive, hypertrophied left ventricle. This reactive fibrosis that is not secondary to myocyte necrosis is progressive over time.[24,30]

Because LVH is not always associated with a rise in collagen volume fraction (CVF), despite comparable pressure or volume overload, nonhemodynamic factors, such as circulating hormones, may represent growth stimuli to cardiac fibroblasts. The importance of various hemodynamic factors and circulating hormones on the fibrous tissue response of the rat right and left ventricles was examined in a number of different models of experimental hypertension[8,31] summarized in Table 1. Morphometric evaluation of interstitial CVF, by videodensitometry, was used to quantitate the reactive fibrous tissue response seen in coronal sections of the myocardium pre-

---

The remodeling of interstitial and perivascular collagen in the normotensive, nonhypertrophied right ventricle for the various models of experimental hypertension was similar to that found in the hypertensive, hypertrophied left ventricle, i.e., irrespective of pre- and afterload conditions. With permission from Brilla et al., Circ Res 1990;67:1355.

Table 1

Interstitial and Perivascular Fibrosis of the Rat Right and Left Ventricles in Various Experimental Models With and Without Systemic Hypertension and Hypertrophy

Model	Fibrosis	HT	LVH	AngII	ALDO
RHT	+	+	+	↑	↑
IRB	−	+	+	→	→
AL/1K/high Na⁺	+	+	+	↓	↑
Vehicle/1K/high Na⁺	−	−	+	→	→
RHT + C	−	−	−	→	→
RHT + S(low)	−	+	+	↑	↕
AL/1K/high Na⁺ + S(low)	−	+	+	↓	↕
AL/1K/high Na⁺ + S(high)	−	−	−	↓	↕

RHT, renovascular hypertension (2-kidney-1-clip model); IRB, infrarenal aortic band; AL, aldosterone infusion via subcutaneously implanted osmotic minipumps; 1K, uninephrectomy; high Na⁺, enhanced dietary sodium; C, Captopril; S, spironolactone in variable dosage, low, a small dose that did not prevent hypertension or LVH in RHT or hyperaldosteronism and a larger dose (high) that did; HT, hypertension; LVH, left ventricular hypertrophy; AngII or ALDO, plasma angiotensin II or aldosterone concentrations, respectively; and ↕, aldosterone receptor blockade (with permission; Weber and Brilla, Circulation 83:1849, 1991).

pared with the collagen-specific stain, Sirius Red F3BA. Microscopic scars, differentiated from the interstitial and perivascular fibrosis on the basis of morphological presentation,[29,32,33] were excluded from the analysis. Systolic and mean carotid artery pressures were determined at the time of sacrifice while the presence of LVH was established from the left to right ventricular weight ratio. Right ventricular weight was not found to be different between the various experimental groups and their respective controls. Plasma concentrations of AngII and ALDO were determined by radioimmunoassay.[8]

Comparable levels of systemic hypertension and LVH were observed with RHT, infrarenal aortic banding (nonrenovascular hypertension), and in uninephrectomized animals receiving enhanced dietary sodium plus the mineralocorticoid ALDO. Control animals included a group with previous uninephrectomy receiving a high sodium diet. A diverse profile for plasma AngII and ALDO, outlined in Table 1, was purposefully created with these models in order to dissociate the importance of elevations in ventricular systolic pressure from circulating AngII and ALDO.

In the hypertrophied left ventricle that accompanied RHT or hyperaldosteronism (uninephrectomized animals receiving ALDO plus enhanced dietary sodium), CVF was significantly increased. CVF was also significantly increased in the normotensive, nonhypertrophied right ventricle in these two experimental groups. CVF was not increased in either ventricle in the nonrenovascular model of hypertension with LVH or the normotensive control group with uninephrectomy and enhanced dietary sodium, who did not receive ALDO but where LVH accompanied the circulatory overload. Thus, despite comparable elevations in left ventricular systolic pressure or increments in LV mass in each of these models of experimental hypertension, the fibrous tissue response was associated with an elevation in plasma AngII and/or ALDO. The relative importance of AngII and ALDO to myocardial fibrosis is discussed below. Hypertension alone did not induce myocardial fibrosis. These findings support the view that ventricular loading is the primary determinant of myocyte growth[3,34] while nonmyocyte growth can occur in the absence of myocyte growth, as was the case with myocardial fibrosis appearing in the normotensive, nonhypertrophied right ventricle in RHT and hyperaldosteronism. Furthermore, arterial hypertension associated with infrarenal aortic banding is accompanied by LVH, but interstitial CVF remains normal in the right and left ventricles.

Thus, it would appear that elevations in arterial or coronary perfusion pressure must be accompanied by elevated plasma AngII and or ALDO in order to mediate the fibrous tissue response and elevation in CVF, as seen with RHT and primary hyperaldosteronism.

Myocardial Fibrosis and Plasma Aldosterone

Potassium Metabolism and Reparative Fibrosis

Acute myocyte necrosis, estimated by antimyosin labeling, has not been observed with the administration of ALDO in rats (unpublished data). On the other hand, a modest degree of reparative fibrosis was observed[8,29] in both the right and left ventricles, in uninephrectomized rats receiving ALDO for 8 weeks, together with enhanced dietary sodium. In this model, circulating AngII was suppressed while plasma ALDO was increased to levels comparable to those seen with RHT. In pretreating rats with spironolactone, an aldosterone receptor antagonist, prior to the induction of hyperaldosteronism, it was possible to prevent this scarring.[31] Mineralocorticoid excess for at least 4 weeks leads to myocyte loss and subsequent scarring that has been related to enhanced potassium excretion and reduced potassium in the myocardium where potassium supplementation has been found to prevent myocyte necrosis and subsequent scarring in animals with chronic mineralocorticoid excess.[35]

Reactive Fibrosis

The chronic administration of d-aldosterone in uninephrectomized animals receiving an enhanced dietary sodium, is associated with a perivascular fibrosis, in the myocardium of the right and left ventricles[8] while fibrosis has also been found in the pancreas, adrenals, and other organs.[36,37] An interaction between the mineralocorticoid ALDO and the heart has not been fully considered despite the fact that steroid receptors have previously been identified in homogenates of the myocardium.[38,39] The relative contribution of elevations in plasma AngII and ALDO to the interstitial and peri-

vascular fibrosis seen in both ventricles in the rat with RHT was considered. Captopril pretreatment in RHT, where plasma AngII and ALDO were each suppressed, prevented myocardial fibrosis.[40]

Further evidence in support of the role of elevated plasma ALDO was obtained in rats with either RHT or hyperaldosteronism, who were pretreated with a small or large dose of spironolactone.[31] The smaller dose did not prevent hypertension or LVH, while the larger dose did. Irrespective of the presence of hypertension or LVH, either dose of spironolactone prevented myocardial fibrosis. Thus, in vivo findings in arterial hypertension strongly implicate the importance of circulating ALDO in contributing to the reactive fibrous tissue response.

These studies confirmed that the adverse remodeling of the myocardial collagen matrix occurred also in the right ventricle in the absence of ventricular hypertrophy, or myocyte growth, suggesting that the signals for myocyte and nonmyocyte growth are independent of each other. Ventricular loading determines myocyte growth, while elevations in plasma AngII and ALDO with reduced intracellular potassium mediate a reparative and reactive fibrosis with different pathogenetic mechanisms. This serves to explain why myocardial collagen concentration is increased in RHT, hyperaldosteronism, and low cardiac output myocardial failure due to rapid ventricular pacing,[41] but not with chronic anemia, an arteriovenous fistula, thyroxine or growth hormone administration, an atrial septal defect, or exercise training,[42] where plasma AngII and ALDO each remain normal. In addition, the chronic administration of another mineralocorticoid, deoxycorticosterone, has likewise been associated with the reactive accumulation of fibrillar collagen within the adventitia of intramyocardial coronary arteries and mural vessels of other organs, such as the pancreas and adrenal glands.[43]

Furthermore, it is widely ignored that vascular complications are not rare in patients with hypertension due to primary hyperaldosteronism. In a larger study of 136 cases, 22.8% of these patients developed vascular events, e.g., stroke or myocardial infarction, over a mean observation time of 5.9 years.[44]

Hormone Fibroblast Interaction and Collagen Metabolism

Collagen Synthesis

A specialized cell can quickly respond (e.g., seconds or minutes) to a given stimulus. Contraction, secretion, movement, and altered metabolism are examples of such short-term cellular responses to hormones. Long-term responses require hours to days and include cell division. The influence of various hormones including AngII on short-term and long-term cellular responses has been studied in cultured Swiss 3T3 cells,

a murine fibroblast cell line.[45–48] AngII, that can be generated either within circulating or tissue compartments interacts with cell surface receptors of the fibroblast. A series of intracellular events that follow are likely to involve inositol triphosphate and proteinkinase C-mediated pathways.

In our laboratory, we have focused on the target cell of myocardial collagen turnover, i.e., the cardiac fibroblast from the same species that we used for our above cited in vivo studies. After AngII incubation, total collagen synthesis of adult rat cardiac fibroblasts, measured by ^{3}H-proline incorporation and normalized per total protein synthesis, was increased in a concentration-dependent manner (Figure 2). This increase could be completely abolished by selective type 1 AngII-receptor antagonists, DuP 753 or ICI D8731, respectively.[49]

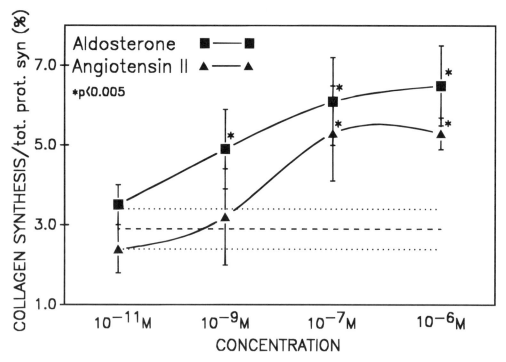

Figure 2. Collagen synthesis measured by ^{3}H-proline incorporation and normalized per total protein synthesis (%) of adult rat cardiac fibroblasts (Fb) in culture at passage 6 to 10 incubated with either angiotensin II (AngII) or aldosterone (ALDO) at different concentrations. A dose-dependent rise in collagen synthesis was found for either hormone compared with untreated control Fb (normal range, mean ± SEM, is indicated). ALDO increased Fb-mediated collagen synthesis at plasma concentrations seen in renovascular hypertension, while higher concentrations of AngII were necessary to raise collagen synthesis, presumably due to simultaneous AngII degradation in culture. With permission from Brilla et al., J Mol Cell Cardiol 1994;26:809.

In contrast to AngII, lower concentrations of aldosterone were needed to significantly increase collagen synthesis (Figure 2). The increase in collagen synthesis mediated by 10^{-9}M ALDO was inhibited by prior incubation with an equimolar concentration of the competitive ALDO receptor antagonist, spironolactone.[50] The twofold rise in collagen synthesis promoted by AngII or ALDO is within the range shown for other stimulated mesenchymal cells, such as normal human skin fibroblasts exposed to serum from scleroderma patients, skin fibroblasts from patients with scleroderma, or human keloid fibroblasts.[51–53] Circulating ALDO is likely to bind to a cytosolic receptor. These short-term effects of ALDO on fibroblasts have not been previously examined and may be explained by the potential presence of high affinity, low capacity steroid receptors to ALDO in cardiac fibroblasts. It has been already shown that the arterial compartment of the vascular system[54] and fibroblasts of the aortic adventitia[55] contain such type I corticoid receptors.[53]

Collagen Degradation

Concentrations between 10^{-11} to 10^{-9}M of AngII had no effect on collagenase or matrix metalloproteinase 1 (MMP-1) activity of cultured adult rat cardiac fibroblast conditioned medium while high concentrations (10^{-7} to 10^{-6}M) significantly decreased MMP-1 activity compared with untreated control cells (Figure 3). This inhibitory effect could be completely abolished by simultaneous incubation with 10^{-5}M of the type II AngII receptor antagonist, PD123177.[50] In contrast, MMP-1 activity remained significantly reduced when fibroblasts were simultaneously incubated with 10^{-7}M AngII and 10^{-5}M DuP 753.[50]

The mineralocorticoid hormone, ALDO, showed no significant effect on MMP-1 activity over the entire range of concentrations (10^{-11} to 10^{-6}M) examined (Fig-

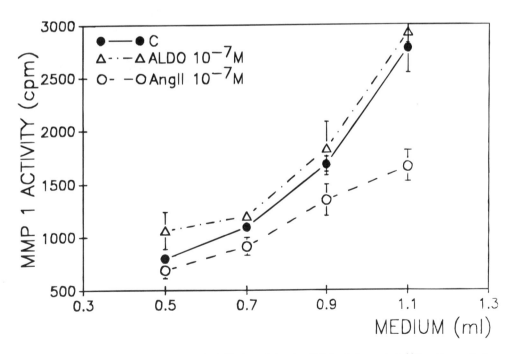

Figure 3. Matrix metalloproteinase 1 (MMP-1) activity in CPM of degraded ^{14}C-collagen/ml medium/mg protein/30 min of adult rat cardiac fibroblasts (Fb) incubated with either 10^{-7}M of angiotensin II (AngII) or aldosterone (ALDO) compared with untreated control Fb (C). ALDO did not effect collagen degradation, while AngII significantly ($P<0.01$) decreased MMP-1 activity.

ure 3). Whether transcriptional, translational, or posttranslational regulatory steps of MMP-1 activity are modulated by AngII is objective of ongoing studies in our laboratory.

Therapeutical Implications

Prevention of Fibrosis

The prevention of arterial hypertension and elevation in circulating AngII and ALDO are logical targets for the prevention of myocardial fibrosis. Our in vivo studies with spironolactone or captopril pretreatment in the rat with either renovascular hypertension or hyperaldosteronism, where it was possible to attenuate the fibrous tissue response suggest that these agents have cardioprotective properties.[31,40] This approach would appear to interrupt the process at the outset of the hormone-mediated response that leads to fibroblast activation.

Regression of Fibrosis

Removal of the interstitial and perivascular fibrosis represents a means by which myocardial failure due to collagen accumulation would be reversible. Agents that would restore myocardial structure to normal and thereby alleviate abnormalities in myocardial stiffness would have cardioreparative properties. The premise of this approach is based on either inhibiting the stimulus to fibrous tissue formation, while retaining the myocardium's proteolytic enzyme system[56,57] for continued gradual collagen degradation, or actively invoking proteolytic digestion for more rapid degradation. At the present time little is known about the regulation of the active or inactive forms of myocardial MMP-1, the key enzyme for collagen degradation. However, Laurent[56] has underscored the fact that it is no longer tenable to view collagen as an inert protein and that its turnover may be more rapid than previously appreciated. In the heart he estimates that collagen degradation may be as high as 5% per day and that a major portion of this proteolysis may occur within lysosomes of fibroblasts. The half-life of collagen which measures be-

tween 80 and 120 days in the normal myocardium has been found to be decreased down to 17 days in the hypertrophied heart.[58]

In two regression trials the angiotensin-converting-enzyme (ACE) inhibitor lisinopril was able to remove excess collagen from the myocardial interstitium. After 12 weeks of lisinopril treatment initially in 14-week-old spontaneously hypertensive rats (SHR) with established LVH, myocardial fibrosis, and abnormal diastolic stiffness, interstitial and perivascular fibrosis could be regressed along with myocardial mass, and myocardial stiffness was restored to values seen in normotensive genetic controls.[59] In advanced hypertensive heart disease in 78-week-old SHR, 32 weeks of lisinopril treatment was able to remove excess fibrous tissue accumulation and to normalize myocardial diastolic stiffness associated with an increase in MMP-1 activity in the myocardium and regression of LVH.[60] In the same study, the development of systolic dysfunction as measured by a significant decrease of the slope of the systolic stress strain relationship of the isovolumetrically beating isolated heart could be prevented by chronic ACE inhibition.[61] Another ACE inhibitor, zofenopril, was likewise able to regress myocardial fibrosis in rats with 2-kidney-1-clip model of renovascular hypertension, while the combined α/β-receptor antagonist labetalol did not.[62] In contrast, in a 45-week treatment trial, the calcium channel blocker verapamil did not reduce collagen concentration or collagen synthesis in initially 10-week-old SHR despite a reduction in LVH and normalization of arterial pressure.[63] Minoxidil, a nonspecific antihypertensive agent, even increased collagen concentration in similarly treated animals. In contrast, Motz and Strauer have reported that 20-weeks treatment with another calcium channel blocker, nifedipine, was able to restore collagen concentration in 20-week-old SHR to values seen in age-matched genetic controls.[64]

These findings indicate that not all agents are associated with an involution in collagen mass. Certain pharmacological agents may therefore prove to have a greater influence on myocardial collagen concentration because of their specific mechanism of action or tissue specificity. The opportunity is at hand to determine which antihypertensive agents have antifibrotic effects and are cardiovascular tissue specific. In so doing, such agents may have the potential to restore myocardial structure and function to normal and eliminate pathological hypertrophy as a major determinant of myocardial failure.[65]

References

1. Kannel WB. Epidemiological aspects of heart failure. In:KT Weber, ed. Congestive Heart Failure. Card Clinics 1989;7:1.
2. Levy D, Garrison RJ, Savage DD, et al. Prognostic implications of echocardiographically determined left ventricular mass in the Framingham heart study. N Engl J Med 1990; 322:1561.
3. Weber KT. Cardiac interstitium in health and disease: the fibrillar collagen network. J Am Coll Cardiol 1989;13:1637.
4. Weber KT, Brilla CG. Pathologic hypertrophy and the cardiac interstitium: fibrosis and the renin-angiotensin-aldosterone system. Circulation 1991;83:1849.
5. Weber KT, Brilla CG, Janicki JS. Structural remodeling of myocardial collagen in systemic hypertension: functional consequences and potential therapy. Heart Failure 1990;6:129.
6. Holubarsch C, et al. Passive elastic properties of myocardium in different models and stages of hypertrophy: a study comparing mechanical, chemical and morphometric parameters. Perspect Cardiovasc Res 1983;7: 323.
7. Marino TA, et al. Structural analysis of pressure versus volume overload hypertrophy of cat right ventricle. Am J Physiol 1985;18: H371.
8. Brilla CG, et al. Remodeling of the rat right and left ventricle in experimental hypertension. Circ Res 1990;67:1355.
9. Zak R. Cell proliferation during cardiac growth. Am J Cardiol 1973;31:211.
10. Frank JS, Langer GA. The myocardial interstitium: its structure and its role in ionic exchange. J Cell Biol 1974;60:586.
11. Eghbali M, et al. Localization of types I, III and IV collagen mRNAs in rat heart cells by in situ hybridization. J Mol Cell Cardiol 1989; 21:103.
12. Medugorac I, Jacob R. Characterization of left ventricular collagen in the rat. Cardiovasc Res 1983;17:15.
13. Weber KT, et al. Collagen remodeling of the pressure-overloaded, hypertrophied nonhuman primate myocardium. Circ Res 1988;62: 757.
14. Whittaker P, Boughner DR, Kloner RA. Analysis of healing after myocardial infarction using polarized light microscopy. Am J Pathol 1989;134:879.
15. Gilbert PL, et al. Cardiac morphology in rats with growth hormone-producing tumours. J Mol Cell Cardiol 1985;17:805.
16. Laks MM, Morady F, Swan MB. Myocardial hypertrophy produced by chronic infusion of subhypertensive doses of norepinephrine in the dog. Chest 1973;64:75.
17. Simpson P, McGrath A, Savion S. Myocyte hypertrophy in neonatal rat heart cultures and its regulation by serum and by catecholamines. Circ Res 1982;51:787.
18. Mann DL, Kent RL, Cooper G. Load regulation of the properties of adult feline cardiocytes: growth induction by cellular deformation. Circ Res 1989;64:1079.
19. Komuro I, et al. Stretching cardiac myocytes stimulates protooncogene expression. J Biol Chem 1990;265:3595.
20. Yamazaki T, et al. Angiotensin II mediates stretch-induced cardiac hypertrophy. (Abstract) Circulation 1993;88:I-474.
21. Lindy S, Turto H, Uitto J. Protocollagen proline hydroxylase activity in rat heart during experimental cardiac hypertrophy. Circ Res 1972;30:205.
22. Chapman D, Weber KT, Eghbali M. Regulation of fibrillar collagen types I and III and basement membrane type IV collagen gene expression in hypertrophied rat myocardium. Circ Res 1990;67:787.
23. Bing OHL, et al. The effect of the lathyrogen B-amino proprionitrile (BAPN) on the mechanical properties of experimentally hypertrophy rat cardiac muscle. Circ Res 1978;43: 632.
24. Doering CW, et al. Collagen network remodeling and diastolic stiffness of the rat left ventricle with pressure overload hypertrophy. Cardiovasc Res 1988;22:686.
25. Jalil JE, et al. Fibrillar collagen and myocardial stiffness in the intact hypertrophied rat left ventricle. Circ Res 1989;64:1041.
26. Brilla CG, Janicki JS, Weber KT. Impaired diastolic function and coronary reserve in genetic hypertension: role of interstitial fibrosis and medial thickening of intramyocardial coronary arteries. Circ Res 1991;69:107.
27. Capasso JM, et al. Left ventricular failure-induced by long term hypertension in rats. Circ Res 1990;66:1400.
28. Tan LB, et al. Cardiac myocyte necrosis in-

duced by angiotensin II. Circ Res 1991;69: 1185.

29. Brilla CG, Weber KT. Reactive and reparative myocardial fibrosis in arterial hypertension. Cardiovasc Res 1992;26:671.

30. Silver MA, et al. Reactive and reparative fibrosis in the hypertrophied rat left ventricle. Cardiovasc Res 1990;24:741.

31. Brilla CG, Matsubara LS, Weber KT. Antialdosterone treatment and the prevention of myocardial fibrosis in primary and secondary hyperaldosteronism. J Mol Cell Cardiol 1993;25:563.

32. Pick R, Janicki JS, Weber KT. Myocardial fibrosis in nonhuman primate with pressure overload hypertrophy. Am J Pathol 1989;135: 771.

33. Weber KT, et al. Patterns of myocardial fibrosis. J Mol Cell Cardiol 1989;21:121.

34. Cooper G. Cardiocyte adaptation to chronically altered load. Annu Rev Physiol 1987; 49:501.

35. Darrow DC, Miller HC. The production of cardiac lesions by repeated injections of desoxycorticosterone acetate. J Clin Invest 1942; 21:601.

36. Hall CE, Hall O. Hypertension and hypersalimentation. Lab Inv 1965;14:285.

37. Campbell SE, Diaz-Arias AA, Weber KT. Fibrosis of the human heart and systemic organs in adrenal adenoma. Blood Pressure 1992;1:149.

38. Funder JW, et al. Mineralocorticoid action: target tissue specificity is enzyme, not receptor, mediated. Science 1988;242:583.

39. Lombes M. Detection of mineralocorticoid receptors in new sites. Abstract Book of the 16th International Aldosterone Conference, Meetings & Events Communications, Evansville, Ind., 1990;5.

40. Jalil JE, et al. Coronary vascular remodeling and myocardial fibrosis in the rat with renovascular hypertension: response to captopril. Am J Hypertens 91;4:51.

41. Weber KT, et al. Fibrillar collagen and the remodeling of the dilated canine left ventricle. Circulation 1990;82:1387.

42. Bartosova D, et al. The growth of the muscular and collagenous parts of the rat heart in various forms of cardiomegaly. J Physiol 1969;200:185.

43. Selye H. The general adaptation syndrome and the diseases of adaptation. J Clin Endo 1946;6:117.

44. Beevers DG, et al. Renal abnormalities and vascular complications in primary hyperaldosteronism. Evidence on tertiary hyperaldosteronism. Quart J Med (N.S.) 1976;179: 401.

45. Rozengurt E. Early signals in the mitogenic response. Science 1986;234:161.

46. Ganten D, et al. Effect of angiotensin and an angiotensin antagonist on iso-renin and cell growth in 3T3 mouse cells. Int Res Commun Med Sci 1975;3:327.

47. Rana RS, Hokin LE. Role of phosphoinositides in transmembrane signaling. Physiol Rev 1990;70:115.

48. Berridge MJ. Inositol triphosphate and diacylglycerol: two interacting second messengers. Annu Rev Biochem 1987;56:159.

49. Brilla CG, Maisch B, Zhou G, Weber KT: Hormonal regulation of cardiac fibroblast function. Euro Heart J 1995;16(Suppl. D):45.

50. Brilla CG, Zhou G, Matsubara L, Weber KT: Collagen metabolism in cultured adult rat cardiac fibroblasts: response to angiotensin II and aldosterone. J Mol Cell Cardiol 1994; 26:809–820.

51. Botstein GR, Sherer GK, Leroy EC. Fibroblast selection in scleroderma: an alternative model of fibrosis. Arthritis and Rheumatism 1982;25:189.

52. Uitto J, Bauer EA, Eisen AZ. Scleroderma: increased biosynthesis of triple-helical type I and type III procollagens associated with unaltered expression of collagenase by skin fibroblasts in culture. J Clin Invest 1979;64: 921.

53. Diegelmann RF, Cohen IK, McKoy BJ. Growth kinetics and collagen synthesis of normal skin, normal scar and keloid fibroblasts in vitro. J Cell Physiol 1979;98:341.

54. Kornel L, Kanamarlapudi N, Ramsay C. Arterial steroid receptors and their putative role in the mechanism of hypertension. J Ster Biochem 1983;19:333.

55. Meyer WJ III, Nichols NR. Mineralocorticoid binding in cultured smooth muscle cells and fibroblasts from rat aorta. J Ster Biochem 1981;14:1157.

56. Laurent GJ. Dynamic state of collagen: pathways of collagen degradation in vivo and their possible role in regulation of collagen mass. Am J Physiol 1987;252(Cell Physiol 21): C1.

57. Chakraborty A, Eghbali M. Collagenase activity in the normal rat myocardium: an immunohistochemical method. Histochemistry 1989;92:391.

58. Turner JE, et al. Collagen metabolism during right ventricular hypertrophy following induced lung injury. Am J Physiol 1986;21: H915.

59. Brilla CG, Janicki JS, Weber KT. Cardioreparative effects of lisinopril in rats with genetic hypertension and left ventricular hypertrophy. Circulation 1991;5:1771.

60. Brilla CG, et al. Advanced hypertensive

heart disease in SHR: lisinopril-mediated regression of myocardial fibrosis. Circulation 1992;86(Suppl. I):I-329.

61. Brilla CG, et al. Prevention of LV systolic dysfunction in hypertensive heart disease due to ACE inhibition. Circulation 1993; 88(Suppl. I):I-8.

62. Brilla CG, Weber KT. Regression of myocardial fibrosis in hypertension by ACE inhibition vs adrenergic blockade. Circulation 1991;84(Suppl. II):II-48.

63. Ruskoaho HJ, Savolainen ER. Effects of long-term verapamil treatment on blood pressure, cardiac hypertrophy and collagen metabolism in spontaneously hypertensive rats. Cardiovasc Res 1985;19:355.

64. Motz W, Strauer BE. Left ventricular function and collagen content after regression of hypertensive hypertrophy. Hypertension 1989;13:43.

65. Brilla CG. Hochdruck und hypertensive Herzkrankheit: Pathophysiologie, Klinik, Diagnostik und Therapie. Berlin: Walter de Gruyter Verlag, 1994.

Chapter 17

Locally Produced Substances and Tissue Repair in Heart

Yao Sun M.D., Ph.D., Karl T. Weber, M.D.

Introduction

A cascade of responses accompany tissue injury, parenchymal cell necrosis, or tissue invasion by foreign material. They constitute exudative, inflammatory, fibroplastic, and fibrogenic phases of healing. It is through healing that wounds or foreign material are contained and injured tissue repaired. Chemical mediators of exudative and inflammatory phases of healing include various hormones, such as bradykinin (BK) and prostaglandins (PG),[1] and more recently discovered regulatory peptides[2] generated within tissue at the site of repair. Mediators of the fibroplastic and fibrogenic phases of healing, likewise produced at the site of repair, are under investigation; they may or may not prove identical to established mediators of inflammation. In this connection, a role for cytokines[2] and locally produced hormones, angiotensin II (AngII), BK, and PG in regulating fibroblast growth and collagen turnover have attracted considerable interest.[3,4] Increasing evidence indicates that locally produced substances play an important role in tissue repair.[5–8] Herein we review recent studies that have addressed the localization and quantitation of angiotensin converting enzyme (ACE), AngII receptors and BK receptors in rat heart by in vitro autoradiography and their relationship to fibrous tissue formation.

Fibrous Tissue and Local Hormones

Angiotensin Converting Enzyme (ACE)

ACE is located in many tissues[9,10] including heart, kidney, brain, and adrenals. It is bound to endothelial cells, epithelial cells, macrophages, or myofibroblasts.[6] These cells likewise appear responsible for ACE generation. Unlike renin, which is a fastidious enzyme acting only on angiotensinogen, ACE is capable of acting on various substrates that include not only AngI but also BK, substance P, enkephalins, neurotensin, and the gonadotropin luteinizing hormone-releasing hormone.[11–13]

In vitro autoradiography has demonstrated that ACE is not uniformly distributed within the rat heart (Figure 1, panels A and B, see page 226A). Heart valves, for example, are a site of high density ACE binding.[14] This includes not only endothelial cells found on the surface of each valve leaflet, but also valvular interstitial cells that reside within the interstices of each leaflet. This was confirmed immunohistochemically with a monoclonal ACE antibody. ACE binding is also marked in the endothelium of the aorta and pulmonary artery, as well as their adventitia and the adventitia of intramyocardial coronary arteries. Low density ACE binding, on the other hand, is present in the ventricles and atria (atria> ventricles).

Only recently has the prospect been

[1] This work was supported in part by NIH Grant R01-HL-31701.

From Weber KT, MD *Wound Healing in Cardiovascular Disease*, Armonk, NY, Futura Publishing Company Inc., © 1995.

raised that connective tissue and its cellular constituents may be a site of peptide hormone generation and degradation and receptor-ligand binding, each of which could serve to regulate fibrillar collagen turnover. This possibility emerged largely from morphological studies wherein in vitro autoradiography, using an iodinated derivative of lisinopril (^{125}I-351A), localized and quantitated ACE binding density.[15] High density ACE binding was observed within subcutaneous connective tissue[16] (Figure 1, panel C), where fibroblasts are metabolically active. This contrasts to quiescent fibrocytes residing in skeletal muscle tendon, where ACE binding was not detected.[16] We therefore preceded to examine the concurrence between ACE and fibrous tissue formation in several different models of tissue injury in the rat heart.

In the scar tissue that appears at sites of cardiac myocyte necrosis, induced by either coronary artery ligation[6] or isoproterenol administration, ACE binding density is markedly increased. The density of ACE binding postinfarction increased (Figure 2, panel A, see page 226A) over the course of 8 weeks in parallel with the progressive accumulation of fibrillar collagen stained with the collagen-specific marker, Sirius red. Sites of high density ACE binding that appeared remote to the infarction were also linked to fibrous tissue formation. This include perivascular fibrosis and microscopic scars which involved the right ventricle, endocardial fibrosis of the interventricular septum, and fibrosis of the visceral pericardium following pericardiotomy (with or without coronary artery ligation).[6,7] The presence of fibrosis at these remote sites have been reported previously in the infarcted rat and human left ventricle.[17,18]

Using a monoclonal ACE antibody,[6] ACE producing cells at the site of infarction were found to include fibroblast-like cells, macrophages, and endothelial cells that included new vessels that appeared with the angiogenic component of tissue repair. Fibroblast-like cells at the site of necrosis and within the fibrosed pericardium were found to be alpha-smooth muscle actin positive by immunolabeling. At each site, where high collagen turnover is high, in situ hybridization identified that these fibroblast-like cells

expressed the transcript for type I collagen.[6] Alpha-smooth muscle actin-containing fibroblasts are likely myofibroblasts. They are contractile and contract in response to AngII and BK.[19]

Chronic administration of AngII or aldosterone (ALDO), (together with uninephrectomy and high salt diet) leads to the appearance of myocardial fibrosis. This includes a perivascular fibrosis of intramyocardial coronary arteries and microscopic scars that follow cardiac myocyte necrosis.[20,21] (Figure 3, see page 226B) depicts collagen-specific staining, Sirius red, and this perivascular fibrosis (Panel A) and microscopic scarring (panel B). High density ACE binding is observed at these sites that appear in the right and left ventricles with the chronic administration of AngII (Figure 2, panel B) or ALDO.

The anatomical coincidence between ACE binding and normal and pathological expressions of collagen formation is evident. However its biological functions and substrate(s) utilization in fibrosis tissue remain to be identified.

Angiotensin II

In addition to its well-described endocrine properties as a circulating hormone, there is now accumulating evidence that locally generated AngII has important autocrine and paracrine functions in a variety of organs that includes less well-appreciated roles in inflammation[22,23] and tissue structure,[4,24] as well as a more widely recognized role in homeostasis.[25] Recent evidence suggests the existence of an intrinsic generation of angiotensin peptides in mammalian hearts. Components required for the generation of AngI and AngII peptides have been localized within inflammatory cells[22] and cardiac tissue.[24,26,27] Expression of angiotensinogen mRNA[25,28] have been detected in the neonatal heart and localized to its fibroblasts and myocytes.[29,30] Intracardiac conversion of AngI to AngII has been confirmed in the isolated, perfused working heart.[31,32] Aspartyl proteases, such as cathepsin D and renin, and serine proteases (e.g., cathepsin G) have been found, as well as ACE.[6,33–36] Each of these cells would appear capable of generating AngII, which in

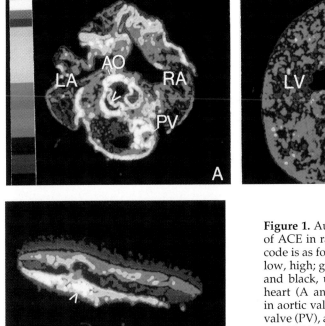

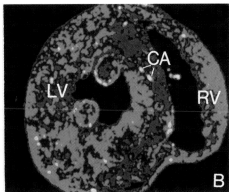

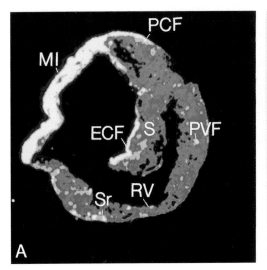

Figure 1. Autoradiographic localization of ACE in rat heart and skin. The color code is as follows: white, very high; yellow, high; green, moderate; purple, low and black, undetectable. In normal rat heart (A and B), ACE binding is high in aortic valve (arrowhead), pulmonary valve (PV), aorta (AO), and coronary artery (CA), moderate in right atrium (RA) and low in left atrium (LA) and both ventricles (RV and LV). High ACE binding is present in subcutaneous tissue (Panel C, arrowhead).

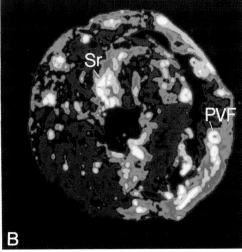

Figure 2. Autoradiographic localization of ACE in myocardial fibrosis. In the rat heart at week 8 postinfarction (Panel A), high ACE binding is observed at the site of infarction (MI), endocardial fibrosis (ECF) of interventricular septum (S), microscopic scar (Sr), and perivascular fibrosis of right ventricle (RV) and septum. High ACE binding is present in perivascular fibrosis and microscopic scar in the rat receiving 6 weeks of AngII (9 μg/hour) (Panel B).

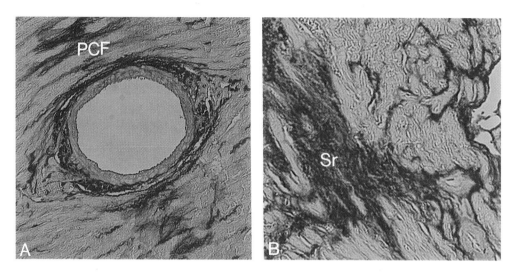

Figure 3. Sirius red staining showing pericardial fibrosis (Panel A) and microscopic scar (Panel B) in the rat receiving 6 weeks of AngII.

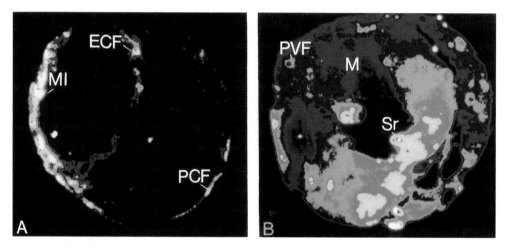

Figure 4. AngII receptor and BK receptor binding in the rat heart with myocardial fibrosis. AngII receptor binding was high at site of myocardial infarction, endocardial fibrosis, and pericardial fibrosis at week 8 postinfarction (Panel A). BK receptor binding in perivascular fibrosis and microscopic scar following AngII infusion was increased compared with normal myocardium (M) (Panel B).

turn may have autocrine properties that regulate collagen turnover. AngII receptors have been identified in cardiac tissue[14,33,37] including its myocytes,[38,39] and fibroblasts.[3,40,41]

Apart from its well-described influences on extracellular electrolyte, fluid balance, and vascular resistance, the biologically active peptide AngII exerts diverse actions on the heart, including positive inotropic and chronotropic effects.[42,43] It may also stimulate myocyte growth[44,45] and modulate myocardial metabolism. A paracrine/autocrine role for AngII in fibroblast collagen turnover has attracted considerable interest.[3,46,47] To date, evidence suggests AngII contributes to tissue repair in the heart,[18] skin,[48] and kidney.[49] Both inflammatory cells and fibroblasts or fibroblast-like cells contain requisite components to generate AngII.[50-52] AngII is reported to stimulate protein synthesis.[44,45,52] Using ^{3}H-proline incorporation, collagen synthesis of confluent adult rat cardiac fibroblasts was found to be increased by AngII in a concentration-dependent manner.[46] Type I collagen synthesis and its transcription in these cells were found to be increased by AngII.[53] AngII also reduced collagenase activity in fibroblast culture medium.[46] Each of these nonclassical responses in these nonclassical target cells suggest that locally generated AngII could have autocrine and/or paracrine effects that would promote fibrous tissue formation. These findings raise the intriguing prospect that AngII generation in tissue contributes to its wound healing response.

Local production of angiotensin peptides is likely influenced by tissue-specific mechanisms of regulation. AngI and AngII may be generated intracellularly from cleavage of either locally synthesized angiotensinogen, angiotensinogen derived from plasma, or which has been taken up by the cell from the interstitial space. On day 5 following coronary artery ligation, the expression of angiotensinogen mRNA was found to be increased in the rat left ventricle.[54] This precedes the morphological appearance of fibrillar collagen in the form of scar tissue.[55,56] During the first 2 weeks postligation, AngII content of infarcted tissue has not been measured. It was found to be in-

creased at 21 days and could be attenuated by delapril treatment initiated at the time of infarction.[57]

Angiotensin II Receptors

The multiple physiological effects of AngII are initiated by binding to specific receptors located on the plasma membrane. The existence of at least two subtypes of AngII receptors (AT_1 and AT_2) has been demonstrated.[58] These two receptor subtypes have been distinguished by the use of peptide and nonpeptide AngII antagonists. The receptor antagonist DuP 753 (now losartan) has been shown to bind selectively to the AT_1 receptor subtype, whereas PD123177 binds selectively to the AT_2 receptor subtype. AT_1 receptors correlates with most known physiological functions of AngII. The functional role of AT_2 receptors in adult tissue is not yet apparent.

The distribution of AngII receptors in the normal rat heart differs markedly from that of ACE. Major vessels, including the aorta and pulmonary artery, contain AngII receptors that are uniformly distributed throughout the media and also in the adventitia.[37] In the rat myocardium, low levels of AngII receptors are found in cardiac muscle present throughout both the atrium and ventricles. In our study, the majority of cardiac AngII receptors are of the AT_1 subtype (more than 90%).[7]

We have previously reported that AngII receptor binding was markedly increased at site of infarction, endocardial fibrosis, and pericardial fibrosis (Figure 4, panel A, see page 226B) following coronary artery ligation for over 8 weeks. The subtype of AngII receptors at each of these sites is AT_1. AngII receptor binding in infarcted heart is anatomically coincident with ACE binding and myocardial fibrosis suggesting AngII is associated with fibrous tissue formation in this model. Further study is needed in support of this concept. AT_1 receptor antagonist losartan prevented fibrosis, but not fibroblast proliferation, at these sites.[59] AngII stimulates collagen synthesis in cultured cardiac fibroblasts and in valvular interstitial cells which can be blocked by AT1 receptor antagonist.[40,60] This again implicates AngII in fibrous tissue formation.

Relation Between Tissue ACE, Plasma ACE, and AngII

Vascular endothelial ACE is subject to negative feedback by circulating AngII.[61] In rats with myocardial infarction, cardiac ACE,[6,62] AngII receptor binding density,[7] angiotensinogen mRNA,[54] and AngII level are increased which indicates that local angiotensin peptide generation is stimulated. However, circulating renin, ACE, AngII, or ALDO concentrations remain normal indicating that circulating angiotensin system is not activated.[63] Our previous findings further corroborated that ACE binding in fibrous tissue is independent of circulating levels of AngII and ALDO.[21] These hormones were administered by implanted minipump thereby raising plasma levels of AngII and ALDO. Plasma renin activity and AngI would be suppressed in each model, whereas with ALDO administration, plasma AngII would also be suppressed or remain normal. ACE binding density was increased within fibrous tissue that appeared in each experimental model. Therefore, elevated ACE in myocardial fibrosis is independent of circulating AngII or ACE. ACE in fibrous tissue may be regulated by local substrates. This requires further study. As an integral feature of fibrous tissue formation, ACE may regulate the extent of fibrosis that appears as part of wound healing.

ACE Inhibition

(ACE) inhibitors have been shown to increase coronary blood flow, improve myocardial metabolism and hemodynamics, and reduce reperfusion arrhythmias.[64–66] Additional cardioprotective effects of ACE inhibitors include significant reduction of myocardial infarct size in dogs[67] and prevention or attenuation of left ventricular geometric remodeling in rats following infarction.[68,69] Perindopril, given 1 week after infarction, decreased the endomyocardial fibrosis that appeared in the non-necrotic segment of left ventricle.[66] Captopril treatment commenced at the time of coronary artery ligation, prevented the expected proliferation of fibroblasts and fibrosis of the right ventricle and septum that appeared at 1 and 2 weeks following infarction.[70] In a model of cardiac myocyte necrosis associated with chronic AngII administration,[71,72] lisinopril attenuated microscopic scarring despite the presence of myocyte injury.[73] In pericardial fibrosis following pericardiotomy without infarction, lisinopril decreased collagen accumulation.[7] These beneficial effects of ACE inhibition on myocardial fibrosis are likely due to attenuated activity of fibrous tissue ACE and reduced AngII generation at sites of healing. There is also evidence that BK accumulation following administration of ACE inhibitor may also contribute to the cardioprotective effects of such an agent. In the ischemic, isolated, perfused rat heart, BK is as effective as an ACE inhibitor in improving cardiac metabolism and hemodynamic performance, whereas a specific BK antagonist blocks these cardiac responses to ACE inhibition.[74]

Bradykinin and Prostaglandins

BK is an important endogenous substrate for ACE. The enzyme kinetics for BK are more favorable than AngI. BK stimulates PG synthesis by endothelial cells and fibroblasts.[75] BK and PG are also endogenous hormones. Their role as chemical mediators of inflammation is well recognized. BK, PGI_2, and PGE_2 have each been detected in coronary sinus drainage. During myocardial ischemia or following infarction, BK in sinus effluent rises severalfold.[76] A similar response is observed for PGE_2.[77] During the acute inflammatory phase that appears during the first several days after infarction, the release of PGE_2 is markedly increased by administration of BK suggesting inflammatory cells may be involved. Both BK and PGE_2 also alter cultured cardiac fibroblast collagen turnover.[78,79] Fibroblast-like cells, isolated from the site of infarction 7 days after coronary ligation, demonstrate increased cyclooxygenase activity and increased prostanoid production, including PGE_2. At 30 days after infarction, BK-induced release of PGE_2 from the heart is increased.[80] Prostaglandin synthesis is increased in microsomes prepared from infarcted myocardium at 3 weeks and 3 months after coronary ligation. Thus there is a persistence of PGE_2 production well beyond the inflammatory phase of tissue repair. Recent studies using a specific BK receptor antagonist suggest that some of the cardiac and antiproliferative actions of ACE inhibition involve BK.[81]

The cellular effects of BK are mediated through specific surface receptors. BK receptors were initially divided into two classes, B1 and B2, based on the activity of selective receptor antagonists.[82] Endothelial cells, epithelial cells, and fibroblasts contain BK receptors.[83] We have previously reported increased BK receptor binding in perivascular fibrosis and microscopic scarring in response to chronic administration of AngII or ALDO (Figure 4, panel B). BK receptor binding density increased progressively as tissue repair became more developed. This suggests that in regions of myocardial fibrosis, BK receptor binding increases in a time-dependent manner in these models. The cellular site of BK receptors requires further study. The subtype of BK receptors at these sites also remains unknown. The coincidence of ACE and BK receptors suggests that ACE in these models may be responsible for metabolizing BK. We have found that fibrous tissue formation seen in response to AngII infusion was attenuated by pretreatment with lisinopril. BK is known to mediate prostaglandin release. Various prostaglandins stimulate fibroblast collagenase expression and collagenase activity. Hence after ACE inhibition, increased concentrations of tissue BK may increase local collagenase activity by stimulating prostaglandins synthesis. Collagenase, in turn, would degrade fibrillar collagen and attenuate fibrous tissue accumulation.

Summary

High ACE binding density is anatomically coincident with myocardial fibrosis irrespective of its location and etiologic basis. This raises the prospect that ACE may be an integral component of tissue repair associated with fibrous tissue formation in the heart. Elevated AngII or BK receptor binding within myocardial fibrosis represents additional circumstantial evidence in favor of this proposition. ACE in fibrous tissue may regulate the local concentration of various peptides, such as AngII and/or BK, which then govern tissue repair in the heart. One potential salutary effect of ACE inhibition would be to attenuate the adverse structural remodeling of the myocardium that is produced by the accumulation of fibrous tissue.

References

1. Whalley ET. Inflammatory and vascular basis of connective tissue disease. In: Gardner DL, ed. Pathological Basis of the Connective Tissue Diseases. Philadelphia, Pa: Lea & Febiger, 1992:282–299.
2. Miller MD, Krangel MS. Biology and biochemistry of the chemokines: a family of chemotactic and inflammatory cytokines. Crit Rev Immunol 1992;12:17–46.
3. Villarreal FJ, Kim NN, Ungab GD, et al. Identification of functional angiotensin II receptors on rat cardiac fibroblasts. Circulation 1993;88:2849–2861.
4. Weber KT, Sun Y, Katwa LC, et al. Connective tissue: a metabolic entity? J Mol Cell Cardiol 1995;27:107–120.
5. Johnston CI. Tissue angiotensin converting enzyme in cardiac and vascular hypertrophy, repair, and remodeling. Hypertension 1994;23:258–268.
6. Sun Y, Cleutjens JPM, Diaz-Arias AA, et al. Cardiac angiotensin converting enzyme and myocardial fibrosis in the rat. Cardiovasc Res 1994;28:1423–1432.
7. Sun Y, Weber KT. Angiotensin II receptor binding following myocardial infarction in the rat. Cardiovasc Res 1994;28:1623–1628.
8. Sun Y, Weber KT. Fibrosis and myocardial ACE: possible substrate and independence from circulating angiotensin II. J Cardiac Failure 1994;1:81–89.
9. Jackson B, Cubela R, Johnston C. Angiotensin converting enzyme (ACE), characterization by ^{125}I-MK351A binding studies of plasma and tissue ACE during variation of salt status in the rat. J Hypertens 1986;4:759–765.
10. Sakaguchi K, Chai SY, Jackson B, et al. Inhibition of tissue angiotensin converting enzyme. Quantitation by autoradiography. Hypertension 1988;11:230–238.
11. Erdös EG. Angiotensin I converting enzyme and the changes in our concepts through the

years. Lewis K. Dahl memorial lecture. Hypertension 1990;16:363–370.

12. Skidgel RA, Erdös EG. The broad substrate specificity of human angiotensin I converting enzyme. Clin Exp Hypertens [A] 1987;9:243–259.

13. Unger T, Gohlke P. Converting enzyme inhibitors in cardiovascular therapy: current status and future potential. Cardiovasc Res 1994;28:146–158.

14. Sun Y, Mendelsohn FAO. Angiotensin converting enzyme inhibition in heart, kidney, and serum studied ex vivo after administration of zofenopril, captopril, and lisinopril. J Cardiovasc Pharmacol 1991;18:478–486.

15. Mendelsohn FAO. Localization of angiotensin converting enzyme in rat forebrain and other tissues by in vitro autoradiography using ^{125}I-labelled MK351A. Clin Exp Pharmacol Physiol 1984;11:431–435.

16. Sun Y, Diaz-Arias AA, Weber KT. Angiotensin-converting enzyme, bradykinin and angiotensin II receptor binding in rat skin, tendon and heart valves: an in vitro quantitative autoradiographic study. J Lab Clin Med 1994;123:372–377.

17. van Krimpen C, Schoemaker RG, Cleutjens JPM, et al. Angiotensin I converting enzyme inhibitors and cardiac remodeling. Basic Res Cardiol 1991;86(Suppl. 1):149–155.

18. Volders PGA, Willems IEMG, Cleutjens JPM, et al. Interstitial collagen is increased in the non-infarcted human myocardium after myocardial infarction. J Mol Cell Cardiol 1993;25:1317–1323.

19. Gabbiani G. The myofibroblast: a key cell for wound healing and fibrocontractive diseases. In: Deyl Z, Adam M, eds. Connective Tissue Research: Chemistry, Biology, and Physiology. New York, NY: Liss, 1981:183–194.

20. Sun Y, Weber KT. Angiotensin II and aldosterone receptor binding in rat heart and kidney: response to chronic angiotensin II or aldosterone administration. J Lab Clin Med 1993;122:404–411.

21. Sun Y, Ratajska A, Zhou G, et al. Angiotensin converting enzyme and myocardial fibrosis in the rat receiving angiotensin II or aldosterone. J Lab Clin Med 1993;122:395–403.

22. Weinstock JV. The significance of angiotensin I converting enzyme in granulomatous inflammation. Functions of ACE in granulomas. Sarcoidosis 1986;3:19–26.

23. Ehlers MRW, Riordan JF. Angiotensin-converting enzyme: new concepts concerning its biological role. Biochemistry 1989;28:5311–5318.

24. Baker KM, Booz GW, Dostal DE. Cardiac ac-

tions of angiotensin II: role of an intracardiac renin-angiotensin system. Annu Rev Physiol 1992;54:227–241.

25. Johnston CI. Biochemistry and pharmacology of the renin-angiotensin system. Drugs 1990;39(Suppl. 1):21–31.

26. Dzau VJ. Cardiac renin-angiotensin system. Molecular and functional aspects. Am J Med 1988;84:22–27.

27. Lindpaintner K, Ganten D. The cardiac renin-angiotensin system: an appraisal of present experimental and clinical evidence. Circ Res 1991;68:905–921.

28. Kunapuli SP, Kumar A. Molecular cloning of human angiotensinogen cDNA and evidence for the presence of its mRNA in rat heart. Circ Res 1987;60:786–790.

29. Dostal DE, Rothblum KN, Chernin MI, et al. Intracardiac detection of angiotensinogen and renin: a localized renin-angiotensin system in neonatal rat heart. Am J Physiol 1992;263:C838-C850.

30. Dostal DE, Rothblum KN, Conrad KM, et al. Detection of angiotensin I and II in cultured rat cardiac myocytes and fibroblasts. Am J Physiol 1992;263:C851-C863.

31. Lindpaintner K, Wilhelm MJ, Jin M, et al. Tissue renin-angiotensin systems: focus on the heart. J Hypertens Suppl 1987;5:S33-S38.

32. Lindpaintner K, Jin M, Niedermaier N, et al. Cardiac angiotensin and its local activation in the isolated perfused beating heart. Circ Res 1990;67:564–573.

33. Yamada H, Fabris B, Allen AM, et al. Localization of angiotensin converting enzyme in rat heart. Circ Res 1991;68:141–149.

34. Pinto JE, Viglione P, Saavedra JM. Autoradiographic localization and quantification of rat heart angiotensin converting enzyme. Am J Hypertens 1991;4:321–326.

35. Klickstein LB, Kaempfer CE, Wintroub BU. The granulocyte-angiotensin system. Angiotensin I-converting activity of cathepsin G. J Biol Chem 1982;257:15042–15046.

36. Pearl LH, Taylor WR. A structural model for the retroviral proteases. (Letter) Nature 1987;329:351–354.

37. Allen AM, Yamada H, Mendelsohn FAO. In vitro autoradiographic localization of binding to angiotensin receptors in the rat heart. Int J Cardiol 1990;28:25–33.

38. Reiss K, Capasso JM, Huang H-E, et al. ANG II receptors, c-*myc*, and c-*jun* in myocytes after myocardial infarction and ventricular failure. Am J Physiol 1993;264:H760-H769.

39. Meggs LG, Coupet J, Huang H, et al. Regulation of angiotensin II receptors on ventricular myocytes after myocardial infarction in rats. Circ Res 1993;72:1149–1162.

40. Brilla CG, Zhou G, Matsubara L, et al. Collagen metabolism in cultured adult rat cardiac fibroblasts: response to angiotensin II and aldosterone. J Mol Cell Cardiol 1994;26:809–820.

41. Sadoshima J, Izumo S. Molecular characterization of angiotensin II-induced hypertrophy of cardiac myocytes and hyperplasia of cardiac fibroblasts. Critical role of the AT_1 receptor subtype. Circ Res 1993;73:413–423.

42. Kobayashi M, Furukawa Y, Chiba S. Positive chronotropic and inotropic effects of angiotensin II in the dog heart. Eur J Pharmacol 1978;50:17–25.

43. Nakashima A, Angus JA, Johnston CI. Chronotropic effects of angiotensin I, angiotensin II, bradykinin and vasopressin in guinea pig atria. Eur J Pharmacol 1982;81:479–485.

44. Schelling P, Fischer H, Ganten D. Angiotensin and cell growth: a link to cardiovascular hypertrophy? J Hypertens 1991;9:3–15.

45. Baker KM, Aceto JF. Angiotensin II stimulation of protein synthesis and cell growth in chick heart cells. Am J Physiol 1990;259:H610-H618.

46. Brilla CG, Matsubara LS, Weber KT. Anti-aldosterone treatment and the prevention of myocardial fibrosis in primary and secondary hyperaldosteronism. J Mol Cell Cardiol 1993;25:563–575.

47. Sano H, Okada H, Kawaguchi H, et al. Increased angiotensin II-stimulated collagen synthesis in cultured cardiac fibroblasts from spontaneously hypertensive rats. (Abstract) Circulation 1991;84(Suppl. II):II-48.

48. Kimura B, Sumners C, Phillips MI. Changes in skin angiotensin II receptors in rats during wound healing. Biochem Biophys Res Commun 1992;187:1083–1090.

49. Wolf G, Neilson EG. Angiotensin II as a renal growth factor. J Am Soc Nephrol 1993;3:1531–1540.

50. Costerousse O, Allegrini J, Lopez M, et al. Angiotensin I-converting enzyme in human circulating mononuclear cells: genetic polymorphism of expression in T-lymphocytes. Biochem J 1993;290:33–40.

51. Weinstock JV, Blum AM. Synthesis of angiotensins by cultured granuloma macrophages in murine schistosomiasis mansoni. Cell Immunol 1987;107:273–280.

52. Aceto JF, Baker KM. [Sar¹]angiotensin II receptor-mediated stimulation of protein synthesis in chick heart cells. Am J Physiol 1990;258:H806-H813.

53. Zhou G, Matsubara L, Brilla CG, et al. Angiotensin II and aldosterone regulate collagen turnover in cultured adult rat cardiac fibro-

54. Lindpaintner K, Lu W, Niedermajer J, et al. Selective activation of cardiac angiotensinogen gene expression in post-infarction ventricular remodeling in the rat. J Mol Cell Cardiol 1993;25:133–143.

55. Pick R, Jalil JE, Janicki JS, et al. The fibrillar nature and structure of isoproterenol-induced myocardial fibrosis in the rat. Am J Pathol 1989;134:365–371.

56. Jugdutt BI, Amy RWM. Healing after myocardial infarction in the dog: changes in infarct hydroxyproline and topography. J Am Coll Cardiol 1986;7:91–102.

57. Yamagishi H, Kim S, Nishikimi T, et al. Contribution of cardiac renin-angiotensin system to ventricular remodelling in myocardial-infarcted rats. J Mol Cell Cardiol 1993;25:1369–1380.

58. Song K, Zhuo J, Allen AM, et al. Angiotensin II receptor subtypes in rat brain and peripheral tissues. Cardiology 1991;79(Suppl. 1):45–54.

59. Smits JFM, van Krimpen C, Schoemaker RG, et al. Angiotensin II receptor blockade after myocardial infarction in rats: effects on hemodynamics, myocardial DNA synthesis, and interstitial collagen content. J Cardiovasc Pharmacol 1992;20:772–778.

60. Katwa LC, Ratajska A, Cleutjens JPM, et al. Angiotensin converting enzyme and kininase-II-like activities in cultured valvular interstitial cells of the rat heart. Cardiovasc Res 1995;29:57–65.

61. Schunkert H, Ingelfinger JR, Hirsch AT, et al. Feedback regulation of angiotensin converting enzyme activity and mRNA levels by angiotensin II. Circ Res 1993;72:312–318.

62. Fabris B, Jackson B, Kohzuki M, et al. Increased cardiac angiotensin-converting enzyme in rats with chronic heart failure. Clin Exp Pharmacol Physiol 1990;17:309–314.

63. Hodsman GP, Kohzuki M, Howes LG, et al. Neurohumoral responses to chronic myocardial infarction in rats. Circulation 1988;78:376–381.

64. van Gilst WH, de Graeff PA, Wesseling H, et al. Reduction of reperfusion arrhythmias in the ischemic isolated rat heart by angiotensin converting enzyme inhibitors: a comparison of captopril, enalapril, and HOE 498. J Cardiovasc Pharmacol 1986;8:722–728.

65. Linz W, Schölkens BA, Han YF. Beneficial effects of the converting enzyme inhibitor, ramipril, in ischemic rat hearts. J Cardiovasc Pharmacol 1986;8(Suppl. 10):S91-S99.

66. Michel J-B, Lattion A-L, Salzmann J-L, et al. Hormonal and cardiac effects of converting

enzyme inhibition in rat myocardial infarction. Circ Res 1988;62:641–650.

67. Ertl G, Kloner RA, Alexander RW, et al. Limitation of experimental infarct size by an angiotensin-converting enzyme inhibitor. Circulation 1982;65:40–48.

68. Pfeffer MA, Lamas GA, Vaughan DE, et al. Effect of captopril on progressive ventricular dilatation after anterior myocardial infarction. N Engl J Med 1988;319:80–86.

69. Pfeffer MA, Braunwald E. Ventricular remodeling after myocardial infarction. Experimental observations and clinical implications. Circulation 1990;81:1161–1172.

70. van Krimpen C, Smits JFM, Cleutjens JPM, et al. DNA synthesis in the non-infarcted cardiac interstitium after left coronary artery ligation in the rat heart: effects of captopril. J Mol Cell Cardiol 1991;23:1245–1253.

71. Tan LB, Jalil JE, Pick R, et al. Cardiac myocyte necrosis induced by angiotensin II. Circ Res 1991;69:1185–1195.

72. Ratajska A, Campbell SE, Cleutjens JPM, et al. Angiotensin II and structural remodeling of coronary vessels in rats. J Lab Clin Med 1994;124:408–415.

73. Sun Y, Ratajska A, Weber KT. Inhibition of angiotensin converting enzyme and attenuation of myocardial fibrosis by lisinopril in rats receiving angiotensin II. J Lab Clin Med. 1995. (In Press).

74. Schölkens BA, Linz W, Konig W. Effects of the angiotensin converting enzyme inhibitor, ramipril, in isolated ischaemic rat heart are abolished by a bradykinin antagonist. J Hypertens Suppl 1988;6:S25-S28.

75. Conklin BR, Burch RM, Steranka LR, et al. Distinct bradykinin receptors mediate stimulation of prostaglandin synthesis by endothelial cells and fibroblasts. J Pharmacol Exp Ther 1988;244:646–649.

76. Baumgarten CR, Linz W, Kunkel G, et al. Ramaprilat increases bradykinin outflow from isolated hearts of rat. Br J Pharmacol 1993;108:293–295.

77. Hashimoto K, Hirose M, Furukawa K, et al. Changes in hemodynamics and bradykinin concentration in coronary sinus blood in experimental coronary artery occlusion. Jpn Heart J 1977;18:679–689.

78. Goldstein RH, Polgar P. The effect and interaction of bradykinin and prostaglandins on protein and collagen production by lung fibroblasts. J Biol Chem 1982;257:8630–8633.

79. Zhou G, Tyagi SC, Weber KT. Bradykinin regulates collagen turnover in cardiac fibroblasts. (Abstract) Clin Res 1993;41:630A.

80. Weber DR, Stroud ED, Prescott SM. Arachidonate metabolism in cultured fibroblasts derived from normal and infarcted canine heart. Circ Res 1989;65:671–683.

81. Linz W, Schölkens BA. A specific B_2-bradykinin receptor antagonist HOE 140 abolishes the antihypertrophic effect of ramipril. Br J Pharmacol 1992;105:771–772.

82. Regoli D, Barabé J. Pharmacology of bradykinin and related kinins. Pharmacol Rev 1980;32:1–46.

83. Roscher AA, Manganiello VC, Jelsema CL, et al. Receptors for bradykinin in intact cultured human fibroblasts. Identification and characterization by direct binding study. J Clin Invest 1983;72:626–635.

Chapter 18

Connective Tissue ACE

Laxmansa C. Katwa, Ph.D., Karl T. Weber, M.D.

Introduction

Angiotensin converting enzyme (ACE) is a chloride-dependent, zinc containing plasma membrane-bound glycoprotein. Bound to vascular endothelial cells, ACE has a dual role: it converts circulating angiotensin (Ang) I to the biologically active octapeptide AngII, which accounts for its most widely recognized function; and a less well-recognized function as a kininase II that metabolizes bradykinin (BK), substance P, and enkephalins.[1,2] An ectoenzyme, ACE is also bound to plasma membrane of other cells, including epithelial cells of the kidney and neuroepithelial cells of the brain.[2–4] The function of ACE at these nonendothelial cell sites is uncertain.

ACE is found in the heart; however, its distribution is nonuniform.[5–7] High density autoradiographic ACE binding, for example, is found at sites where collagen turnover is normally high, such as heart valve leaflets[5,7,8] and adventitia of intramyocardial coronary arteries.[9] Such is also the case at sites of fibrous tissue formation that appear in the myocardium secondary to diverse etiologic causes.[8,10] The presence of ACE protein at these sites, demonstrated by monoclonal antibody, was largely confined to α-smooth muscle actin containing valvular interstitial cells, pericytes, and myofibroblasts, respectively. In addition, endothelial cells that cover valve leaflets and which line the luminal surface of blood vessels are positively immunolabeled for ACE. These findings led us to hypothesize that the function of ACE in nonendothelial cells that reside at these sites of high collagen turnover may be related to local regulation of peptides (e.g., AngII and BK)[11] and that such peptides contribute to collagen synthesis and/or degradation. The observation that ACE inhibition attenuates normal fibrillar collagen formation in the developing heart and vasculature of young rats[12] and that found at fibrous tissue sites[13] further supports this proposition.

To more rigorously address our hypothesis, an experimental model was needed. One that would permit characterization of nonendothelial ACE, its expression, substrate specificity, and potential involvement in collagen turnover. Toward this end, valvular interstitial cells (VIC) were isolated and cultured from the distal portion of rat heart valve leaflets.[14] Studies of cultured VIC have been reported previously.[15–18] We used intact VIC or extracts of their cell membrane to determine their phenotypic characteristics, document the presence of ACE, its mRNA expression and activity, substrate specificity, and the presence of AngII and BK receptors. To address the potential for collagen turnover in VIC, in situ hybridization was used to detect the presence of type I collagen mRNA, while zymography of VIC culture media was used to detect collagenase activity. Finally, the influence of AngII on type I collagen synthesis and mRNA expression of serum-deprived VIC was determined.

[1] This work was supported in part by NIH Grant R01-HL-31701.

From Weber KT, MD *Wound Healing in Cardiovascular Disease*, Armonk, NY, Futura Publishing Company Inc., © 1995.

Characterization of VIC Phenotype

Rhodamine phalloidin demonstrated VIC from each valve contained actin microfilaments organized in bundles. In the majority of VIC these actin bundles were oriented in a "fan-like" structure suggesting they are not smooth muscle or myofibroblast-like cells. Actin filaments were oriented along the long axis of the cell in remaining cells. Desmin, a histochemical marker typical for smooth muscle cells and some myofibroblasts,[19] was not found in VIC. Griffonia simplicifolia lectin, a marker of endothelial cells,[20] was likewise absent in VIC. Our VIC preparation would therefore appear similar to VIC obtained from similar valve explants of the mouse, rat and rabbit reported by Filip et al.[15] Smooth muscle cells are typically found in the proximal and middle portions of the atrioventricular valve leaflet. The distal portion of valve leaflets, on the other hand, contains mostly VIC.[15] Our findings confirm these anatomical features of leaflet tissue. Actin microfilaments present in VIC contribute to the contractile behavior of VIC that appears in response to AngII or L-epinephrine.[15]

Angiotensin Converting Enzyme

Human anti-ACE monoclonal antibody labeling revealed the presence of ACE on VIC membrane obtained from each valve. By contrast, cultured rat cardiac fibroblasts were negatively labeled while endothelial cells of frozen rat heart sections were positively labeled for this antibody.

Autoradiographic localization of ACE by ^{125}I-351A binding in cultured VIC further confirmed the presence of this ectoenzyme. ACE binding was observed in VIC from all four valves. Differences in ^{125}I-351A binding were found between VIC membrane preparations and rat cardiac fibroblast membranes. Membrane ACE binding in VIC was statistically ($P<0.05$) greater compared to rat cardiac fibroblast membranes.[14] Average ^{125}I-351A binding in VIC for all four leaflets versus cardiac Fb membranes was 1.32 ± 0.31 and 0.26 ± 0.19 pmol/mg protein, respectively.

To amplify and analyze ACE mRNA

expression in VIC, we used RT-PCR. The housekeeping gene GAPDH, whose levels of mRNA expression are not expected to vary greatly among cell types, was used as internal standard. Total cellular RNA was isolated from VIC, cDNA synthesized, and used for PCR with GAPDH primers. The amount of cDNA that produced the same amount of GAPDH PCR product was chosen among different VIC samples and used for PCR amplification of ACE cDNA. The results of PCR analysis in VIC indicate a PCR product corresponding to the predicted size for ACE (403 bp, Figure 1, lane 2) and GAPDH (195 bp, Figure 1, lane 3) sequences. ACE mRNA was detected in VIC from all four valves.

As there is no published sequence available for rat ACE cDNA, we used published mouse cDNA[21] probe for Northern blot and cDNA sequences to synthesize 5' and 3' oligonucleotide primers for our rat ACE RT-PCR studies. Our inability to detect mRNA for ACE in VIC using the Northern filter hybridization technique may have been due to the low levels of ACE mRNA.

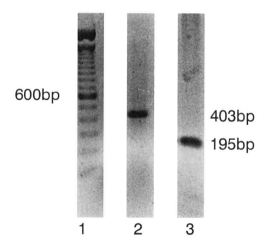

Figure 1. RT-PCR analysis of ACE mRNA in cultured mitral VIC. Lane 1, size markers (100-bp ladder); lane 2, ACE; lane 3, GAPDH. Total RNA was reverse-transcribed into cDNA and then amplified with ACE-specific primers. PCR reactions generated a product of 403 bp (lane 2) for ACE, which corresponds to the predicted size based on published cDNA sequences. GAPDH (195 bp, lane 3) was used as an internal control. Reproduced from reference 14 with permission.

However, ACE mRNA was detected in all four VIC with the more sensitive RT-PCR technique. As already noted, ACE was observed in VIC by immunolabeling, using an ACE monoclonal antibody, and autoradiographic detection of [125]I-351A binding of intact VIC, and their cell membrane preparations. This contrasts to cultured adult rat cardiac fibroblast membranes, where low ACE binding density was observed.

ACE binding activity ([125]I-351A/mg protein) in VIC (1.32 ± 0.31 pmol/mg protein) was found to be much higher than reported[5,7] for right atrium, left atrium, right ventricle, and left ventricle, while aortic wall (1.352 pmol/mg protein)[7] and lung membrane preparation activity (1.13 ± 0.091 pmol/mg protein)[5] approximated that seen for VIC membranes. Yamada et al.[5] reported no difference in ACE binding density between aortic, pulmonary, mitral, and tricuspid valves of the rat heart, whereas Pinto et al.[7] reported differences in mitral, tricuspid, aortic, and pulmonary valves ACE binding in the rat heart. Whether differences in VIC ACE binding density truly exist to represent true biologi-

cal variability rather than culture conditions or variations in the rate of enzyme enrichment during VIC membrane preparation requires further study.

Substrate Specificity

ACE and kininase II-like activities were determined in VIC membrane preparations using AngI, BK, Leu-enkephalin, and substance P as substrates, with and without 50-μM lisinopril. ACE activity (conversion of AngI to AngII) in VIC membranes was partially (30% to 60%) blocked by 0.1 to 3 μM lisinopril and completely blocked by 10 to 50-μM lisinopril. Kininase II activity, on the other hand, exceeded ACE activity and was not effectively inhibited by 50 μM lisinopril (Figure 2).

Substrates for ACE bound to vascular endothelial cells include AngI, BK, enkephalins, and substance P.[1-3] VIC membrane ACE utilized these substrates as well. Based on lisinopril (50 μM) inhibition, ACE activity in VIC appears to have potent kininase II-like activity and is not a chymase.[22] However, the ACE used in this study was a crude

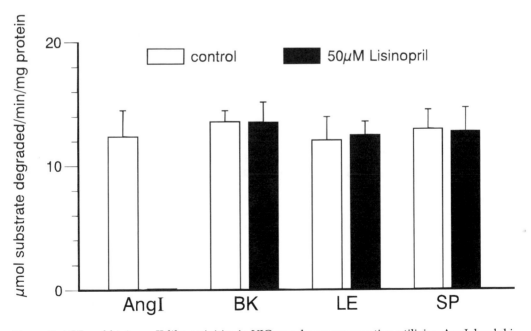

Figure 2. ACE and kininase II-like activities in VIC membrane preparation utilizing AngI, bradykinin, leucine enkephalin, and substance P as substrates. Results are mean ± SEM from three experiments performed as described under Methods. Reproduced from reference 14 with permission.

membrane preparation and at this stage we do not know whether ACE and kininase II-like activity exists on the same molecule. Since the enzyme is tightly bound to cell membranes, it must be solubilized prior to purification either with detergent or by trypsin cleavage.[4] Future studies will need to address solubilization and purification of ACE in VIC and its molecular characterization.

Inhibition by lisinopril, as well as EDTA, further suggests that ACE found in VIC could be similar to endothelial ACE in its catalytic function. However, minor differences in substrate specificity, molecular weight and perhaps carbohydrate moieties may exist between VIC and endothelial cell ACE and could determine the concentrations of locally generated substrates.

Angiotensin II and Bradykinin Receptors

AngII and BK receptor binding were demonstrated using ^{125}I-[Sar^1, Ile^8]-AngII and ^{125}I-BK as radioligands, respectively. Receptor binding studies were found for both AngII and BK receptors in VIC membranes obtained from all four heart valves.[14]

Angiotensin II type I (AT$_1$) receptor subtype was further detected by Western immunoblotting using rat AT$_1$ receptor antibody. A major 60-kDa band of AT$_1$ receptors was found in VIC, cardiac endothelial cells, and cardiac fibroblasts. This antibody also crossreacted with a minor 55-kDa band. Similar results were obtained with aortic, pulmonic, and tricuspid VIC.

We observed high receptor binding densities for AngII and BK in VIC membranes. Even though these receptor binding experiments were performed under identical conditions, differences in binding densities were observed and could be due to the differential distribution of receptor population in the respective membrane preparations. Both AngII and BK receptor binding activities may, in turn, depend upon local concentrations of AngII and BK, respectively. ACE activity may play an important role in regulating local concentrations of these hormones. Further study is required.

Collagen Turnover

Fibroblasts and fibroblast-like cells are widely recognized as contributing to tissue repair.[23] VIC contributes to the healing response of valve leaflets.[16] The contribution of substances produced by VIC[24] in promoting connective tissue formation is uncertain. Nevertheless, the potential autocrine and/or paracrine responses of such locally produced substances require high affinity receptors for binding; receptor-ligand binding leads to transcriptional and/or posttranslational alteration in collagen turnover.

Previous studies indicated the presence of AT$_1$ receptor and receptors for endothelins (ET)-1 and -3 in cardiac fibroblasts. Both AngII and the endothelins increase collagen synthesis and the expression of type I collagen mRNA in cultured adult rat cardiac fibroblasts while both AngII and ET-1 reduce collagenase activity of fibroblast culture medium.[25–29] AngII-mediated alterations in collagen turnover of cardiac fibroblasts is mediated by AT$_1$ receptor.[26,28]

AngII (10^{-7}M and 10^{-9}M) significantly ($P<0.05$) increased the synthesis of VIC type I collagen as determined by ELISA. AngII also increased the expression of type I collagen mRNA in VIC. Both 10^{-7}M and 10^{-9}M AngII increased the expression of 5.8-kb and 4.8-kb mRNA for type I collagen and both β-actin and 18S rRNA probes were used as internal controls and results for VIC are shown in Figure 3. VIC were also found to produce abundant type I collagen mRNA. Type I collagen gene expression in VIC was demonstrated by in situ hybridization suggesting that VIC are capable of producing type I collagen mRNA. The response of serum-deprived VIC collagen turnover to incubation with endothelins-1 and -3 is presently unknown.

Collagenolytic activity present in the culture media from VIC, cardiac fibroblasts, and rat heart endothelial cells were determined by zymography. Results indicate the presence of high collagenolytic activity (matrix metalloproteinase [MMP]: MMP-1, 55 kDa and 62 kDa; and MMP-9, 92 kDa) in the culture media obtained from all three cell lines. This high collagenolytic activity observed in VIC and other cell lines sug-

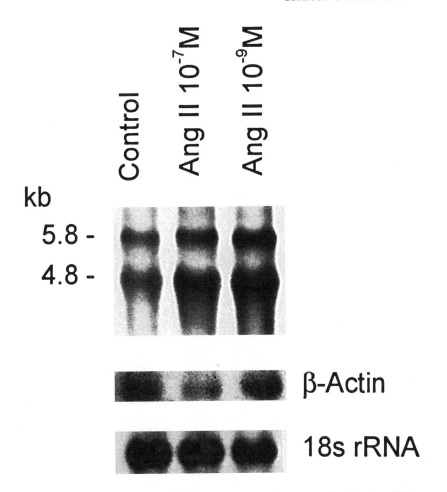

Figure 3. Northern hybridization showing the effect of AngII on type I collagen mRNA expression in pulmonic VIC (n = 5). Lane 1, control; lane 2, with 10^{-7}M AngII; and lane 3, with 10^{-9}M AngII. Equal amounts of RNA (5 μg) were used in each case. The blot was exposed to film for 24 hours, developed, and photographed. Both β-actin and 18S rRNA were used as internal controls. Reproduced from reference 14 with permission.

gests that they express MMPs and are actively involved in collagen degradation.

Overall Implications

ACE activity of VIC could play a major role in heart valves by maintaining normal structure of a metabolically active tissue compartment where high collagen synthesis and deposition and high collagenolytic activity are present. Differences in this balance between synthesis and degradation could lead to fibrous tissue formation based on a paradigm of reciprocal regulation mediated by AngII and BK. Our current understanding of VIC suggests they express ACE and type I collagen mRNA and have collagenolytic activity. AngII stimulates VIC type I collagen gene expression at the mRNA and protein levels and promotes VIC contraction. ACE may regulate local concentrations of AngII and BK which could serve to influence VIC collagen turnover under normal and pathological states, such as valvular heart disease and carcinoid syndrome. This requires further investigation. Activation of the circulating renin-angiotensin-aldosterone system could, in like manner, contribute to increased DNA synthesis and mRNA expression for type I and III collagens and which have been observed in mitral, aortic, and tricuspid valves following suprarenal aortic banding.

References

1. Soubrier F, Hubert C, Testut P, et al. Molecular biology of the angiotensin I converting enzyme. I. Biochemistry and structure of the gene. J Hypertens 1993;11:471–476.
2. Skidgel RA, Erdös EG. Biochemistry of angiotensin I converting enzyme. In: Robertson JIS, Nicholls MG, eds. The Renin Angiotensin System. Vol. 1. London: Gower, 1993: 10.1–10.10.
3. Ehlers MRW, Riordan JF. Angiotensin-converting enzyme: new concepts concerning its biological role. Biochemistry 1989;28: 5311–5318.
4. Skidgel RA, Defendini R, Erdös EG. Angiotensin I converting enzyme and its role as neuropeptidase. In: Turner AJ, ed. Neuropeptides and Their Peptidases. Chichester, UK: Ellis Horwood, 1987:165–177.
5. Yamada H, Fabris B, Allen AM, et al. Localization of angiotensin converting enzyme in rat heart. Circ Res 1991;68:141–149.
6. Schunkert H, Ingelfinger JR, Hirsch AT, et al. Feedback regulation of angiotensin converting enzyme activity and mRNA levels by angiotensin II. Circ Res 1993;72:312–318.
7. Pinto JE, Viglione P, Saavedra JM. Autoradiographic localization and quantification of rat heart angiotensin converting enzyme. Am J Hypertens 1991;4:321–326.
8. Sun Y, Ratajska A, Zhou G, et al. Angiotensin converting enzyme and myocardial fibrosis in the rat receiving angiotensin II or aldosterone. J Lab Clin Med 1993;122:395–403.
9. Rogerson FM, Chai SY, Schlawe I, et al. Presence of angiotensin converting enzyme in the adventitia of large blood vessels. J Hypertens 1992;10:615–620.
10. Johnston CI, Mooser V, Sun Y, et al. Changes in cardiac angiotensin converting enzyme after myocardial infarction and hypertrophy in rats. Clin Exp Pharmacol Physiol 1991;18: 107–110.
11. Sun Y, Ratajska A, Weber KT. Bradykinin receptor and tissue ACE binding in myocardial fibrosis: response to chronic angiotensin II or aldosterone administration in rats. J Mol Cell Cardiol 1995;27:813–822.
12. Keeley FW, Elmoselhi A, Leenan FHH. Enalapril suppresses normal accumulation of elastin and collagen in cardiovascular tissues of growing rats. Am J Physiol 1992;262: H1013-H1021.
13. Sun Y, Ratajska A, Weber KT. Inhibition of angiotensin converting enzyme and attenuation of myocardial fibrosis by lisinopril in rats receiving angiotensin II. J Lab Clin Med 1995 (In Press).
14. Katwa LC, Ratajska A, Cleutjens JPM, et al. Angiotensin converting enzyme and kininase II-like activities in cultured valvular interstitial cells of the rat heart. Cardiovasc Res 1995;29:57–64.
15. Filip DA, Radu A, Simionescu M. Interstitial cells of the heart valves possess characteristics similar to smooth muscle cells. Circ Res 1986;59:310–320.
16. Lester WM, Gotlieb AI. In vitro repair of the wounded porcine mitral valve. Circ Res 1988;62:833–845.
17. Lester W, Rosenthal A, Granton B, et al. Porcine mitral valve interstitial cells in culture. Lab Invest 1988;59:710–719.
18. Zacks S, Rosenthal A, Granton B, et al. Characterization of cobblestone mitral valve interstitial cells. Arch Pathol Lab Med 1991; 115:774–779.
19. Yusuf S, Pepine CJ, Garces C, et al. Effect of enalapril on myocardial infarction and unstable angina in patients with low ejection fractions. Lancet 1992;340:1173–1178.
20. Hansen-Smith FM, Watson L, Lu DY, et al. Griffonia simplicifolia I: fluorescent tracer for microcirculatory vessels in nonperfused thin muscles and sectioned muscle. Microvasc Res 1988;36:199–215.
21. Bernstein KE, Martin BM, Edwards AS, et al. Mouse angiotensin-converting enzyme is a protein composed of two homologous domains. J Biol Chem 1989;264:11945–11951.
22. Kinoshita A, Urata H, Bumpus FM, et al. Measurement of angiotensin I converting enzyme inhibition in the heart. Circ Res 1993; 73:51–60.
23. Skalli O, Schürch W, Seemayer T, et al. Myofibroblasts from diverse pathologic settings are heterogenous in their content of actin isoforms and intermediate filament proteins. Lab Invest 1989;60:275–285.
24. Johnson CM, Hanson MN, Helgeson SC. Porcine cardiac valvular subendothelial cells in culture: cell isolation and growth characteristics. J Mol Cell Cardiol 1987;19: 1185–1193.
25. Katwa LC, Weber KT. Angiotensin type I and type II receptors in cultured adult rat cardiac fibroblasts. (Abstract) J Mol Cell Cardiol 1993;25(Suppl. III):S89.
26. Villarreal FJ, Kim NN, Ungab GD, et al. Identification of functional angiotensin II receptors on rat cardiac fibroblasts. Circulation 1993;88:2849–2861.

27. Katwa LC, Guarda E, Weber KT. Endothelin receptors in cultured adult rat cardiac fibroblasts. Cardiovasc Res 1993;27:2125–2129.

28. Brilla CG, Zhou G, Matsubara L, et al. Collagen metabolism in cultured adult rat cardiac fibroblasts: response to angiotensin II and aldosterone. J Mol Cell Cardiol 1994;26: 809–820.

29. Guarda E, Katwa LC, Myers PR, et al. Effects of endothelins on collagen turnover in cardiac fibroblasts. Cardiovasc Res 1993;27: 2130–2134.

30. Willems IEMG, Havenith MG, et al. Structural alterations in heart valves during left ventricular pressure overload in the rat. Lab Invest 1994;71:127–133.

Chapter 19

Role of Endothelial-Derived Signals

Eduardo Guarda, M.D., Karl T. Weber, M.D.

Introduction

Recent evidence indicates that endothelial cells modulate vascular structure. This is evident with the reparative wound healing response that follows vessel injury[1,2] or with increments in intraluminal pressure.[3] Growth and function of cells that compose the vasculature, specifically vascular smooth muscle cells and fibroblasts, can be regulated by soluble peptides secreted by endothelial cells. In some cases, this interaction is mediated by intercellular communications and gap junction molecular transfer that mandates cell-cell contact.[4] This is exemplified by the physical relationship that exists between endothelial cells and pericytes in the microcirculation and which promotes intracellular signaling, such as pericyte-mediated capillary growth through contact inhibition of endothelial cell proliferation.[5] Co-culture methodology, where direct contact appears between cells, is useful to demonstrate such events. In other cases, a substance released by one given member of this vascular cell population will provide extracellular signaling and paracrine effects that promote the growth and/or alter the metabolic behavior of its neighboring cells. Such events can be demonstrated in co-culture where cells are physically separated from one another, but where conditioned media gains access to another population of cells from microporous wells.

Previous studies from this[6] and other[7] laboratories identified that an abnormal ac-cumulation of fibrous tissue appears within systemic and intramyocardial coronary arteries and arterioles when the renin-angiotensin-aldosterone system (RAAS) is activated or when its effector hormones, angiotensin II (AngII) and aldosterone (ALDO), are chronically administered. This fibrosis tissue response appears first within the adventitia of intramural coronary vessels and subsequently extends into neighboring interstitial spaces. This wound healing-like response led to the hypothesis that substances produced by endothelial cells could modulate the function of fibroblasts present in the adventitia of coronary vessels and thus contribute to the pathological accumulation of fibrillar collagen, expressed as perivascular fibrosis. Using co-culture methodology where cells were physically separated from one another, and where confounding variables, such as arterial hypertension and left ventricular hypertrophy could be eliminated, we addressed this hypothesis.[8] We examined: 1) the effect of cultured vascular endothelial cells on cultured rat cardiac fibroblast collagen synthesis and collagenase activity; 2) whether angiotensin II or aldosterone, influenced endothelial cells induced modulation of fibroblast collagen metabolism and; 3) whether the substance released in endothelial cell conditioned medium was angiotensin II or aldosterone.

Endothelial Cells and Fibroblast Collagen Synthesis

In Figure 1 the results of endothelial cell conditioned media on cardiac fibroblast

---

[1] This work was supported in part by NIH Grant R01-HL-31701.

From Weber KT, MD *Wound Healing in Cardiovascular Disease*, Armonk, NY, Futura Publishing Company Inc., © 1995.

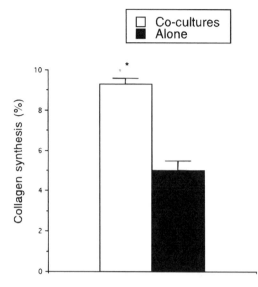

Figure 1. Collagen synthesis in fibroblasts alone and in co-cultured fibroblasts at 48 hours (n = 6). *$P<0.01$ vs. fibroblasts alone. Reproduced with permission from ref. 8.

collagen synthesis is shown. There was a 1.9-fold increase in collagen synthesis in fibroblasts co-cultured with endothelial cells compared to fibroblasts alone ($P<0.001$). There were no differences in the rate of collagen synthesis when fibroblasts were co-cultured with fibroblasts alone at 6 or 12 hours of co-culture. A trend toward greater collagen synthesis in co-cultured fibroblasts compared with fibroblasts alone was observed at 24 hours, with differences between each group reaching statistical significance ($P<0.001$) at 48 hours, when fibroblast collagen synthesis had risen 1.9-fold.

Effects of Angiotensin II and Aldosterone on Collagen Synthesis

We considered the effects of aldosterone and angiotensin II as potential contributors to the increased collagen synthesis seen in co-culture. Accordingly, in one group of experiments, cardiac fibroblasts (not in co-culture) were incubated with either angiotensin II (10^{-7} M) or aldosterone (10^{-8} M). Both hormones were able to increase collagen synthesis in cardiac fibroblasts ($P<0.05$) compared to fibroblast cultured without these hormones.

In an attempt to disclose the nature of the stimulatory substance produced by endothelial cells, we supplemented the endothelial cell medium for 24 hours with ALDO (10^{-8} M) or AngII (10^{-7} M), in a second group of experiments where co-culture preparation was again used. These hormones did not increase fibroblast collagen synthesis over co-cultures alone.

To explore the possibility that the collagen synthesis enhancing substance released by the endothelial cells was ALDO or AngII, co-cultured endothelial cells and fibroblasts were incubated for 24 hours with the aldosterone receptor antagonist spironolactone (10^{-8} M), or a type I (DuP 753, 10^{-8} M) or type II (PD123319, 10^{-8} M) AngII receptor antagonist. Neither spironolactone nor the AT_1 or AT_2 receptor antagonists were able to prevent the increase on fibroblast collagen production induced by endothelial cells, indicating that neither AngII nor ALDO influence the response in cardiac fibroblast collagen metabolism to endothelial cells conditioned medium. These findings indicate that it is not these hormones that are produced by endothelial cells and released into their conditioned medium to augment fibroblast collagen metabolism.

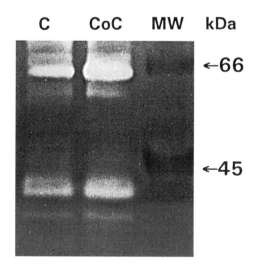

Figure 2. Collagenolytic activity in co-cultured fibroblast-conditioned medium (CoC) and in fibroblasts alone-conditioned medium (C). Reproduced with permission from ref. 8.

Collagenolytic Activity

Experiments were also conducted under similar conditions to quantitate collagenolytic activity in conditioned medium from fibroblasts co-cultured for 24 hours with endothelial cells. Figure 2 is a representative example of these zymographic studies. Collagenolytic activity was markedly increased in co-cultured fibroblasts relative to collagenolytic activity of fibroblasts alone. We also studied the effects of AngII or ALDO on collagenase activity in fibroblasts alone (Figure 3). We consistently observed that AngII (10^{-8} M) markedly decreased collagenolytic activity on cardiac fibroblasts alone, while aldosterone (10^{-8} M) produced only a slight decrement in collagenolytic activity.

Thus, in these co-culture studies, we were unable to demonstrate that either AngII or ALDO augmented the influence of endothelial cell conditioned medium on fibroblast collagen synthesis or collagenolytic activity beyond that observed for the co-culture preparation. We did not, however, incubate endothelial cells with a mixture of these hormones, as would exist in

vivo when the (RAAS) is activated.[9] Thus, based on these findings, we cannot support the proposition that this peptide and steroid hormone lead to a perivascular fibrosis of intramyocardial vessels because of their ability to enhance the normal interaction that exists between the endothelium and neighboring fibroblasts. These studies, however, have not considered the elaborate interplay that exists between these effector hormones of the renin-angiotensin-aldosterone system (RAAS) and endothelins, a family of peptide hormones released by vascular endothelial cells with diverse biological action.[10]

Endothelins and Fibroblast Collagen Synthesis

Endothelins have been found to alter collagen synthesis of mesenchymal cells.[11] ET-1 induces proliferation of fibroblast-like cells,[12] while it increases collagen synthesis of skin fibroblasts[13] and bone organ cultures.[14] The influence of ET-3 on collagen turnover and cellular proliferation had not been reported. We tested the hypothesis that endothelins regulate collagen turnover and DNA synthesis of cultured adult rat cardiac fibroblasts through differential modulation of collagen synthesis, specifically its type I and III collagen phenotypes and collagenolytic activity. Potential differences in the effects of these endothelins on these cells were analyzed by using ET-1, ET-3, and an ET_A receptor antagonist, since ET-1 acts through both ET_A and ET_B receptors while the influence of ET-3 is thought to be mediated by ET_B receptors.[15]

Endothelins and Collagen Synthesis, Collagen Phenotypes, and DNA Synthesis

Previous reports using the ^{3}H-proline incorporation method have demonstrated that ET-1 increases collagen synthesis in cultured human dermal fibroblasts.[16] Using a similar approach, we found both ET-1 and ET-3 increased collagen synthesis in adult rat cardiac fibroblasts.[17] The effect of ET-1 was 10 times more potent than ET-3 (Figure

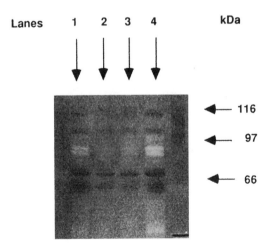

Lanes   1   2   3   4   kDa

← 116

← 97

← 66

Figure 3. Effects of aldosterone (lane 1, 10^{-8} M) or angiotensin II (lane 3, 10^{-8} M) supplementation for 24 h on collagenolytic activity estimated by zymography in medium obtained from fibroblasts alone. Lane 4, fibroblasts alone without hormonal supplementation. Reproduced with permission from ref. 8.

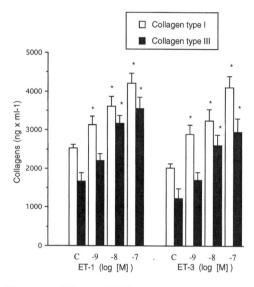

Figure 4. Effects of different concentrations of ET-1 and ET-3 upon the release of collagens types I and III from rat cardiac fibroblasts. Aliquots (100 μL) of conditioned medium were tested using an ELISA method. *$P < 0.01$ vs. controls. Reproduced with permission from ref. 17.

4). The 1.7-fold maximal increase in collagen synthesis in response to endothelins found in our study fall within the range shown by others in dermal fibroblasts[13] and is also comparable to the synthesis of collagen found in response to ALDO or AngII.[18,19]

Although collagen type I is the major fibrillar collagen found in different species and in disease states, type III collagen increased in parallel with the early development of ventricular hypertrophy.[20] In our study, using an ELISA method to analyze collagen phenotypes secreted by cultured rat cardiac fibroblasts, we found that the relative ratio of type I:III collagens under basal conditions was 60%:40%. ET-1 and ET-3 induced increments in both collagen phenotypes in similar proportion.

In addition to its action on collagen synthesis, we found that endothelins increase DNA synthesis in cardiac fibroblasts. ET-1 has been shown to increase DNA synthesis and total collagen synthesis in human dermal fibroblasts[13] and in transformed fibroblast 3T3 cells.[12] In this study, we demonstrated that ET-1 and ET-3 induced a significant increase in ^{3}H-thymidine incorporation in cultured adult rat cardiac fibroblasts. Overall, our findings support the general concept that ET-1 and ET-3 are mitogens for fibroblasts and that endothelins released during pathological states may play a role in the proliferation and turnover of collagen by fibroblasts.

Endothelins and Collagenase

We found ET-1, but not ET-3, decreased collagenolytic activity in cardiac fibroblasts (Figure 5). These results suggested that ET_A, but not ET_B receptors, mediate the effect of endothelin on collagenolytic activity. This observation was further supported by our experiments showing inhibition of the ET-1–dependent decrease in collagenolytic activity with the ET_A receptor antagonist PED-3512-PI. The modulation of collagenolytic activity has important implications regarding the dynamic regulation of collagen synthesis and collagen breakdown and the relative amounts of collagen in the extracellular matrix. Collagenase, a metalloproteinase, can be regulated by the action of several inhibitors, the best characterized being the tissue inhibitor of metalloproteinases (TIMP). TIMP, a glycoprotein which forms a tight complex with active collagen-

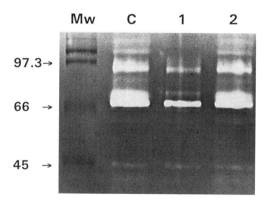

Figure 5. Collagenolytic activity determined by zymography in cardiac fibroblast conditioned medium. Lane C, control fibroblasts; Lane 1, fibroblasts incubated with ET-1 (10^{-7} M); Lane 2, fibroblasts incubated with ET-1 (10^{-7} M) plus PED-3512-PI (10^{-6} M). Reproduced with permission from ref. 17.

ase,[21] may be important in the overall regulation of collagenolytic activity. However, its relationship to endothelin and the actions of endothelin reported in this study remains to be determined.

Endothelin Receptor Subtypes

The cellular responses to endothelins are mediated by the interaction of endothelins with specific cell surface receptors, namely ET_A and ET_B receptors. The ET_A receptor is specific for ET-1, while the ET_B receptor shows no selectivity for ET isoforms.[15] We found the effects of ET-1 and ET-3 were similar in their ability to increase the synthesis of fibrillar collagens and fibroblast DNA synthesis, which suggest these effects were mediated by the ET_A and ET_B receptor subtypes. We were not able to block the effects of ET-1-mediated increases in collagen synthesis with the ET_A receptor antagonist PED-3512-PI. Thus, it is possible ET-1–dependent increases in collagen synthesis could be mediated through both ET receptor subtypes in similar proportions. The presence of both ET_A and ET_B receptor subtypes in adult rat cardiac fibroblasts has recently been reported.[22]

Regulation of Endothelin Levels: Relationship to the RAAS

Several factors contribute to ET-1 and ET-3 regulation.[23] In advanced heart failure, circulating ET-1 is increased, which could contribute to the maintenance of blood pressure in the presence of low cardiac output.[24] A complex relationship exits between the RAAS and ET-1. On the one hand, ET-1 increases endothelial angiotensin converting enzyme (ACE) activity and the conversion of AngI to AngII.[25] ET-1 and ET-3 each increase ALDO synthesis in cultured glomerulosa cells.[26,27] On the other hand, AngII increase ET-1 secretion from vascular endothelial cells in vivo.[28,29] It has recently been demonstrated that ET-1 and AngII work synergistically to raise blood pressure in rats.[30] Combining these observations with our present findings, it is possible that endothelins and AngII act synergistically to modify the extracellular matrix by increasing fibrillar collagen deposition in certain disease states. Furthermore, the beneficial effects of ACE inhibitors to decrease perivascular collagen accumulation[31] could be related, in part, to the recently described effect of angiotensin converting enzyme inhibitors to suppress endothelin secretion.[29]

Thus, perivascular fibrosis found in human[32] and experimental animal is associated with activation of the circulating RAAS.[6] However, using co-culture methodology of vascular endothelial cells and cardiac fibroblasts, we demonstrated the stimulation of collagen synthesis through mechanisms independent of AngII or ALDO. Furthermore, we demonstrated that ET-1 and ET-3 increased total collagen synthesis and the expression of both type I and III collagens in cardiac fibroblasts. Interestingly, ET-1, but not ET-3, reduced collagenolytic activity. Therefore, our data support the hypothesis that a locally produced or circulating substance, such as endothelins could play an important role in the perivascular fibrosis seen in specific pathophysiological states, such as renovascular hypertension. Furthermore, the disparate effects of endothelins on collagen and collagenase are consistent with an important role of endothelins in the dynamic regulation of the synthesis and breakdown of collagen. Our findings that endothelins may also be involved in the mitogenic response with subsequent proliferation of fibroblasts adds further credence to the hypothesis that endothelins may be functional in vascular and perivascular remodeling. Pathological states that result in an increase of endothelins—promoters of collagen accumulation, relative to substances (e.g., nitric oxide) that serve as inhibitors of collagen synthesis—may provoke fibrous tissue formation that ultimately impairs tissue and organ function. This concept emphasizes the importance of the relative balance between opposing factors that regulate vascular and tissue structure and thereby overall organ function.

Summary

Beyond the regulation of vasomotor reactivity in both the arterial and venous circulation, vascular endothelial cells play an important role in modulating vascular structure. This includes the reparative wound healing response that follows injury. An emerging body of evidence implicates a complex reciprocal interaction between cells that compose the vasculature, specifically endothelial cells, vascular smooth muscle cells, pericytes, and fibroblasts, and which is mediated at least in part by soluble peptides secreted by endothelial cells. Because these peptides can have paracrine properties on neighboring cells, vascular structure will be altered. This may include a perivascular fibrosis of coronary arterioles such as appears in various disease states. This wound healing-like response led us to the hypothesis that substances produced by endothelial cells are involved in fibroblast collagen metabolism and the pathological accumulation of fibrillar collagen that was expressed as perivascular fibrosis. We focused on the interplay that exists between effector hormones of the RAAS and endothelins, a family of peptide hormones with diverse biological action, released by vascular endothelial cells.

References

1. Munro JM, Cotran RS. The pathogenesis of atherosclerosis: atherogenesis and inflammation. Lab Invest 1988;58:249–261.
2. Madri JM, Bell L, Marx M, et al. Effects of soluble factors and extracellular matrix components on vascular cell behavior in vitro and in vivo: models of de-endothelialization and repair. J Cell Biochem 1991;45:123–130.
3. Iwatsuki K, Cardinale GJ, Spector S, et al. Hypertension: increase of collagen biosynthesis in arteries but not in veins. Science 1977;198:403–405.
4. Sheridan JD, Larson DM. Junctional communication in the peripheral vasculature. In: Pitts JD, Finbow ME, eds. The Functional Integration of Cells in Animal Tissues. New York, NY: Cambridge University Press, 1982: 263–283.
5. Orlidge A, D'Amore PA. Inhibition of capillary endothelial cell growth by pericytes and smooth muscle cells. J Cell Biol 1987;105: 1455–1462.
6. Weber KT, Brilla CG. Pathological hypertrophy and cardiac interstitium: fibrosis and renin-angiotensin-aldosterone system. Circulation 1991;83:1849–1865.
7. Michel JB, Salzmann JL, Ossondo Nlom M, et al. Morphometric analysis of collagen network and plasma perfused capillary bed in the myocardium of rats during evolution of cardiac hypertrophy. Basic Res Cardiol 1986; 81:142–154.
8. Guarda E, Myers PR, Brilla CG, et al. Endothelial cell induced modulation of cardiac fibroblast collagen metabolism. Cardiovasc Res 1993;27:1004–1008.
9. Kawaguchi H, Sawa H, Yasuda H. Endothelin stimulates angiotensin I to angiotensin II conversion in cultured pulmonary artery endothelial cells. J Mol Cell Cardiol 1990;22: 839–842.
10. Lerman A, Hildebrand FL Jr, Margulies KB, et al. Endothelin: a new cardiovascular regulatory peptide. Mayo Clin Proc 1990;65: 1441–1455.
11. Schrey MP, Patel KV, Tezapsidis N. Bombesin and glucocorticoids stimulate human breast cancer cells to produce endothelin, a paracrine mitogen for breast stromal cells. Cancer Res 1992;52:1786–1790.
12. Takuwa N, Takuwa Y, Yanagisawa M, et al. A novel vasoactive peptide endothelin stimulates mitogenesis through inositol lipid turnover in Swiss 3T3 fibroblasts. J Biol Chem 1989;264:7856–7861.
13. Kahaleh MB. Endothelin, an endothelial-dependent vasoconstrictor in scleroderma: enhanced production and profibrotic action. Arthritis Rheum 1991;34:978–983.
14. Tatrai A, Foster S, Lakatos P, et al. Endothelin-1 actions on resorption, collagen and noncollagen protein synthesis, and phosphatidylinositol turnover in bone organ cultures. Endocrinology 1992;131:603–607.
15. Thomas CP, Simonson M, Dunn MJ. Endothelin: receptors and transmembrane signals. News Physiol Sci 1992;7:207–211.
16. Botstein GR, Sherer GK, Leroy EC. Fibroblast selection in scleroderma: an alternative model of fibrosis. Arthritis Rheum 1982;25: 189–195.
17. Guarda E, Katwa LC, Myers PR, et al. Effects of endothelins on collagen turnover in cardiac fibroblasts. Cardiovasc Res 1993;27: 2130–2134.
18. Brilla CG, Zhou G, Weber KT. Aldosterone and collagen synthesis in cultured adult rat cardiac fibroblasts. (Abstract) FASEB J 1992; 6:A1914.
19. Zhou G, Brilla CG, Weber KT. Angiotensin II-mediated stimulation of collagen synthesis in cultured cardiac fibroblasts. (Abstract) FASEB J 1992;6:A1914.
20. Chapman D, Weber KT, Eghbali M. Regulation of fibrillar collagen types I and III and basement membrane type IV collagen gene

expression in pressure overloaded rat myocardium. Circ Res 1990;67:787–794.

21. Woessner JF Jr. Matrix metalloproteinases and their inhibitors in connective tissue remodeling. FASEB J 1991;5:2145–2154.

22. Katwa LC, Guarda E, Weber KT. Endothelin receptors in cultured adult rat cardiac fibroblasts. Cardiovasc Res 1993;27:2125–2129.

23. Inoue A, Yanagisawa M, Kimura S, et al. The human endothelin family: three structurally and pharmacologically distinct isopeptides predicted by three separate genes. Proc Natl Acad Sci USA 1989;86:2863–2867.

24. Rodeheffer RJ, Lerman A, Heublein DM, et al. Increased plasma concentrations of endothelin in congestive heart failure in humans. Mayo Clin Proc 1992;67:719–724.

25. Kawaguchi H, Sawa H, Yasuda H. Effect of endothelin on angiotensin converting enzyme activity in cultured pulmonary artery endothelial cells. J Hypertens 1991;9:171–174.

26. Cozza EN, Gomez-Sanchez CE, Foecking MF, et al. Endothelin binding to cultured calf adrenal zona glomerulosa cells and stimulation of aldosterone secretion. J Clin Invest 1989;84:1032–1035.

27. Hinson JP, Kapas S, Teja R, et al. Effect of the endothelins on aldosterone secretion by rat zona glomerulosa cells in vitro. J Steroid Biochem Mol Biol 1991;40:437–439.

28. Emori T, Hirata Y, Ohta K, et al. Secretory mechanism of immunoreactive endothelin in cultured bovine endothelial cells. Biochem Biophys Res Commun 1989;160:93–100.

29. Kohno M, Yokokawa K, Horio T, Yasunari K, Murakawa K, Takeda T. Atrial and brain natriuretic peptides inhibit the endothelin-1 secretory response to angiotensin II in porcine aorta. Circ Res 1992;70:241–247.

30. Yoshida K, Yasujima M, Kohzuki M, et al. Endothelin-1 augments pressor response to angiotensin II infusion in rats. Hypertension 1992;20:292–297.

31. Brilla CG, Janicki JS, Weber KT. Impaired diastolic function and coronary reserve in genetic hypertension: role of interstitial fibrosis and medial thickening of intramyocardial coronary arteries. Circ Res 1991;69:107–115.

32. Campbell SE, Diaz-Arias AA, Weber KT. Fibrosis of the human heart and systemic organs in adrenal adenoma. Blood Pressure 1992;1:149–156.

Chapter 20

Activation of Angiotensin II Receptors in the Postinfarcted Heart and Myocyte Growth Processes

Leonard G. Meggs, M.D., Piero Anversa, M.D.

Myocardial Infarction and Reactive Myocyte Growth

A sudden occlusion of a coronary artery leads in 1 minute to loss of function in the supplied myocardium, affecting ventricular pump performance in proportion to the magnitude of tissue involved in the ischemic event.[1,2] This phenomenon results in a redistribution of cardiac loading and the remaining viable myocardium is called upon to maintain cardiac output and blood flow to the peripheral circulation. Recent work, concerning the effects of partial and total occlusion of the coronary artery, has demonstrated that the immediate reaction of the left ventricle to an impairment in cardiac dynamics consists of chamber dilation and thinning of the wall.[1,2] Mural thinning occurs in the nonischemic region of the wall through an architectural rearrangement of the myocyte compartment of the myocardium without involving the Starling mechanism and sarcomere stretching. This anatomical adaptation, consisting of side-to-side slippage of cells within the wall, appears to be the major determinant of the decrease in wall thickness-to-chamber radius ratio and ventricular dilation, acutely following myocardial infarction.[3] Such an effect, in combination with the early modifications in the necrotic portion of the wall, expands cavitary volume resulting in an abnormal increase in diastolic wall stress and, to a lesser degree, systolic wall stress.[1-3] Thus, a segmental loss of myocardium alters ventricular loading acutely and this mechanical stimulus may be the initiating event of ventricular remodeling after infarction.

The long-term consequences of cardiac restructuring after infarction are mandated by the acute events which establish the initial load on the viable tissue and the magnitude and nature of the growth reaction of the remaining myocytes. In essence, ventricular dilation after the acute phase may occur only by lengthening of myocytes and/or the in-series addition of newly formed cells. Although thinning of the infarcted myocardium also takes place until healing is completed,[4] contributing to the expansion in cavitary volume, myocyte lengthening may have to be considered the major determinant of the cardiac size and shape after infarction. This process may be further amplified by myocyte proliferation when it occurs.[5] In contrast, the rigid collagen of the scar region may stretch very little over periods of months, contributing minimally to chronic remodeling.

Any loss of cardiac mass from ischemic necrosis can be expected to result in a proportional loss of myocyte nuclei and, subse-

[1]This work was supported by Grants HL-38132, HL-39902, and HL-40561 from the National Heart, Lung, and Blood Institute.

quently, a proportional accumulation of connective tissue scar in the ventricle. In addition, the initial volume of spared tissue can be assumed to be proportional to the number of myocyte nuclei remaining in the ventricular myocardium. Such a relationship has been demonstrated in rats at the completion of healing, approximately 1 month after coronary artery occlusion.[1] The graphical comparison of the percent of scarred tissue in the whole ventricle versus the total number of myocyte nuclei measured in the spared myocardium was found to be inversely related. This association is consistent with the notion that smaller residual numbers of myocyte nuclei are present with larger infarcts and can be applied in the estimation of infarct size. Conversely, the magnitude of myocyte reactive hypertrophy was shown to be a function of infarct size. In this regard, muscle cell volume in the spared myocardium of infarcted hearts, when plotted against the percent of scarred tissue in the ventricle, demonstrated a highly significant positive correlation. This relationship documented that larger infarcts were accompanied by greater average myocyte cell volume in the remaining non-infarcted region of the wall.[1] Importantly, these findings indicate that the consequences of myocardial infarction on cardiac remodeling can be characterized only by the determination of the changes in myocyte size and number.

The dimensional changes of ventricular myocytes after myocardial infarction which involve increases in myocyte cross-sectional area and length are consistent with cellular shape changes characteristic of concentric and eccentric hypertrophy in the intact ventricular wall.[1,2,5] Loss of cardiac cells in the ventricle results in a greater stress on the remaining viable myocytes. To reduce the magnitude of systolic stress, myocytes would tend to hypertrophy by increasing their diameter, as shown in several reports.[1,2,5] On this basis, infarction-induced hypertrophy may be viewed, at least in part, as pressure overload hypertrophy, despite the presence of a normal or decreased pressure.[5]

Physiological studies performed over several weeks in the dog heart have documented a progressive increase of the end-diastolic segment lengths in the normal regions of infarcted ventricles.[6–8] Similar adaptations have been observed in chronic volume-overloaded left ventricles[9] in which lengthening of the myocyte population would have the effect of counteracting the greater end-diastolic wall stress by contributing to the enlargement in chamber volume, as suggested by Grossman, et al.[10,11] Therefore, cardiac hypertrophy associated with myocardial infarction appears to be the result of both pressure and volume overload, consonant with the increases in myocyte diameter and length measured morphologically.[1,5] Derivations of systolic and diastolic wall stress after infarction have supported these conclusions.[2] In summary, myocyte reactive hypertrophy after infarction induces changes in myocyte shape which, together with myocyte loss, are the major determinants of chronic ventricular remodeling in the cardiomyopathic heart of ischemic origin.[5]

Cardiac Renin-Angiotensin System and Myocardial Infarction

A growing body of evidence supports the concept of an intracardiac renin-angiotensin system (RAS),[12,13] which operates via an autocrine/paracrine signaling pathway.[14] Activation of this local cardiac RAS promotes the generation of angiotensin II (AngII)[12,14] which is believed to be an early event in the adaptive growth response of ventricular myocytes.[15,16] The trophic influence of AngII is also supported by in vivo studies demonstrating a selective effect of angiotensin-converting-enzyme (ACE) inhibitors on the hypertrophic response of myocytes in genetic hypertension[17] and experimental models of pressure overload.[18,19] Although these investigations do not provide direct documentation that cardiac muscle cells can synthesize AngII or that this peptide is a growth factor for these cells, several laboratories have demonstrated that myocytes possess the molecular components required for the local generation of AngII.[16,20] In addition, mechanical stretch of neonatal myocytes in culture causes release of AngII, which acts as the proximate mediator of the stretch-induced hypertrophic response.[16] Thus, these observations are consistent with the notion that the cardiac RAS is activated by work overload and induces myocyte growth.

Acute occlusion of the left coronary artery in rats has served not only as a useful model to examine the morphological and functional consequences of myocardial infarction,[21-23] but also the expression of the molecular constituents of RAS. In this regard, an up-regulation in angiotensinogen[24] and ACE mRNAs[25] in myocytes has been reported as well as an increase in the density of AngII binding sites.[26] The latter alteration in binding capacity was temporally correlated with the phase of intense reactive myocyte growth in the immediate postinfarction period. Additional support for activation of an AngII autocrine signaling mechanism after myocardial infarction can be inferred from studies in which administration of ACE inhibitors has been shown to reduce myocyte hypertrophy[27] and left ventricular dilation,[28] while improving survival in both animals[29] and man.[30,31]

The observations summarized above provide the construct for the hypothesis that AngII may participate in the changes of cardiac size and shape which characterize the postinfarcted heart. In this scheme of events, the activation of surface AngII receptors may play a key role in the adaptive and maladaptive processes which constitute ventricular remodeling.[1,2,5,30-34] However, other mechanisms may influence this process, such as myocardial fibrosis and rearrangement in the architecture of the extracellular matrix.[34] Of note, a picture closely resembling the infarcted heart has been shown following prolonged exposure of myocardial tissue to suppressor doses of AngII.[35] In addition, focal myocyte necrosis was a prominent feature in this model. Therefore, AngII appears capable of inducing a spectrum of biological responses ranging from cell growth to cell death which may involve regulatory modifications in the expression and density of AngII binding sites. However, until recently, evidence that adult rat cardiac muscle cells possess pharmacologically distinct AngII receptors has been lacking. The inability to demonstrate AngII binding sites has been a limiting factor in the characterization of the events by which AngII signals are transmitted to the nucleus activating growth-promoting pathways in normal and infarcted heart.

Identification and Characterization of Angiotensin II (ANGII) Receptors on Adult Rat Ventricular Myocytes

A prerequisite for establishing the proposed role of AngII as a cardiac growth factor was the identification of discrete binding sites on the surface of myocytes. With the exception of the presence of AngII receptors in neonatal myocytes,[36] attempts at characterization of these receptors in adult rat hearts proved to be technically difficult. This was due to high levels of nonspecific binding and contamination of crude membrane preparations with nonmyocyte cells. The latter concern is underscored by recent reports confirming that vascular smooth cells and cardiac fibroblasts exhibit a high binding capacity for AngII.[37-39] To address these problems our laboratory adopted a methodology that provided a homogenous population of adult rat ventricular myocytes. This was accomplished through enzymatic dissociation of muscle cells by retrograde collagenase perfusion. Intact cardiac cells were then enriched by centrifugation through Percoll and the extent of nonmyocytes present in each preparation determined. Consistent with previous results in our laboratory,[40] the degree of contamination was found to be very low, ranging from 1% to 3%. Subsequently, a membrane fraction was prepared from these purified myocytes[41] and AngII receptors were immediately labeled with the antagonist $[^{125}I]Sar^1$-Ile^8 AngII. Since membranes were made by discarding a preliminary 14,000-g pellet to eliminate cellular debris and nuclear particles, the possibility had to be raised that binding sites could have been lost in this fraction. Extensive studies on the discarded 14,000-g pellets documented the presence of β-adrenoreceptors[42] but AngII receptors

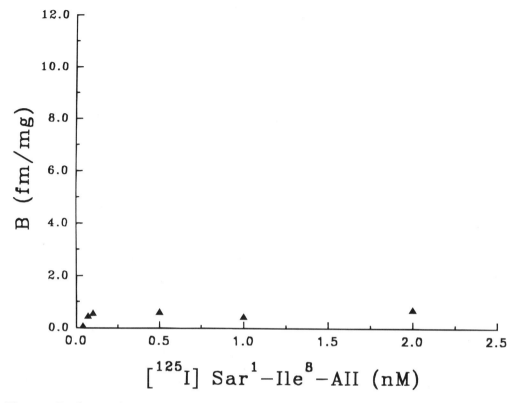

Figure 1. Binding isotherm performed utilizing the resuspended 14,000-g fraction which was discarded during the membrane preparation procedure. No AT_1 receptor binding sites are detected in this fraction.

were repeatedly found to be absent (Figure 1). Utilization of lower speeds to purify the homogenate resulted in barely detectable binding sites or poorly reproducible data. Finally, the use of a radiolabeled antagonist offered the advantage of identifying a homogenous population of binding sites. Radiolabeled agonists may recognize multiple receptor affinities complicating analysis of binding data by Scatchard transformation.[37,43]

In preliminary studies, the specificity and selectivity of the radioligand [^{125}I]Sar[1]-Ile[8] AngII to label AngII receptors on ventricular myocytes were demonstrated by performing a series of competition curves with peptide and nonpeptide competitors of AngII.[44] The nonpeptide receptor subtype antagonists, DuP753 and PD123319, were used to identify AT_1 and AT_2 receptor

subtypes (Figure. 2). The Hill coefficient for displacement of the radioligand by DuP753 was 0.98, consistent with the recognition of a uniform set of binding sites. The calculated K_i for DuP753 was 0.62 nM. In contrast, PD123319 failed to displace the radioligand, and the Hill coefficient (0.16) indicated the absence of recognizable AT_2 binding sites. In addition, K_i was >1000 nM. On the other hand, the nonselective peptide analog Sar[1]Ile[8] AngII displaced the radioligand as expected. The Hill coefficient and calculated K_i[45] for this partial agonist were 0.73 and 0.1 nM, respectively. In addition, binding isotherms indicated that AngII binding sites were saturable and Scatchard transformation documented a homogenous set of binding sites with high affinity (Figure 3). Thus, based on these cumulative results, adult rat ventricular myocytes were

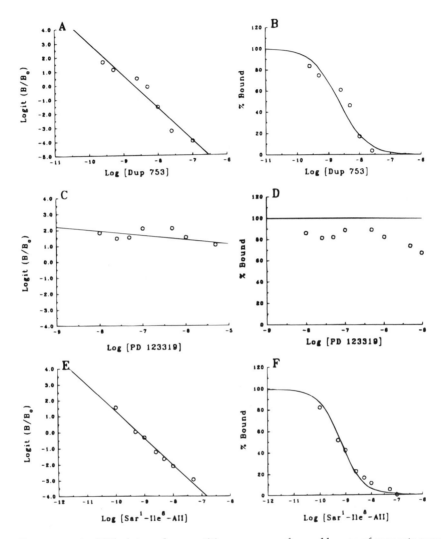

Figure 2. Representative Hill plots and competition curves performed by use of myocyte membranes from unoperated rats and the radioligand $[^{125}I]Sar^1Ile^8$ AngII. Panel A: Analysis of AT_1 receptor antagonist DuP753 displacement of $[^{125}I]Sar^1Ile^8$ AngII by Hill conversion. The Hill coefficient approaches unity (-0.98), consistent with the recognition of a single set of binding sites. Panel B: Competition binding profile of DuP753 demonstrating total displacement of bound counts by the AT_1 selective antagonist ($K_i = 0.62$ nM). Panel C: Analysis of AT_2 receptor antagonist PD123319 displacement of $[^{125}I]Sar^1Ile^8$ AngII by Hill conversion. The Hill coefficient (0.16) indicates that PD123319 does not recognize a uniform population of binding sites. Panel D: Competition binding profile of PD123319 demonstrating minimal displacement of bound counts by the AT_2 selective antagonist ($K_i \geq 1000$ nM). Panel E: Analysis of Sar^1Ile^8 AngII displacement of $[^{125}I]Sar^1Ile^8$ AngII by Hill conversion. The Hill coefficient (-0.73) indicates that Sar^1Ile^8 AngII is not a selective AngII receptor antagonist and recognized more than one binding site. Panel F, competition binding profile of Sar^1Ile^8 AngII demonstrating total displacement of bound counts by the nonselective peptide analog ($K_i = 0.1$ nM).

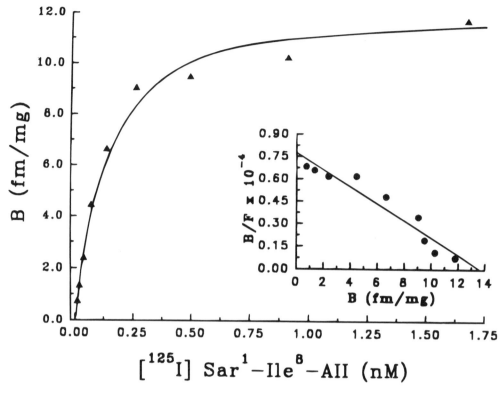

Figure 3. Binding isotherm and Scatchard transformation of [^{125}I]Sar^{1}Ile^8 AngII binding to membranes prepared from isolated ventricular myocytes of unoperated rats. The inset shows Scatchard transformation of saturation isotherm data indicating a homogeneous set of binding sites with high affinity.

demonstrated to possess AT$_1$ receptor subtypes exclusively.[41]

Regulation of AT$_1$ Receptors and Myocardial Infarction

In a recent communication,[26] our laboratory has documented that enhanced expression of AngII receptor mRNA occurred two to three days after myocardial infarction and this phenomenon was temporally coupled with induction of the early growth-related genes *c-myc* and *c-jun* in myocytes. Furthermore, a comparable increase in surface AngII receptors was detected suggesting that regulatory modifications of this receptor were induced by myocardial infarction and most likely at the level of transcription. These molecular adaptations were more prominent on the left side of the heart possibly reflecting differences in myo-

cardial loading between the ventricles. The 48 to 72 hour postinfarction interval corresponded to the initial phases of myocyte hypertrophy,[3] raising the possibility of a link between the mechanical stimulus on the surface of the cells and the activation of the AngII receptor gene (Figure 4).

Subsequently, at 7 days after myocardial infarction,[41] cellular hypertrophy was documented by increases in cell length and width, which were greater in the left ventricle. Reactive hypertrophy was accompanied by a 1.84-fold and 1.85-fold increase in AngII binding sites on left and right ventricular myocytes, respectively. In addition, AngII-stimulated phosphoinositol turnover was enhanced 3.7-fold and 2.5-fold in left and right ventricular muscle cells (Figure 5), suggesting that this signaling pathway may have initiated molecular responses leading to myocyte hypertrophy. In this regard, re-

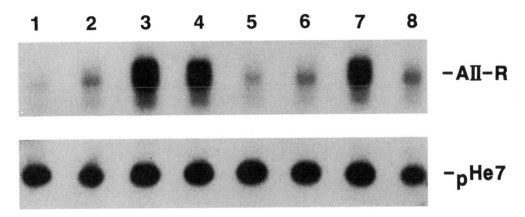

Figure 4. Detection of AngII-R mRNA by RTPCR in myocytes isolated from sham operated animals, lanes 1, 2, 5, and 6, and infarcted rats, lanes 3, 4, 7, and 8. Note high level of AngII-R mRNA expression after acute myocardial infarction. Corresponding pHe7 bands are illustrated.

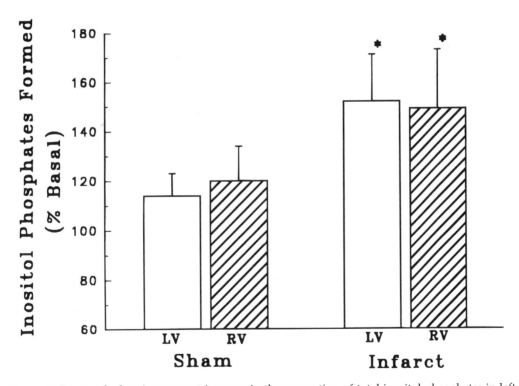

Figure 5. Bar graph showing percent increase in the generation of total inositol phosphates in left ventricular (LV) and right ventricular (RV) myocytes after exposure to 100 μM AngII. The formation of inositol phosphates is increased in LV and RV myocytes after infarction. Results are presented as mean $\pm$ SD. *Statistically significant at $P<0.05$.

cent studies confirm that AT_1 receptors are coupled to several phospholipid second messengers including inositol 1,4,5 triphosphate (IP_3), diacylglycerol (DAG), phosphatidic acid (PA,) and arachidonic acid metabolites.[15] Although it is generally agreed that a putative guanine nucleotide binding protein (G protein) couples the AT_1 receptor to phospholipase C (PLC) with the subsequent hydrolysis of bis 4,5 phosphatidylinositol, it is not known if the generation of PA and arachidonic acid metabolites in cardiocytes is mediated via G protein activation of phospholipase D (PLD) and phospholipase A_2 (PLA_2), respectively.

Activation of the phosphorylating enzyme protein Kinase C (PKC) has been shown to play a central role in the trophic influence of AngII on myocytes.[15] As mentioned above, DAG, an intermediate of phosphoinositide hydrolysis, is the physiological activator of PKC. Cardiocytes also possess alternate pathways to generate DAG through the hydrolysis of phosphatidylcholine (PC) by PLC, PLD, and PLA_2 leading to the formation of PA. The latter substrate is converted by PA phosphohydrolase to DAG. Although the exact sequence of events by which PKC induces growth in ventricular myocytes is not known, effects on cell pH and expression of immediate early genes have been reported.[15,46] The Na/H antiporter, which promotes alkalinization of the cell, an early event in the growth process, is a substrate for PKC.[46] In addition, induction of c-fos by AngII is PLC and PKC dependent and the AngII response sequence of this gene has been detected on the PKC-dependent portion of the serum response element.[15] The available evidence appears to suggest that AngII promotes cardiocyte growth via a signaling pathway of PKC and the expression of early immediate genes.

The proto-oncogenes c-myc and c-jun belong to a family of early growth-related genes whose mRNAs markedly increase soon after stimulation of quiescent cells with growth factors.[47,48] The expression of these genes has been found to be transient and to return rapidly to baseline levels.[49,50] In vivo models of pressure overload hypertrophy have repeatedly indicated that the immediate induction of early growth-related genes, including c-myc and c-jun, is followed by progressive reduction of their message, which becomes undetectable shortly after the imposition of the overload.[50] Acute elevations in systolic stress also correlate linearly with the expression of c-fos mRNA in the stressed myocardium.[51] These observations have led to the conclusion that the increase in systolic stress is coupled with the induction of early growth-related genes that participate in the modulation of myocyte growth. With lateral expansion of myocytes and mural thickening, systolic wall stress declines and concentric ventricular hypertrophy in its compensated stage typically occurs.[1] The mechanical stimulus generated by the increase in afterload may be fully counteracted by these adaptive processes, abolishing the signal for proto-oncogene activation. Systolic wall stress is biventricularly elevated 2 to 3 days after coronary occlusion, and this condition may be responsible for the enhanced c-myc and c-jun mRNA levels in myocytes (Figure 6) and the active growth reaction of the viable cells. The AngII receptors may be the proximate mediator in this sequence of events coupling mechanical stress with transcription of genes modulating myocyte reactive hypertrophy.

It should be recognized that stimulation of AngII receptors by ambient and/or circulating AngII may exert a positive inotropic effect on myocytes by increasing transmembrane calcium conductance.[51,52] AngII may also affect voltage-dependent sodium channels,[53] enhancing the contractile ability of myocytes through an increase in the rate of tension development of these cells.[54] It should also be acknowledged that AngII may exert its action on the myocardium indirectly by increasing the release of neurotransmitters from adrenergic cardiac presynaptic nerve terminals.[55] On the other hand, a negative inotropic effect of AngII has also been documented in adult rat myocytes.[56,57] In summary, the bifunctional role of AngII receptors on myocytes has been only partially characterized, and future studies remain to be performed to clarify their influence on myocyte hypertrophy and contractility in normal and pathological conditions.

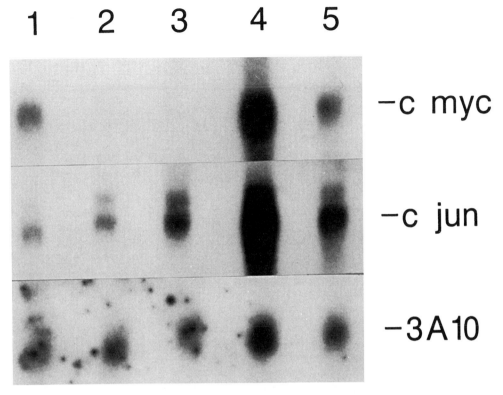

Figure 6. Northern blot analysis of *c-myc* and *c-jun* proto-oncogene expression in fetal myocardium (lane 1), left (lane 2) and right (lane 3) myocytes isolated from sham-operated rat, and left (lane 4) and right (lane 5) myocytes isolated from an infarcted rat. Note that proto-oncogene expression is markedly higher in myocytes from infarcted hearts. 3A10 was used as an internal standard.

Non-AngII Growth-Promoting Pathways and Myocardial Infarction

Stimulation of surface α_1-adrenoreceptors in vitro induces hypertrophy of neonatal and adult myocytes.[58-63] Activation of these receptors increases the rate of myosin light chain-2 transcription and mediates a transcriptional change in sarcomeric actin isoforms, reinducing the expression of α-skeletal actin.[61] Intracellular signals by which α_1-adrenoreceptors mediate myocyte growth and selective increases in the transcription of genes encoding contractile proteins have not been identified. Recent evidence favors an effector pathway that involves phospholipase C-mediated hydrolysis of phosphatidylinositol 4,5 bisphosphate which leads to formation of diacylglycerol

and inositol 1,4,5 triphosphate (IP_3), both of which may act as intracellular second messengers.[63] The reactive hypertrophic response of viable myocytes after infarction has been found to be accompanied by enhanced norepinephrine-stimulated phosphoinositol turnover and up-regulation of α-skeletal actin[64] which support a role of α_1-adrenoreceptors and effector pathways associated with these receptors in myocyte hypertrophy.

At least four subtypes of α_1-adrenergic receptors, α_{1a}, α_{1b}, α_{1c}, and α_{1d}, have been identified.[65-69] However, only the α_{1a} and α_{1b} subtypes have been characterized pharmacologically in the myocardium.[70] Different effector pathways appear to be linked to the α_{1a} and α_{1b} subtypes.[71] In vascular tissue the α_{1a} subtype may be involved in the regulation of calcium influx across the plasma membrane whereas the α_{1b} subtype is associated with the generation of IP_3 and diacylglycerol.[71] On the other hand, recent studies on cardiac myocytes tend to suggest that the α_{1a} subtype may be implicated in the formation of IP_3 and DAG and consequently myocyte growth and hypertrophy.[70,72] Thus, the functional significance of the α_{1a}- and α_{1b}-adrenergic receptor subtypes on adult rat ventricular myocytes remains to be determined. However, the availability of selective α_{1a} and α_{1b}-receptor subtype antagonists[65,67] have made these investigations feasible. A relevant aspect of a recent study performed in our laboratory[73] involved the characterization of the α_{1a} and α_{1b}-receptor subtypes in terms of their functional role in myocytes. Findings indicate that the α_{1a}-receptor subtype is coupled to PLC, leading to the generation of inositol phosphates. The coupling between α_{1a} subtype and phospholipase C was documented by the ability of the selective α_{1a}-adrenergic receptor subtype antagonist WB 4101 to inhibit agonist stimulated inositol phosphate formation at low concentrations. In contrast, inactivation of α_{1b}-binding sites by CEC did not produce a comparable effect. In addition, stimulation of α_{1a}-receptor subtypes improved myocyte mechanics, whereas activation of α_{1b}-receptor subtypes had no effect on the mechanical properties of the cells. Importantly, α_{1a}-receptor subtypes were found to influence myocardial contractility through increases in intracellular calcium. This did not occur following stimulation of the α_{1b}-receptor subtype. Thus, regulatory modifications of α_{1a}-receptor subtypes may positively or negatively modulate effector responses coupled with single cell function, calcium transient, and growth processes in myocytes.[73] On the assumption that the α_{1a}-adrenergic receptors are implicated in myocyte hypertrophy, the question concerns the mechanisms dictating the characteristics of this cellular enlargement, i.e., lengthening and/or lateral expansion. These cellular shape changes are the major determinants of wall thickness and chamber volume[1,2] which represent 2 of the 3 critical variables of ventricular loading.[1-3] Myocardial infarction-induced left ventricular hypertrophy is accomplished by a prevailing increase in myocyte length than in diameter, since the diastolic component

exceeds the systolic portion of the overload.[1-3] In contrast, infarction-induced right ventricular hypertrophy is generated by the lateral expansion of myocytes, reflecting an afterload stress on the myocardium.[1] Moreover, the possibility may be advanced that different mechanical stimuli on myocytes selectively activate specific surface receptors which may engender the addition in parallel of newly formed myofibrillar units, i.e., pressure hypertrophy, or the in-series addition of sarcomeres, i.e., volume hypertrophy, or the synthesis of contractile elements in parallel and in series, i.e., a combination of pressure and volume hypertrophy.[1] Recent results have demonstrated that cardiac hypertrophy produced by renal and mechanical hypertension which involves a lateral expansion of myocytes may be fully prevented by the administration of ACE inhibitors at doses which do not affect the magnitude of the afterload.[17,18] In a parallel manner, α_1-adrenergic receptor blockade has been claimed to reduce the extent of hypertrophic response of surviving myocytes after infarction[74] and in the cardiomyopathic Syrian hamster.[75] Thus, α_{1a}-adrenergic receptors and AngII receptors may be both involved in the modulation of ventricular remodeling after infarction.[26,41,64]

An active area of investigation concerns whether AngII acts independently or in concert with other growth factors. For example, AngII induces the synthesis of platelet-derived growth factor-A (PDGF-A), B-fibroblast growth factor (B-FGF), and transforming growth factor-β (TGF-β) in vascular smooth muscle cells.[76] In addition, it has been shown that the balance between B-FGF and TGF-β determines whether these cells divide or hypertrophy under basal conditions and in response to AngII stimulation. Although similar data are as yet lacking in myocytes, TGF-β has been detected in adult rat ventricles following aortic banding and myocardial infarction.[77] Furthermore, the vasoconstrictor/vasopressor peptide endothelin-1 (ET-1) promotes growth in myocytes and other cell lines.[77-82] In cardiac myocytes, both AngII and ET-1 have been shown to up-regulate the expression of pre-pro ET-1 (ppET-1) in a dose- and time-dependent manner.[80] This effect appears to be PKC-dependent as it was completely abolished by the PKC inhibitor H-7 or by down-regulation of endogenous PKC activity by pretreatment with phorbol ester. Finally, introduction of antisense sequence against the coding region of ppET-1 mRNA into myocytes, inhibited AngII induction of ppET-1 mRNA and blocked [³H] leucine incorporation.[80]

Non ACE-Dependent Cardiac AngII Generation: Therapeutic Implications

Recent investigations have provided strong evidence for an alternate enzymatic pathway of AngII synthesis in the myocardium.[83] AngII formation by a cardiac serine proteinase localized in interstitial cells was found to account for 80% of the local AngII, whereas ACE-dependent AngII generation was approximately 10%.[83] Moreover, this cardiac serine proteinase is a member of the chymase group of enzymes and is the most efficient and specific AngII-forming system described.[84] Importantly, ACE inhibitors do not block the synthesis of AngII via this pathway raising some questions as to how these agents confer a salutary effect in ischemic heart disease and heart failure. Chronic treatment with ACE inhibitors results in only a partial decrease in circulating AngII levels,[85] and there is no consensus on whether these drugs inactivate myocardial ACE activity.[84] On the other hand, AngII formation through the chymase-dependent pathway may conceivably increase with these therapeutic interventions, as a result of the enhanced availability and uptake of AngI.[84] If such a mechanism were operative, the availability of a selective AT₁ receptor antagonist may offer a decisive advantage, bypassing ACE-dependent and alternate pathways of AngII synthesis.

Myocyte Proliferation and Myocardial Infarction

Although a number of in vitro and in vivo studies have indicated that adult ventricular myocytes may undergo DNA synthesis and possibly mitotic division and cell proliferation, this fundamental issue is still a matter of controversy.[86–97] However, it has been demonstrated that myocyte cellular hyperplasia by mitotic division occurs in the senescent rat heart[92,93] in association with cardiac dysfunction and failure.[92] Importantly, observations in animals[90-92,94] and humans[95–97] indicate that myocyte hyperplasia is accompanied by little[91] or no[92,94,95] myocyte hypertrophy, raising the possibility that myocyte enlargement may be self limiting. Recent results obtained in our laboratory indicate that myocyte mitotic division is a relatively early event in the reactive growth response of the myocardium to ischemic injury.[98] These findings are at variance with the contention that considered myocyte mitotic division a late phenomenon characterizing the end stage of the disease. On the basis of this unexpected observation, myocyte cellular hyperplasia may be considered to play a more prominent role than recognized in the pathological heart.

Work on the infarct model[99] has provided additional insights in support of myocyte hyperplasia. By employing flow cytometry, it has been documented that acute myocardial infarction (AMI) is characterized by DNA synthesis in the surviving myocytes of the left and right ventricles at 1 week.[99] This phenomenon was found to be load-dependent and to become attenuated with the regeneration of tissue mass and amelioration of ventricular function.[99] Such a phase of decreased DNA synthesis corresponds to the development of the maximal cellular hypertrophic response.[1] Similarly, aging of the heart has been observed to be coupled with marked elevations in diastolic wall stress and increases in the percentage of myocyte nuclei in the S + G₂M phase of the cell cycle in both ventricles. Linear regression analyses revealed a correlation between the fraction of myocytes which enter the cell cycle and diastolic pressure and wall stress.[100]

In summary, ventricular myocytes appear to respond to abnormalities in diastolic loading produced by different pathological conditions by reexpressing their ability first to synthesize DNA and secondly to proliferate. This phenomenon requires the induction of late growth-related genes, such as proliferating cell nuclear antigen (PCNA) and histone-H_3 which are essential for DNA replication to occur.[100–102] The question then concerns the mechanism by which the mechanical stimulus on the cell surface is translated into mitogenic signals at the nucleus, initiating DNA synthesis. One potential candidate is insulin-like growth factor-1 receptor (IGF_1-R) which has been shown to be up-regulated in various cell types during phases of active cell growth and proliferation.[103–107] In addition, this receptor has been documented in neonatal cardiac myocytes[108] which are known to undergo intense mitotic division.[109] Stressed muscle cells may also generate the corresponding IGF_1 ligand which may activate surface receptors via an autocrine signaling system.

Studies have been recently performed to determine whether short-term coronary constriction was associated with activation of the myocyte IGF_1 autocrine system and induction of genes implicated in DNA synthesis.[98] Results showed that coronary stenosis led to an enhanced expression of PCNA and histone-H_3 genes in myocytes. PCNA protein was also detected in the stressed cells. These molecular responses were associated with an increase in mRNA for IGF_1 and IGF_1-R in combination with enhanced DNA synthesis and appearance of myocyte nuclear mitotic division.[98] Thus, cardiac myocytes may respond to the elevation in wall and myocyte stress by activating an IGF_1-IGF_1-R autocrine system which may modulate the induction of late growth-related genes, DNA replication, and myocyte cellular hyperplasia.[98] Work has also been completed in the infarct model to document the temporal sequence of molecular events involving the changes in the expression of IGF_1 and IGF_1-R in the surviving myocytes from 12 hours to 7 days after coronary occlusion.[110] Additionally, induction of PCNA mRNA and its protein in these cells was evaluated in combination with the measurement of BrdU labeling of myocyte nuclei and the detection of mitotic images. The collected findings indicate that left ventricular failure produced by AMI evoked reactive growth adaptations in the spared nonischemic tissue which involved DNA synthesis and mitotic division of the remaining viable myocytes. These cellular processes were coupled with molecular responses represented by increase in mRNA for IGF_1-R and IGF_1 ligand which preceded the up-regulation of the message for the cell cycle-related gene PCNA, and the appearance of its protein in the unaffected myocytes. Thus, these observations[98,110] suggest that the IGF_1 autocrine system is activated acutely in the failing heart, leading to the expression of PCNA and its protein which may engender DNA replication and mitosis, potentially evoking myocyte cellular hyperplasia and regeneration of tissue mass after infarction.

Acknowledgment

The expert technical assistance of Maria Feliciano is greatly appreciated.

References

1. Anversa P, Sonnenblick EH. Ischemic cardiomyopathy: pathophysiologic mechanisms. Prog Cardiovasc Dis 1990;33:49.
2. Anversa P, Li P, Zhang X, et al. Ischemic myocardial injury and ventricular remodeling. Cardiovasc Res 1993;27:145.
3. Olivetti G, Capasso JM, Sonnenblick EH, et al. Side-to-side slippage of myocytes participates in ventricular wall remodeling acutely after myocardial infarction in rats. Circ Res 1990;67:23.
4. Weisman HF, Bush DE, Mannisi JA, et al. Cellular mechanisms of myocardial infarct expansion. Circulation 1988;78:186.
5. Anversa P, Olivetti G, Meggs LG, et al. Cardiac anatomy and ventricular loading after myocardial infarction. Circulation 1993;87: VII-22.
6. Theroux P, Franklin D, Ross J Jr, et al. Regional myocardial function during acute coronary artery occlusion and its modification by pharmacologic agents in the dog. Circ Res 1974;35:896.
7. Theroux P, Ross J Jr, Kemper WS, et al. Regional myocardial function in the conscious dog during acute coronary occlusion and responses to morphine, propranolol, nitroglycerin and lidocaine. Circulation 1976;53: 302.
8. Theroux P, Ross J Jr, Franklin D, et al. Regional myocardial function and dimensions early and late after myocardial infarctions in the unanesthetized dog. Circ Res 1977; 40:158.
9. Ross J Jr, McCullagh WH. Nature of en-

hanced performance of the dilated left ventricle in the dog during chronic volume overloading. Circ Res 1972;30:549.

10. Grossman W, Jones D, McLaurin LP. Wall stress and patterns of hypertrophy in the human left ventricle. J Clin Invest 1975;56:56.

11. Grossman W, Carabello BA, Gunther S, et al. Ventricular wall stress and the development of cardiac hypertrophy and failure. In: NR Alpert, ed. Perspectives in Cardiovascular Research: Myocardial Hypertrophy and Failure. Vol 7. New York, NY: Raven Press, 1983:1.

12. Lindpaintner K, Jin M, Niedermeyer N, et al. Cardiac angiotensinogen and its local activation in the isolated perfused beating heart. Circ Res 1990;67:564.

13. Lindpaintner K, Wilhelm MJ, Jin M, et al. Tissue renin-angiotensin system: focus on the heart. J Hypertens 1987;5:33.

14. Lindpaintner K, Ganten D. The cardiac renin-angiotensin system. Circ Res 1991;68:905.

15. Sadoshima J, Izumo S. Signal transduction pathways of angiotensin II-induced c-fos gene expression in cardiac myocytes in vitro. Roles of phospholipid-derived second messengers. Circ Res 1993;73:424.

16. Sadoshima J, Xu J, Slayter HS, et al. Autocrine release of angiotensin II mediates stretch-induced hypertrophy of cardiac myocytes in vitro. Cell 1993;75:977.

17. Linz W, Scholkens BA, Ganten D. Converting enzyme inhibition specifically prevents the development and induces regression of cardiac hypertrophy in rats. Clin Exp Hypertens 1989;11:1325.

18. Baker KM, Chernin MI, Wixson SK, et al. Renin-angiotensin system involvement in pressure-overload cardiac hypertrophy in rats. Am J Physiol 1990;259:H324.

19. Baker KM, Booz GW, Dostal DE. Cardiac actions of angiotensin II: role of an intracardiac renin-angiotensin system. Annu Rev Physiol 1992;54:227.

20. Dostal DE, Rothblum KN, Chernin MI, et al. Intracardiac detection of angiotensinogen and renin: a localized renin-angiotensin system in neonatal rat heart. Am J Physiol 1992;263:C838.

21. Pfeffer MA, Pfeffer JM, Fishbein MC, et al. Myocardial infarct size and ventricular function in rats. Circ Res 1979;44:503.

22. Fletcher PJ, Pfeffer JM, Pfeffer MA, et al. Left ventricular diastolic pressure-volume relations in rats with healed myocardial infarction. Circ Res 1981;49:618.

23. Anversa P, Loud AV, Levicky V, et al. Left ventricular failure induced by myocardial infarction: I. Myocyte hypertrophy. Am J Physiol 1985;248:H876.

24. Drexler H, Lindpaintner K, Lu W, et al. Transient increase in the expression of cardiac angiotensin in a rat model of myocardial infarction and failure. Circulation 1989; 80(Suppl. II):II-450.

25. Hirsch T, Talsness CE, Schunkert H, et al. Tissue-specific activation of cardiac angiotensin converting enzyme in experimental heart failure. Circ Res 1991;69:47.

26. Reiss K, Capasso JM, Huang H, et al. Angiotensin II receptors, c-myc and c-jun in myocytes after myocardial infarction and ventricular failure. Am J Physiol 1993;164:H760.

27. Capasso JM, Anversa P. Mechanical performance of spared myocytes after acute myocardial infarction in rats: effects of captopril treatment. Am J Physiol 1992;263:H841.

28. Pfeffer JM, Pfeffer MA, Braunwald E. Influence of chronic captopril therapy on the infarcted left ventricle of the rat. Circ Res 1985;57:84.

29. Pfeffer MA, Pfeffer JM, Steinberg C, et al. Survival after an experimental myocardial infarction: beneficial effects of long-term therapy with captopril. Circulation 1985;72:406.

30. Pfeffer MA, Lamas GA, Vaughan DE, et al. Effect of captopril on progressive ventricular dilation after anterior myocardial infarction. N Engl J Med 1988;319:80.

31. Pfeffer MA, Braunwald E. Ventricular remodeling after myocardial infarction. Circulation 1990;81:1161.

32. Lamas GA, Pfeffer MA. Increased left ventricular volume following myocardial infarction in man. Am Heart J 1986;111:30.

33. Weber KT, Janicki JS. Angiotensin and the remodeling of the myocardium. Br J Clin Pharmacol 1989;28:141S.

34. Carroll EP, Janicki JS, Pick R, et al. Myocardial stiffness and reparative fibrosis following coronary embolization in the rat. Cardiovasc Res 1989;23:655.

35. Tan LB, Jalil JE, Pick R, et al. Cardiac myocyte necrosis induced by angiotensin II. Circ Res 1991;69:1185.

36. Rogers TB, Gaa ST, Allen IS. Identification and characterization of functional angiotensin II receptors on cultured heart myocytes. J Pharmacol Exp Ther 1986;236:438.

37. Griendling KK, Delafontaine P, Ritterhouse SE, et al. Correlation of receptor sequestration with sustained diacylglycerol accumulation in angiotensin II stimulated cultured

vascular smooth muscle cells. J Biol Chem 1987;262:14555.

38. Socorro L, Alexander RW, Griendling KK. Cholera toxin modulation of angiotensin II-stimulated inositol phosphate production in cultured vascular smooth muscle cells. Biochem J 1990;265:799.

39. Matsubara H, Kanasaki M, Murasawa S, et al. Differential gene expression and regulation of angiotensin II receptor subtypes in rat cardiac fibroblasts and cardiomyocytes in culture. J Clin Invest 1994;93:1592.

40. Anversa P, Fitzpatrick D, Argani S, et al. Myocyte mitotic division in the aging mammalian rat heart. Circ Res 1991;69:1159.

41. Meggs LG, Coupet J, Huang H, et al. Regulation of angiotensin II receptors on ventricular myocytes after myocardial infarction in rats. Circ Res 1993;72:1149.

42. Muntz KH, Zhao M, Miller JC. Downregulation of myocardial β-adrenergic receptors. Receptor subtype selectivity. Circ Res 1994;74:369.

43. Scatchard G. The attraction of protein for small molecules and ions. Ann NY Acad Sci 1949;51:600.

44. Timmermans PBMWM, Wong PC, Chiu AT, et al. Nonpeptide angiotensin II receptor antagonists. Trends Pharmacol Sci 1991; 12:55.

45. Cheng Y, Prusoff WH. Relationship between the inhibition constant (K_1) and the concentration of inhibitor which causes 50 percent inhibition (I_{50}) of an enzymatic reaction. Biochem Pharmacol 1973;22:3099.

46. Nishizuta Y. The molecular heterogeneity of protein kinase C and its implications for cellular regulation. Nature 1988;334:661.

47. Lamph WW, Wamsley P, Sassone-Corsi P, et al. Induction of protooncogene JUN/AP-1 by serum and TPA. Nature (Lond) 1988; 334:629.

48. Travali S, Koniecki J, Petralla S, et al. Oncogenes in growth and development. FASEB J 1990;4:3209.

49. Chien KR, Knowlton KU, Zhu H, et al. Regulation of cardiac gene expression during myocardial growth and hypertrophy: molecular studies of an adaptive physiologic response. FASEB 1991;55:3037.

50. Nadal-Ginard B, Mahdavi V. Molecular basis of cardiac performance. Plasticity of the myocardium generated through protein isoform switches. J Clin Invest 1989;84:1693.

51. Schunkert H, Hoahn L, Izumo S, et al. Localization and regulation of c-fos and c-jun protooncogene induction by systolic wall stress in normal and hypertrophied rat

hearts. Proc Natl Acad Sci USA 1991;88: 11480.

52. Bonnardeuz JL, Regoli D. Action of angiotensin and analogues on the heart. Can J Physiol Pharmacol 1974;52:50.

53. Moorman JR, Kirsch GE, Lacerda AE, et al. Angiotensin II modulates cardiac Na$^+$ channels in neonatal rat. Circ Res 1989;65: 1804.

54. Dempsey PJ, McCallum ZT, Kent KM, et al. Direct myocardial effects of angiotensin II. Am J Physiol 1971;220:447.

55. Malik UK, Nasjiletti A. Facilitation of adrenergic transmitter by locally generated AII in rat mesenteric arteries. Circ Res 1975; 38:26.

56. Downing SE, Sonnenblick EH. Effects of continuous administration of angiotensin II on ventricular performance. J Appl Physiol 1963;18:585.

57. Frank MJ, Nadimi M, Casanergra P, et al. Effect of angiotensin on myocardial function. Am J Physiol 1970;218:1267.

58. Simpson P. Norepinephrine-stimulated hypertrophy of cultured rat myocardial cells is an α_1-adrenergic response. J Clin Invest 1983;72:732.

59. Ikeda U, Tsuruya Y, Yaginuma T. α_1-adrenergic stimulation is coupled to cardiac myocyte hypertrophy. Am J Physiol 1991;260: H953.

60. Bishopric NH, Simpson PC, Ordahl CP. Induction of the skeletal α-actin gene in α_1-adrenoceptor-mediated hypertrophy of rat cardiac myocytes. J Clin Invest 1987;80: 1194.

61. Chien KR, Zhu H, Knowlton KU, et al. Transcriptional regulation during cardiac growth and development. Annu Rev Physiol 1993;55:77.

62. Cockcroft S, Gomperts BD. Role of guanine nucleotide binding protein in the activation of polyphosphoinositide phosphodiesterase. Nature 1985;314:534.

63. Rana RS, Hokin LE. Role of phosphoinositides in transmembrane signaling. Phys Rev 1990;70:115.

64. Meggs LG, Tillotson J, Huang H, et al. Noncoordinate regulation of alpha-1 adrenoreceptor coupling and reexpression of alpha skeletal actin in myocardial infarction-induced left ventricular failure in rats. J Clin Invest 1990;86:1451.

65. Han C, Abel PW, Minnenman KP. Heterogeneity of α_1-adrenergic receptor revealed by chlorethylclonidine. Mol Pharmacol 1987;32:505.

66. Johnson RD, Minneman DP. Differentiation of α_1-adrenergic receptors linked to phos-

phatidylinositol turnover and cyclic AMP accumulation in rat brain. Mol Pharmacol 1987;32:239.

67. Minneman KP, Han C, Abell PW. Comparison of α_1-adrenergic receptor subtypes distinguished by chlorethylclonidine and WB 4101. Mol Pharmacol 1988;33:509.

68. Klijn K, Slivka SR, Bell K, et al. Renal α_1-adrenergic receptor subtypes: MDCK-D1 cells, but not rat cortical membranes possess a single population of receptors. Mol Pharmacol 1991;39:407.

69. Perez DM, Piascik MT, Graham RM. Solution-phase library screening for the identification of rare clones: isolation of an α_{1D}-adrenergic receptor cDNA. Mol Pharmacol 1991;40:876.

70. del Balzo U, Rosen MC, Malfatto G, et al. Specific α_1-adrenergic receptor subtypes modulate catecholamine-induced increases and decreases in ventricular automaticity. Circ Res 1990;67:1535.

71. Han C, Abel PW, Minneman KP. α_1-adrenoceptor subtypes linked to different mechanisms for increasing intracellular Ca^{2+} in smooth muscle. Nature 1987;329:333.

72. Michel MC, Knowlton KU, Gross G, et al. α_1-adrenergic receptor subtypes mediate distinct functions in adult and neonatal rat heart. Circulation 1990;82(Suppl. III):III-561.

73. Cheng W, Coupet J, Li P, et al. Coronary artery constriction in rats impairs the mechanical behavior and the expression and activation of α_1-adrenergic receptors in cardiac myocytes. Cardiovasc Res 1994;28:1070.

74. Itagaki T, Toma Y, Umemoto S, et al. α_1-blockade reduced myocyte hypertrophy in nonischemic region after myocardial infarct. Circulation 1989;80:501.

75. Kagiya T, Hori M, Iwakura K, et al. Role of increased α_1-adrenergic activity in cardiomyopathic Syrian hamster. Am J Physiol 1991;260:H80.

76. Gibbons GH, Pratt RE, Dzau VJ. Vascular smooth muscle hypertrophy vs hyperplasia: autocrine growth factor β_1 expression determines growth response to angiotensin II. J Clin Invest 1992;90:456.

77. MacLellan WR, Brand T, Schneider MD. Transforming growth factor-β in cardiac ontogeny and adaptation. Circ Res 1993;73:783.

78. Suzuki T, Hoshi H, Mitsui Y. Endothelin stimulates hypertrophy and contractility of neonatal rat cardiac myocytes in a serum-free medium. FEBS 1990;268:149.

79. Shubeita H, McDonough P, Harris A, et al. Endothelin induction of inositol phospholipid hydrolysis, sarcomere assembly, and cardiac gene expression in ventricular myocytes. A paracrine mechanism for myocardial cell hypertrophy. J Biol Chem 1990;265:20555.

80. Ito H, Hirata Y, Adachi S, et al. Endothelin-1 is an autocrine/paracrine factor in mechanism of angiotensin II-induced hypertrophy in cultured rat cardiomyocytes. J Clin Invest 1993;92:398.

81. Hirata Y, Takagi Y, Fukuda Y, et al. Endothelin is a potent mitogen for rat vascular smooth muscle cells. Atherosclerosis 1989;78:225.

82. Takuwa N, Takuwa Y, Yanagisawa M, et al. A novel vasoactive peptide endothelin stimulates mitogenesis through inositol lipid turnover in Swiss 3T3 fibroblasts. J Biol Chem 1989;264:7865.

83. Urata H, Healy B, Stewart RW, et al. Angiotensin II-forming pathways in normal and failing human hearts. Circ Res 1990;66:883.

84. Urata H, Boehm KD, Philip A, et al. Cellular localization and regional distribution of an angiotensin II-forming chymase in the heart. J Clin Invest 1993;91:1269.

85. Mento PF, Wilkes BM. Plasma angiotensin and blood pressure during converting enzyme inhibition. Hypertension 1987;9(Suppl III):III-42.

86. Rakusan K. Cardiac growth, maturation and aging. In: Zak R, ed. Growth of the Heart in Health and Disease. New York, NY: Raven Press, 1984:131–164.

87. Claycomb WC, Moses RL. Culture of atrial and ventricular cardiac muscle cells from the adult squirrel monkey Saimiri Sciureus. Exp Cell Res 1985;161:95.

88. Claycomb WC, Moses RL. Growth factor and TPA stimulate DNA synthesis and alter the morphology of cultured terminally differentiated adult rat cardiac muscle cells. Dev Biol 1988;127:257.

89. Marino TA, Haldar S, Williamson EC, et al. Proliferating cell nuclear antigen in developing and adult rat cardiac muscle cells. Circ Res 1991;69:1353.

90. Olivetti G, Ricci R, Anversa P. Hyperplasia of myocyte nuclei in long-term cardiac hypertrophy in rats. J Clin Invest 1987;80:1818.

91. Olivetti G, Ricci R, Lagrasta C, et al. Cellular basis of wall remodeling in long-term pressure overload-induced right ventricular hypertrophy in rats. Circ Res 1988;63:648.

92. Anversa P, Palackal T, Sonnenblick EH, et al. Myocyte cell loss and myocyte cellular hyperplasia in the hypertrophied aging rat heart. Circ Res 1990;67:871.

93. Anversa P, Fitzpatrick D, Argani S, et al. Myocyte mitotic division in the aging mammalian rat heart. Circ Res 1991;69:1159.

94. Anversa P, Palackal T, Sonnenblick EH, et al. Hypertensive cardiomyopathy: myocyte nuclei hyperplasia in the mammalian heart. J Clin Invest 1990;85:994.

95. Linzbach AJ. Heart failure from the point of view of quantitative anatomy. Am J Cardiol 1960;5:370.

96. Astorri E, Chizzola A, Visioli O, et al. Right ventricular hypertrophy: a cytometric study on 55 human hearts. J Mol Cell Cardiol 1971;2:99.

97. Astorri E, Bolognesi R, Colla B, et al. Left ventricular hypertrophy: a cytometric study of 42 human hearts. J Mol Cell Cardiol 1977;9:763.

98. Reiss K, Kajstura J, Capasso JM, et al. Impairment of myocyte contractility following coronary artery narrowing is associated with activation of the myocyte IGF$_1$ autocrine system, enhanced expression of late growth related genes, DNA synthesis and myocyte nuclear mitotic division in rats. Exp Cell Res 1993;207:348.

99. Capasso JM, Bruno S, Cheng W, et al. Ventricular loading is coupled with DNA synthesis in adult cardiac myocytes after acute and chronic myocardial infarction in rats. Circ Res 1992;71:1379.

100. Capasso JM, Bruno S, Li P, et al. Myocyte DNA synthesis with aging: correlation with ventricular loading in rats. J Cell Physiol 1993;155:635.

101. Rittling SR, Baserga R. Regulatory mechanisms in the expression of cell cycle dependent genes. Anticancer Res 1987;7:541.

102. Chang CD, Ottavio L, Travali S, et al. Transcriptional and post-transcriptional regulation of the proliferating cell nuclear antigene gene. Mol Cell Biol 1990;10:3289.

103. Werner H, Woloschak M, Adamo M, et al. Developmental regulation of the rat insulin-like growth factor I gene. Proc Natl Acad Sci USA 1989;86:7451.

104. McCubry JA, Steelman LA, Mayo MW, et al. Growth-promoting effects of insulin-like growth factor-1 (IGF-1) on hematopoietic cells: overexpression of introduced IGF-1 receptor abrogates interleukin-3 dependency of murine factor-dependent cells by a ligand-dependent mechanism. Blood 1991;78:921.

105. Rosenthal SM, Brunetti A, Brown EJ, et al. Regulation of insulin-like growth factor (IGF) I receptor expression during muscle differentiation. Potential autocrine role of IGF-1. J Clin Invest 1991;87:1212.

106. Travali S, Reiss K, Ferber A, et al. Constitutively expressed *c-myb* abrogates the requirement for insulin-like growth factor 1 in 3T3 fibroblasts. Mol Cell Biol 1991;11:731.

107. Reiss K, Ferber A, Travali S, et al. The protooncogene *c-myb* increases the expression of insulin-like growth factor 1 and insulin-like growth factor 1 receptor messenger RNAs by transcriptional mechanism. Cancer Res 1991;51:5997.

108. Engelmann GL, Boehm KD, Haskell JF. Insulin-like growth factors and neonatal cardiomyocyte development: ventricular gene expression and membrane receptor variations in normotensive and hypertensive rats. Mol Cell Endocrinol 1989;63:1.

109. Anversa P, Olivetti G, Loud AV. Morphometric study of early postnatal development in the left and right ventricular myocardium of the rat. I. Hypertrophy, hyperplasia, and binucleation of myocytes. Circ Res 1980;46:495.

110. Reiss K, Kajstura J, Zhang X, et al. Acute myocardial infarction leads to upregulation of the IGF-1 autocrine system, DNA replication and nuclear mitotic division in the remaining viable cardiac myocytes. Exp Cell Res 1995; *In press*.

Chapter 21

The Human Angiotensin I-Converting Enzyme Polymorphism and its Implication in Cardiovascular Diseases

Florent Soubrier, M.D. Ph.D., François Cambien, M.D.

Introduction

Until recently the main interest on angiotensin-Converting enzyme (ACE) was based on the therapeutic interest of ACE inhibitors in hypertension, and more recently in cardiac failure. New fields of interest on ACE recently emerged after the original structure and expression of the gene was disclosed by molecular cloning of the gene and after a polymorphism of the gene was proposed to be associated with cardiovascular diseases.

In this chapter, we will present the biochemical features of ACE, its localization and regulation, and the data concerning the polymorphism of the gene.

Molecular Biology of ACE

Biochemistry of ACE

ACE is a cell-membrane peptidase, working as an ectoenzyme, with its catalytic site exposed at the extracellular surface of the cell. ACE is a zinc metallopeptidase with a wide substrate specificity but was initially described for its catalytic properties on two vasoactive peptides, angiotensin I (AngI) and bradykinin (BK). On these two peptides, ACE acts as a dipeptidyl carboxypeptidase, processing angiotensin I into the active octapeptide AngII and degrading BK into inactive peptides by two successive cleavages.[1] ACE is able to hydrolyze a wide range of oligopeptides in vitro, such as enkephalins, neurotensins, and the chemotactic peptide FMet-Leu-Phe via its dipeptidyl carboxypeptidase activity.[1] However, on some substrates, ACE can also act as an endopeptidase, releasing predominantly C-terminal tripeptide from amidated substrates such as substance P[2] or amidated C-terminal dipeptides from cholecystokinin-8 and various gastrin analogs.[3] On LH-RH, ACE releases a tripeptide from the amidated C-terminus and in addition an N-terminal tripeptide.[4] The K_m for these substrates is usually high, resulting, even with high K_{cat}, in low K_{cat}/K_m ratios, which seem unfavorable for metabolism in vivo.[5] However, conditions for hydrolysis of these peptides could be fulfilled in some particular tissular environments.

The widely distributed form of ACE, present in endothelial and epithelial cells, is called the somatic form by contrast to the germinal isoform of ACE found in male spermatids. These two forms differ by their primary structures which have been determined in humans by molecular cloning of the two cDNAs.[6–8]

The somatic form has a molecular mass of 170 kDa and has a repetitive structure with two homologous domains. A consensus sequence for zinc metallopeptidase (H-E-X-X-H) is found in each homologous domain. In this sequence, by analogy to the

From Weber KT, MD *Wound Healing in Cardiovascular Disease*, Armonk, NY, Futura Publishing Company Inc., © 1995.

structure of thermolysin, the two histidine residues are co-ordinated to the zinc atom and the glutamic acid is the base donor. The presence of the zinc binding consensus sequence in each domain of ACE suggests the presence of two active sites in each enzyme molecule and this was further supported by the presence of two zinc atoms per mole of enzyme and the binding of two competitive ACE inhibitor molecules per mole of enzyme.[9,10]

Monovalent anions, especially chloride, enhance the activity of ACE towards all known substrates although the presence of chloride is not always essential[11]; for example, BK is hydrolyzed in the absence of chloride. This activation is thought to be a consequence of a change in protein conformation occurring on chloride binding to a putative lysine residue located in the region of the active site.[12]

Many other residues implicated in catalysis have not yet been identified, among them His 231 of thermolysin, which stabilizes the transition state of the substrate, and Glu 166, which provides the third zinc co-ordinating ligand.[13] A tyrosine and a lysine residue have also been identified as essential residues in rabbit lung ACE by inactivation of the purified enzyme with 1-fluoro-2,4,-dinitrobenzene (Dnp-F),[14] confirming previous findings.[15] By peptide mapping and sequencing, these amino acids have been identified as lysine 694 and tyrosine 776 in the C-domain. Separate mutagenesis of the Dnp-F reactive Lys or Tyr did not produce any changes in the enzymatic properties. In contrast, combined mutagenesis of both residues altered several enzymatic characteristics, which suggests a slight modification of the three-dimensional structure.[16]

The germinal form of ACE has a smaller molecular mass of 100 kDa in humans but was known to possess the same enzymatic properties as the somatic enzyme.[17] Its primary structure, deduced from the cDNA sequence, is completely identical to the C-terminal moiety of the somatic enzyme, but it possesses an N-terminal-specific peptide, 67 amino acids long, which includes a signal peptide and a serine threonine rich region, corresponding to potential O-glycosylation sites.[8,18] The germinal isoform thus contains only one potential active site, corresponding to the C-domain of the somatic isoform (Figure 1). The substrate of the germinal ACE is not known and the importance of its physiological role in reproduction has not been determined. The activity of the germinal ACE is preserved during chronic treatment oral treatment by ACE inhibitors, as these molecules usually do not cross the blood testis barrier.[19]

ACE is synthesized as a precursor with a signal peptide at its N-terminal extremity, which is cleaved during biosynthesis, as this peptide is no longer present in the mature molecule.[6] ACE is anchored to the cell membrane by a hydrophobic peptide, 17 amino acids long, which is located at its C-terminus.[20,21] This mechanism of anchoring was demonstrated by several studies.[20] The anchored form of ACE is found on endothelial cells and on several epithelia. A secreted form of ACE is also found in biological fluids, such as the plasma, the cerebro spinal fluid, the amniotic fluid,[22] and the semen.[23] The release of ACE from the cell membrane probably results from a proteolytic process which cleaves the C-terminal part of the enzyme as suggested by the fact that plasma ACE is not recognized by an antiserum raised against the C-terminal extremity of the enzyme.[20] The sequence of the carboxyl-terminus of ACE secreted by CHO cells and of human plasma ACE was determined by carboxyl-terminal microsequencing.[24] This sequence corresponds to a cleavage between Arg-1137 and Leu-1138 of human ACE. Site directed mutagenesis of Arg-1137 into glutamine did not prevent the secretion of ACE in CHO cells, showing that this amino acid does not confer any specificity of the cleavage site by the putative cleaving enzyme. Indeed, a secretase activity from pig kidney microvilli, able to convert the amphipathic membrane-bound enzyme into the soluble form, was characterized.[25] The secretase activity is inhibited by the metal chelator EDTA, and is not sensitive to inhibitors of serine-, thiol-, or aspartic proteases and not affected by reducing agents.

Several types of experiments have assessed the activity of each putative catalytic site present in each homologous domain of

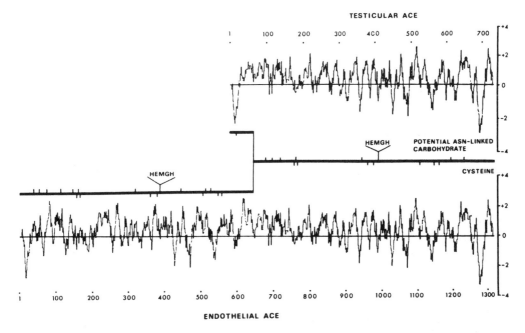

Figure 1. Schematic representation of the testicular and endothelial ACE enzymes. *Middle*: Diagram showing the cysteine positions, the potential asparagine-linked glycosylation sites, and the positions of the putative residues of the active site of the two enzymes. Beyond the point of divergence, the testicular enzyme is figured on the upper line and the endothelial enzyme on the lower line. *Top* and *bottom*: Hydropathy plots of the predicted testicular (*top*) and endothelial (*bottom*) amino acid sequences. Amino acid numbering are presented above and under the hydropathy plots. From Lattion et al., with permission.[18]

ACE. The catalytic properties of the N-domain and the C-domain were assessed by transfecting, in CHO cells, cDNA constructs of the somatic ACE in which 1 of the 2 active sites were either inactivated or deleted.[26] These experiments showed that the two active sites have similar K_m for the two main substrates, AngI and BK, but they show striking differences in the K_{cat}. At optimal chloride concentration, the active site of the N-domain has a K_{cat} 3 and 10 times lower than the C-domain active site for AngI and the specific synthetic substrate Hip-His-Leu, respectively.[26] In all these experiments, both domains appeared to function independently since the activity of the wild type enzyme was equal to the sum of the activities of the N- and C-domains.[26] These studies established that ACE possesses two functional catalytic sites, which were both dependent on a zinc cofactor.

It is well established that chloride has a marked influence on ACE activity[12] and it is interesting to note that the catalytic activity of the two domains was affected differently by chloride.[26] For AngI hydrolysis, the N-active site exhibited low levels of activity in the absence of chloride and optimal activity at a concentration of 10-mM chloride. In contrast, the C-active site was essentially inactive in the absence of chloride and required much higher chloride concentrations for optimal activity ($\geq$800 mM). BK was hydrolyzed efficiently by both active sites with similar K_{cat} values in the presence of NaCl but again with different chloride activation profiles.

The interaction of the two active sites of ACE with competitive ACE inhibitors was also investigated.[27] Both the N- and the C-domains contain a high affinity binding site for ^{3}H-trandolaprilat, a potent ACE inhibitor. Chloride stabilizes the enzyme inhibitor complex and slows the dissociation rate, an effect which is more marked for the C-domain than for the N-domain.

As the N-domain cleaves less efficiently the main substrates of ACE, AngI, and BK, one can hypothesize that the N-domain has another substrate specificity. Although no specific substrate was found for the N-active site, it was shown that the release of the amino-terminal tripeptide of LH-RH was more efficiently performed by the N-domain than by the C-domain.[28]

Tissular Localization of ACE

ACE displays an ubiquitous tissue distribution, due to its association with the plasma membrane of vascular endothelial cells. In addition to an endothelial location, high levels of ACE are also found in the brush borders of absorptive epithelia, such as the apical microvillisities of the small intestine and the kidney proximal convoluted tubule.[29] Other epithelial locations of ACE include the choroid plexus, where the enzyme is found at a high concentration and is probably the source of ACE in the cerebrospinal fluid,[30,31] and the prostate and epididymis of the male genital tract.[32,33] ACE is also found in mononuclear cells, such as monocytes after macrophage differentiation and T-lymphocytes, and in fibroblasts.[34–36]

In vitro autoradiography, employing radiolabeled-specific ACE inhibitors, and immunohistochemical studies have mapped the locations of ACE in brain, mainly in the rat, the monkey, and in humans. ACE was found primarily in the choroid plexus, ependyma, subfornical organ, basal ganglia (caudate-putamen and globus pallidus) but, most notably, the enzyme was found to be highly concentrated in the striato-nigral neuronal pathway.[37,38] High levels of ACE were found in neurosecretory nuclei, paraventricular nucleus and supraoptic nuclei, the median eminence, and posterior pituitary. In these regions, the level of AngII is also high.[39] High concentrations are also found in the hippocampus and in the Purkinje cell layer of the cerebellum. In the monkey, high levels are also found throughout the monkey cerebral cortex and in the interpeduncular and suprachiasmatic nuclei.[40]

In the rat heart, ACE was localized by in vitro quantitative autoradiography with a iodinated ACE inhibitor.[41] High densities of binding sites were found on valve leaflets (aortic, pulmonary, mitral, and tricuspid), but the binding was low on the endocardium. A dense labeling was observed in the coronary arteries, and the labeling was more dense in the right atrium than in the other parts. In the aorta, the labeling was high both in the endothelial and adventitial layers, and low in the media. Immunohistochemical localization showed that ACE is synthesized by fibroblasts and by monocytes in the interstitial tissue of the myocardium.[42]

Structure, Expression, and Evolution of the ACE Gene

There is a single ACE gene per haploid genome, and that was also shown for other mammalian species. It contains 26 exons and the somatic and germinal ACE mRNAs are transcribed from this unique gene.[43]

Several studies have demonstrated the presence of two functional promoters in the ACE gene allowing the transcription of the somatic and germinal mRNAs, each having its own regulation and being expressed with its own cell specificity. The somatic ACE mRNA seems to be constitutively expressed and in the human kidney, the low level of ACE mRNA contrasts with the high concentration of the enzyme. The somatic promoter is located on the 5' side of the first exon of the gene and leads to the transcription of all exons. In the mature somatic ACE mRNA, exons 1 to 26 are found, except exon 13 which is spliced. Fusions of various size fragments of the somatic ACE promoter to a reporter gene in transfection experiments showed the presence of positive regulatory elements inside the 132-bp region upstream the transcription start site and also suggested the presence of negative regulatory elements between -132 and -343 and between position -472 bp and -754.[44] Similarly, a strong negative element was identified in the rabbit ACE gene promoter between nucleotide positions -692 and -610.[45] The negative effect on transcription of this element was shown to be independent of its position, orientation, and to be dose dependent. The transacting factor which putatively binds this element has not yet been identified.

The presence of an internal alternative promoter was suggested by the transcription of another mRNA, with a completely different pattern of expression and regulation from the somatic transcript. The germinal transcript of ACE is expressed exclusively by spermatogenic cells with a precise stage-specific pattern, after the meiosis, starting in round spermatids and finishing in spermatozoa.[46] The germinal mRNA contains exon 13 to exon 26 of the gene.

The location of the germinal promoter on the 5'-flanking region of exon 12, the germinal-specific exon was suggested by several experiments. Primer extension and RNase protection assays on testicular RNAs were performed in rabbits and humans.[43,47] In all species investigated, the 5' extremity of the germinal ACE mRNA corresponded to the 5' end of exon 13. Therefore, intron 12, corresponding to the genomic sequence flanking the 5' region of the testicular-specific exon 13, as deduced from the complete analysis of the ACE gene in humans, was proposed as the putative germinal ACE promoter.[43,47]

The promoter function of this sequence was firmly established by using intron 12 to drive the transcription of a reporter gene in a germinal-specific fashion.[48] A 689-bp fragment, containing intron 12, exon 13, and a part of intron 12 of the mouse ACE gene fused to the beta-galactosidase coding sequence, was used to construct transgenic mice. A histochemical analysis of the transgenic mice revealed that the beta-galactosidase was only expressed, together with the ACE gene, in elongating spermato-

zoa. In another series of transgenic mice, a 91-bp fragment of intron 12 of the ACE gene was used as promoter and was able to confer to the transgene a germinal cell restricted pattern of transcription.[49] Further mapping of elements controlling transcription by DNAse footprint experiments and gel mobility shift assays showed that a sequence between position -42 and -62 specifically binds to nuclear factors from testicular extracts and contains a consensus cAMP responsive element (CRE).[49]

To our knowledge, this is the only example of an intragenic, alternative promoter, present inside a duplicated gene and driving transcription of the ancestral nonduplicated form of the gene.

The structure of the human ACE gene provides further support for the duplication of an ancestral ACE gene (Figure 2). Exons 4 to 11 and 17 to 24, encoding the two homologous domains of the ACE molecule are highly similar both in size and in sequence.[43] In contrast, intron size separating homologous exons is not conserved. The ACE gene duplication appears to have occurred early in evolution. In all mammalian species where the ACE gene has been cloned, that is, rabbits, mice, and humans, the ACE gene appears to be duplicated. A dipeptidyl carboxypeptidase, affinity purified from the electric organ of torpedo marmorata, was recognized by a polyclonal antiserum raised against pig kidney ACE and was activated by chloride.[50] The molecular mass of torpedo ACE is 190 kDa, and therefore this enzyme would also appear to be transcribed from a duplicated ACE gene. If this is the case, then the duplication of the ACE gene must have occurred more than

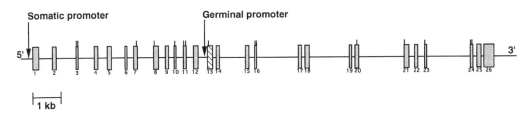

Figure 2. Organization of the human ACE gene. Location of the 26 numbered exons (vertical bars). Exon 13 (open bar) is specific to the testicular ACE mRNA. The two promoters are indicated by vertical arrows. Vertical bars above the exon boxes indicate the location of the cysteine residues. Adapted from Hubert et al.[43]

300 million years ago. Conservation in remote species of the two transcription units inside the ACE duplicated gene reflects their physiological significance, although a local and specific substrate of testicular ACE, which would definitively signify its function, is not yet known.

An ACE-like enzyme has been characterized in the housefly, Musca Domestica.[51] This enzyme is able to cleave the ACE substrate Hip-His-Leu and is inhibited by captopril with an IC_{50} of 0.4 mM. A cDNA coding for an enzyme with high sequence similarity to ACE has been also cloned in drosophila.[52] The amino acid identity reaches 65% in the region of the zinc-binding motif. Interestingly, the D.meganoster ACE-like enzyme gene does not seem to be duplicated as the full length cDNA is 2.1 kb, an observation which is in agreement with the 87 kDa found for the ACE-like enzyme from Musca Domestica.

Hormonal and Pharmacological Control of ACE Expression and Secretion

Pharmacological Stimulation of ACE Secretion and Expression

Several agents, such as cAMP analogues,[53] methylxanthines, calcium ionophore A23187, and sodium ionophore monensin[54] have been shown to induce ACE secretion from cultured bovine endothelial cells. ACE secretion is also increased by glucocorticoid hormones on cultured endothelial cells,[55] cultured rabbit alveolar macrophages,[56] and human monocytes.[34] Glucocorticoid responsive elements are indeed present in the somatic promoter of the ACE gene and an increased ACE gene expression might be responsible for the increased ACE secretion.[43] However, studies using the ACE promoter driving transcription of a reporter gene transfected in various cell types were unable to detect any effect of glucocorticoids on transcription, suggesting that these responsive elements are not functional and that glucocorticoids act through responsive elements located elsewhere or by another mechanism.[44] ACE secretion is also increased in cultured endothelial cells

by thyroid hormones, a result which is in accordance with the observation that ACE is increased during hyperthyroidism in humans.[57]

Serum ACE level and ACE concentrations in tissues are increased after ACE inhibitor treatment in rats.[58,59] The increase of plasma ACE was also observed in patients treated with the ACE inhibitor captopril in humans.[60] On cultured human endothelial cells, the ACE inhibitor captopril was able to increase ACE concentration inside the cell and in the medium.[61] In another study on porcine cultured pulmonary artery endothelial cells, it was shown that ACE mRNA and ACE transcription was increased by captopril treatment of the cells at a comparable level to the increased ACE activity.[62] This result was confirmed by in vivo experiments which showed an increase of rat lung ACE mRNA after treatment of the animals during 3 days with an ACE inhibitor.[63] Interestingly, this work also showed a decrease of ACE mRNA level in the lung of rats receiving angiotensin II infusion, which was associated with a moderate change in pulmonary ACE activity and no change in serum and testicular ACE concentrations.

ACE Expression in Experimental Models of Hypertension and Cardiac Failure

The expression of the ACE gene was studied during experimental overload of the heart by aortic stenosis in the rat.[64] Both ACE activity and ACE mRNA were increased in the left ventricle wall. In the experimental model of heart failure by left coronary ligature in the rat, the ACE activity was also increased in the right ventricle which was unaffected by experimental myocardial infarction.[65] The aortic ACE mRNA was also studied in the two kidney, one clip model of rat hypertension at 4 and 12 weeks after clipping.[66] At both stages an increase of the ACE mRNA was observed, together with an increase of the ACE activity in this tissue. In contrast, no modification of ACE mRNA was observed in other tissues, such as the lung, and the plasma ACE concentration was unchanged. The local expression of ACE is increased in the fibrous scar of myocardial infarction as shown in several experiments performed in the rat.[42]

The Genetic Control and Polymorphism of ACE Expression in Humans

When measured in the same individual several times, the level of plasma ACE is stable. In contrast, large interindividual differences for plasma ACE levels were observed by many investigators. These two observations taken together suggest a strong long-term control of plasma ACE level, and different types of studies have shown it was of genetic origin. Interestingly, the level of plasma ACE is also developmentally regulated since the level of plasma ACE is temporarily increased during adolescence.

Genetic Control of Plasma ACE

In a large study involving 434 healthy, middle aged, Caucasian men, a large interindividual variability was observed for plasma level, since this level can differ up to 5.7 times among subjects. No association was found with candidate environmental or hormonal parameters to explain the interindividual variability in plasma ACE level.[67] In a first study, the level of plasma ACE was measured in 100 normal nuclear families. Statistical analyses were performed to assess the familial correlations of the enzyme and the compatibility of the levels observed with the presence of a major gene segregating in the families.[68] Higher plasma levels were observed in offspring than in parents. Significant correlations were found between parents and their offspring, after adjustment for age, but not between parents. A major gene transmission was better supported by the data than a polygenic or a nongenetic transmission. The frequencies of alleles S/s associated with high/low plasma ACE levels were 0.24/0.76. The effect of S was codominant and stronger in offspring than in parents. In parents, the level of plasma ACE was approximately 1 standard deviation (SD) higher in Ss heterozygotes and 2 SD higher in SS homozygotes

than in ss homozygotes. In offspring, the effects were twofold more important. No residual familial correlation was present after taking into account the major gene effect. According to the segregation analysis, the postulated polymorphism S/s accounted for 29% and 75% of the variance of plasma ACE in parents and offspring, respectively.

These results strongly suggested that plasma ACE level was largely determined by the effect of a single major gene; however the identity of this gene was unknown.

The Insertion/Deletion Polymorphism of the ACE Gene and its Relation with Plasma ACE Level

A frequent insertion (I)/deletion (D) polymorphism (ACE I/D), due to the presence or absence of a 287-bp fragment corresponding to an *alu* sequence in intron 16 of the gene was identified.[69]

The relationship between the ACE I/D polymorphism and plasma ACE level was studied in a sample of 80 healthy adults.[69] The concentration of plasma ACE, measured by radioimmunoassay (RIA), was strongly associated with the genetic polymorphism. In II homozygotes, ID heterozygotes, and DD homozygotes, the mean levels of ACE were 299, 393, and 494 μg/L, respectively (p<0.001). The effect of the gene was strictly codominant and accounted for 47% of the interindividual variability of plasma ACE (Figure 3).

Costerousse et al. have recently studied ACE activity in human circulating mononuclear cells. The highest enzyme level was found in T lymphocytes in which ACE activity was approximately 30 times higher than in monocytes. No detectable activity could be found in B lymphocytes. ACE activity in T lymphocytes was measured in 35 healthy individuals. As for plasma ACE, the cellular level was very stable within individuals but highly variable between individuals. The correlation between the plasma and T lymphocyte levels of ACE was 0.42 (p<0.01). The ACE I/D polymorphism was also investigated in these subjects. Mean ACE levels in T lymphocytes of II, ID, and individuals were significantly different, but this difference was slighter than for plasma ACE values.

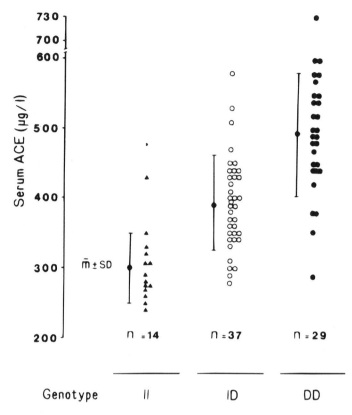

Figure 3. Serum immunoreactive ACE concentrations (μg/L) of individual with the II, ID, and D genotypes, on the left, middle, and right panels, respectively. Solid vertical bars indicate mean concentration and standard deviation for each group. Reproduced from Rigat et al. with permission.[69]

Thus not only plasma ACE, but also ACE in T lymphocytes is largely determined by a polymorphism probably affecting the ACE gene. From these results, it is tempting to extrapolate that the polymorphism could also affect ACE expression in other types of cells; this could have important consequences, in particular in the vessel wall or in the heart.

In a subsequent family study comprising 98 normal nuclear families, plasma ACE activity was measured and the I/D polymorphism was typed by PCR.[70,71] The aim of this study was to establish whether the S/s polymorphism, deduced from the first Nancy study but not identified at the gene and molecular level, and the ACE I/D polymorphism were a single entity. For that purpose, a statistical analysis by combined linkage and segregation was used, essentially

introducing the I/D polymorphism in the analysis. The aim of the statistical analysis was to test whether the S allele postulated from the segregation analysis was in linkage disequilibrium with the marker or even in complete association, suggesting in this latter case that the I/D polymorphism was responsible by itself for the effect on ACE gene expression. The best fitting model for the linkage segregation analysis performed on age-adjusted ACE level yielded a frequency of 0.57 for the D allele and frequencies of S on alleles I and D of 0 and 0.78, respectively. These results suggested that the postulated S/s polymorphism was present within or near the ACE gene and that the ACE I/D polymorphism was a marker of ACE S/s. Allele S was always found on the D allele but the two alleles were not identical since a significant fraction (0.22) of

Table 1

Linkage-Segregation Analysis of Plasma ACE and the ACE/ID Polymorphism in the 98 Nuclear Families Included in the Nancy Study 2

Parameters Estimated in the Linkage-Segregation Analysis	Parameter Estimates (se) for the Best Fitting Model
Frequency of D/I	0.57/0.43
Frequency of S/I	(0)*
Frequency of S/D	0.78
m ss	−0.888
m sS	0.137
m SS	1.07
residual sd	0.745
residual h2	(0)*

ACE levels were adjusted on age and standardized before analysis, so the means and residual sd are expressed in term of sd of the crude level of ACE.
* not significantly different from the specified value. ALL other estimates are significant (p < 0.05). Adapted from Tiret et al.[71]

the D alleles were carrying the s allele. In this study, the S/s susceptibility polymorphism and the I/D marker explained 44% and 28% of the interindividual variance of plasma ACE level, respectively (Table 1).

The ACE Gene Polymorphism in Cardiovascular Disease

The ACE Gene and Blood Pressure

In the rat, a positional cloning strategy enabled the identification of a locus, called BP/1, responsible for part of blood pressure variance in a cross between SHR/SP rats and WKY rats.[72,73] The genetic linkage between BP/1 and blood pressure was stronger when using the BP values measured after the rats were salt loaded. The importance of this locus was also demonstrated in other strains of rats, such as the Dahl hypertensive strain of rats.[74] The BP/1 locus, as defined by the confidence interval for linkage in this cross, is located on chromosome 10 of the rat and belongs to a synteny group with a locus on chromosome 17q23 in humans, inside which the ACE

gene is located. From statistical computations, it is not possible to further define the location of the gene within a 10 centimorgan genetic distance (representing about 10^7 base pairs). New crosses between SHR/SP and WKY rats will be required to map the gene more precisely. Several genetic studies were designed to evaluate the importance of the ACE gene in human essential hypertension. A study, performed on hypertensive subjects from Utah, was based on the affected sib-pair method. This method tests the cosegregation of the marker locus and the disease locus by comparing the observed resemblance for marker genotypes between affected sibs to the expected resemblance under the hypothesis of independent segregation of the locus and the disease. A linkage is indicated by an excess of resemblance for marker genotypes. A highly polymorphic marker was used in this study, located close to the ACE gene, on the GH locus.[75] This study did not show any linkage between hypertension and the GH marker. Similarly, no relation between the ACE genotype and blood pressure was found in the family study on ACE phenotype and genotype.[71] In another study which used the four corner approach, that compared four groups of subjects selected according to the blood pressure level of their parents and to their own blood pressure, no significant difference in ACE genotype frequency was found between the different groups.[76] From these studies it can be concluded that the ACE gene polymorphism itself does not influence BP in Caucasians. Two studies performed in Caucasians were able to find an association of the I allele of the ACE gene I/D polymorphism with hypertension.[77,78] A study performed in Japanese hypertensive and normotensive subjects confirmed the association of the I/D polymorphism with plasma level of the enzyme in this ethnic group, but failed to find an association between the I/D polymorphism and hypertension.[79] The possibility remains that an as yet unidentified gene inside locus BP/1 on chromosome 10 of the rat, at distance from the ACE gene, would be involved both in rat and human hypertension.

ACE Gene Polymorphism and Myocardial Infarction

Investigation of the role of the ACE gene in the genetic predisposition to myocardial infarction was based on several arguments. Various mechanisms have been implicated in the pathogenesis of coronary artery disease, including lipid accumulation and atheroma formation, thrombosis, vasoconstriction, and neointimal proliferation of smooth muscle cells, which are modulated by humoral factors.[80] Experimental studies have shown the role of angiotensin II on proliferation of smooth muscle cells and on vascular tone.[81] Using the balloon-induced injury model of the carotid artery in the rat, it was shown that administration of ACE inhibitors is able to decrease neointimal proliferation.[82] These results suggested a deleterious role of ACE on this process and that the ACE gene was a candidate for myocardial infarction.

The I/D polymorphism was studied in the ECTIM study which includes patients with myocardial infarction and controls recruited in four centers in Europe.[83]

In the total population of controls and patients, the relative risk associated with the DD genotype was 1.34 (95% confidence interval: 1.05 to 1.70). The relative risk was even stronger when the study population was stratified according to a risk status taking into account body mass index (BMI) and apoB level. In patients with low apo B level and low BMI, the relative risk associated with the DD genotype reached 3.2. In contrast, in the high risk population, the DD genotype was no longer associated with any significant increase of the relative risk. This type of epidemiologic result requires confirmation by other groups to be validated and raises many questions. The first concerns the physiopathological mechanism underlying this association and this will be discussed later. The second question concerns the significance of the apparent increased risk related to DD genotype in low risk individuals. At least three main explanations can be proposed. The first explanation assumes that the risk associated with the DD genotype is unmasked by the elimination of other risk factors. According to a second

hypothesis, an unknown pathological mechanism could underlie the statistical difference found between high and low risk patients. A third hypothesis is related with the design of the study, and would imply a selection process which leads to the disappearance of some subjects from the study. In fact, patients were recruited 3 to 9 months after the myocardial infarction. It is conceivable that patients with a high risk and with the DD genotype have an increased risk of early mortality from MI which could reduce their proportion among the survivors.

This hypothesis is further supported by data reported by Bohn et al.[84] and by Tiret et al.[85] in two different reports. In the study by Tiret et al.,[85] an association was investigated between a parental history of myocardial infarction in the control population of the ECTIM study and the presence of the deletion allele in the offspring. This type of association is weakened by the dilution of the informative genotype from the affected parent with the genotype of the nonaffected parent. However, using this study design, Tiret et al. observed an increased frequency of the DD and ID genotype frequencies, as compared to II genotype frequency in offspring of parents with myocardial infarction.[85] Bohn et al. compared the frequency of the alleles of the I/D polymorphism in myocardial infarction survivors and they found an increase of the I allele in patients with MI.[84] These results were in complete discrepancy with the results of Cambien et al.,[83] but in the same study they confirmed the association of a parental history of premature MI with the D allele, with an odds ratio which suggests a codominant effect of the D allele for the increased MI risk.[86]

In noninsulin-dependent diabetic (NIDDM) patients, a significant association was found between the D allele and coronary heart disease (CHD).[87] The DD genotype was associated with early onset CHD, independently of other factors, such as hypertension or lipid values. The progressive increase of the relative risk in individuals heterozygous and homozygous for the D allele suggested a codominant effect on the cardiovascular risk.

The discrepancy between some results obtained from survivors of myocardial infarction and the results obtained using parental history, which include all MI cases, including early fatal events, suggests a negative selection of the DD genotype among MI survivors. These data taken together might suggest that the DD genotype is associated with increased premature death after MI, a hypothesis which is supported by the increased risk of CHD death in subjects carrying the ACE D allele, observed in an autopsy study in Belfast, but which requires confirmation by prospective studies.[88]

The ACE Genotype and Other Pathologies

Some reports have shown an association of the ACE polymorphism with various cardiac pathologies. Marian et al. reported an increased D allele frequency in patients affected by hypertrophic cardiomyopathies (0.69) as compared to their normal relatives (0.57).[89] In 25 hypertrophic cardiomyopathy patients with a strong family history of sudden cardiac death the D allele frequency was even higher reaching 0.82. In another study Raynolds et al. showed a higher frequency of the DD genotype in idiopathic dilated cardiomyopathy patients (35.7%) and in idiopathic ischemic cardiomyopathy patients (39.2%) as compared to their controls (24%).[90]

In a preliminary study, Ohishi et al. found an increased frequency of the DD genotype in patients with restenosis after coronary percutaneous transluminal angioplasty (PTCA) as compared with patients without restenosis.[91]

In a large epidemiologic survey, Schunkert et al. found an association of the D allele with left ventricle hypertrophy using three electrocardiographic criteria.[92] They observed a relative risk associated of 1.22 in women, and of 2.63 in men with the DD genotype and this relative risk was even stronger in individuals with normal blood pressure, reaching 4.05.

ACE inhibition might be more complete in patients with the II genotype as their plasma level of ACE is lower, and this could induce more severe side effects related to this inhibition. As cough is the most frequent side effect of ACE inhibitors therapy, Furuya et al. have tested its possible association with the ACE I/D genotype.[93] A difference in the distribution of the ACE genotypes was found between the groups of patient with and without cough under ACE inhibitor treatment.

Although some of these studies are somewhat preliminary and deserve methodological criticisms, they attest the possible implication of the I/D polymorphism in various pathologies.

Mechanisms Proposed for the Physiopathological Effects of the ACE Gene Polymorphism in Heart Diseases

ACE is one of the major enzymes of the renin-angiotensin system but its concentration is not considered to be critical for the level of activation of the system, since it appears to be nonlimiting for AngII generation, at least in the plasma and in physiological conditions.[94] This statement has underestimated the importance of the tissue generation of AngII, where there is no demonstration that the ACE concentration is not limiting.

According to a "vascular or endothelial" hypothesis, the ACE gene polymorphism would predominantly act at the vascular level. The D allele, associated with an increased vascular enzyme concentration, would lead to a local increase of AngII generation and bradykinin degradation. Bradykinin acts on endothelial B2-kinin receptors and is able to stimulate nitric oxide (NO) formation by endothelial NO synthase and prostacyclin synthesis.[95] Modifying this local hormonal equilibrium might result in an increased neointimal proliferation, increased cellular matrix formation, and chronic or acute vasospasm, all favoring MI occurrence.

The "myocardial" hypothesis is an alternative or additive mechanism which might explain the associations which were found between the D allele and cardiac hypertrophy. ACE is expressed in the heart, predominantly by fibroblasts and other interstitial cells and is thus important for the tissular generation of AngII. Indeed, as mentioned above, the ACE mRNA is increased in the ventricles in rat models of cardiac hypertrophy by aortic banding, and in the model of low output cardiac failure by coronary ligature.[64,65] The cellular importance of AngII for cardiomyocyte hypertrophy is now well characterized. AngII was shown to induce hypertrophy in chicken heart cells in vitro and to be involved in cardiac hypertrophy in the pressure overload model.[96,97] Using an in vitro primary culture model of rat neonatal ventricular cardiomyocytes, Sadoshima et al. recently demonstrated the importance of AngII in the stretch-induced hypertrophy.[98] They observed an increased release of AngII from in vitro stretched cardiomyocytes and the suppression of the effects of AngII on the expression of early genes with the AngII-AT$_1$ receptor antagonist, losartan. Myocardial hypertrophy increases oxygen consumption of the myocardium and diminishes O$_2$ reserve, this would favor myocardial ischemia, especially if coronary flow is impaired by atheromatous plaques.[99,100] ACE inhibitors are able to improve left ventricular diastolic relaxation in response to low flow ischemia in the hypertrophied heart.[101]

It is now important to create an in vivo model of ACE overexpression to confirm these effects.

Conclusion

The polymorphism of expression of ACE, which is due to an unknown structural variation of the ACE gene, may play a role in the predisposition to various cardiovascular diseases. New studies in humans and the creation of adequate experimental models will help to definitively establish the pathological role of the permanent increase of ACE expression associated with this polymorphism. It also represents a paradigm for the studies on the role of common polymorphisms in multifactorial diseases.

References

1. Erdös EG. Angiotensin I converting enzyme and the changes in our concepts through the years, Lewis K. Dahl memorial lecture. Hypertension 1990;16:363.
2. Yokosawa H, Endo S, Ogura Y, et al. A new feature of angiotensin-converting enzyme in the brain: hydrolysis of substance P. Biochem Biophys Res Commun 1983;116:735.
3. Dubreuil P, Fulcrand P, Rodriguez M, et al. Novel activity of angiotensin-converting enzyme hydrolysis of cholecystokinin and gastrin analogues with release of the amidated carboxy-terminal dipeptide. Biochem J 1989;262:125.
4. Skidgel RA, Erdös EG. Novel activity of human angiotensin I converting enzyme: release of the NH2- and COOH-terminal tripeptides from the luteinizing hormone-releasing hormone. Proc Natl Acad Sci USA 1985;82:1025.
5. Skidgel RA, Erdös EG. Angiotensin I converting enzyme and its role in neuropeptide metabolism. In: Turner AJ, ed. Neuropeptides and their Peptidases. Chichester UK. Ellis Horwood, 1967;165.
6. Soubrier F, Alhenc-Gelas F, Hubert C, et al. Two putative active centers in human angiotensin I-converting enzyme revealed by molecular cloning. Proc Natl Acad Sci USA 1988;85:9386.
7. Lattion AL, Michel JB, Arnault E, et al. Recruitment of all the myocardium for ANF mRNA increase during volume overload in the rat. Am J Physiol 1986;251:H890.
8. Ehlers MRW, Fox EA, Strydom DJ, et al. Molecular cloning of human testicular angiotensin-converting enzyme: the testis isozyme is identical to the C-terminal half of endothelial angiotensin-converting enzyme. Proc Natl Acad Sci USA 1989;86:7741.
9. Williams TA, Barnes K, Kenny AJ, et al. A comparison of the zinc content and substrate specificity of the endothelial and testicular forms of porcine angiotensin converting enzyme, and the isolation of isoenzyme specific antisera. Biochem J 1992;288:878.
10. Perich RB, Jackson B, Rogerson F, et al. Two ligand sites on angiotensin-converting enzyme: evidence from radioligand binding studies. Mol Pharmacol 1992;42:286.
11. Bunning P, Riordan JF. Activation of angiotensin converting enzyme by monovalent anions. Biochemistry 1983;22:110.
12. Shapiro R, Holmquist B, Riordan JF. Anion activation of angiotensin-converting enzyme: dependence on nature of substrate. Biochemistry 1983;22:3850.
13. Kester WR, Matthews BW. Crystallographic study of the binding of dipeptide inhibitors to thermolysin: implications for the mechanism of catalysis. Biochemistry 1977;16:2506.
14. Bunning P, Kleemann SG, Riordan JF. Es-

sential residues in angiotensin converting enzyme: modification with 1–fluoro-2,4-dinitrobenzene. Biochemistry 1990;29:10488.

15. Bunning P, Holmquist B, Riordan JF. Functional residues of the active site of angiotensin-converting enzyme. Biochem Biophys Res Commun 1978;83:1442.

16. Sen I, Kasturi S, Jabbar MA, et al. Mutations in two specific residues of testicular angiotensin-converting enzyme change its catalytic properties. J Biol Chem 1993;268:25748.

17. Lanzillo JJ, Stevens J, Dasarathy Y, et al. Angiotensin-converting enzyme from human tissues. Physicochemical, catalytic and immunological properties. J Biol Chem 1985; 260:14938.

18. Lattion AL, Soubrier F, Allegrini J, et al. The testicular transcript of the angiotensin I-converting enzyme encodes for the ancestral, nonduplicated form of the enzyme. FEBS Lett 1989;252:99.

19. Jackson B, Cubela RB, Sakaguchi K, et al. Characterization of angiotensin converting enzyme (ACE) in the testis and assessment of the in vivo effects of the ACE inhibitor. Endocrinology 1988;122:50.

20. Wei L, Alhenc-Gelas F, Soubrier F, et al. Expression and characterization of recombinant human angiotensin I-converting enzyme. Evidence for a C-terminal transmembrane anchor and for a proteolytic processing of the secreted recombinant and plasma enzymes. J Biol Chem 1991;266:5540.

21. Ehlers MRW, Riordan J. Angiotensin-converting enzyme: zinc- and inhibitor binding stoichiometries of the somatic and testis isozymes. Biochemistry 1991;30:7118.

22. Yasui T, Alhenc-Gelas F, Corvol P, et al. Angiotensin I-converting enzyme in amniotic fluid. J Lab Clin Med 1984;104:741.

23. El-Dorry HA, MacGregor JS, Soffer RL. Dipeptidyl carboxypeptidase from seminal fluid resembles the pulmonary rather than the testicular isoenzyme. Biochem Biophys Res Commun 1983;115:1096.

24. Beldent V, A. M, Wei L, et al. Proteolytic release of human angiotensin-converting enzyme. Localization of the cleavage site. J Biol Chem 1993;268:26428.

25. Oppong SY, Hooper NM. Characterization of a secretase activity which releases angiotensin-converting enzyme from the membrane. Biochem J 1993;292:597.

26. Wei L, Alhenc-Gelas F, Corvol P, et al. The two homologous domains of the human angiotensin I-converting enzyme are both catalytically active. J Biol Chem 1991;266:9002.

27. Wei L, Clauser E, Alhenc-Gelas F, et al. The two homologous domains of human angiotensin I-converting enzyme interact differently with competitive inhibitors. J Biol Chem 1992;267:13398.

28. Jaspard E, Wei L, Alhenc-Gelas F. Differences in properties and enzymatic specificities between the two active sites of angiotensin I-converting enzyme. Studies with bradykinin and other natural peptides. J Biol Chem 1993;268:9496.

29. Bruneval P, Hinglais N, Alhenc-Gelas F, et al. Angiotensin I converting enzyme in human intestine and kidney. Ultrastructural immunohistochemical localization. Histochemistry 1986;85:73.

30. Arregui A, AIversen LL. Angiotensin-converting enzyme: presence of high activity in choroid plexus of mammalian brain. Eur J Pharmacol 1978;52:147.

31. Schweisfurth H, Schioberg-Schiegnitz S. Assay and biochemical characterization of angiotensin I-converting enzyme in cerebrospinal fluid. Enzyme 1984;32:12.

32. Yokoyama M, Takada Y, Iwata H, et al. Correlation between angiotensin-converting enzyme activity and histologic patterns in benign prostatic hypertrophy tissue. J Urol 1982;127:368.

33. Cushman DW, Cheung HS. Concentrations of angiotensin-converting enzyme in tissues of rat. Biochim Biophys Acta 1971;250: 261.

34. Friedland J, Setton C, Silverstein E. Induction of angiotensin-converting enzyme in human monocytes in culture. Biochem Biophys Res Commun 1978;83:843.

35. Costerousse O, Allegrini J, Lopez M, et al. Angiotensin I-converting enzyme in human circulating mononuclear cells: genetic polymorphism of expression in T-lymphocytes. Biochem J 1993;290:33.

36. Weinberg KS, Douglas WHJ, MacNamee DR, et al. Angiotensin I-converting enzyme localization on cultured fibroblasts by immunofluorescence. In Vitro 1982;18:400.

37. Defendini R, Zimmerman EA, Weare JA, et al. Angiotensin-converting enzyme in epithelial and neuroepithelial cells. Neuroendocrinology 1983;37:32.

38. Barnes K, Matsas R, Hooper NM, et al. Endopeptidase 24.11 is striosomally ordered in pig brain and, in contrast to aminopeptidase N and dipeptidyl dipeptidase, an angiotensin converting enzyme, is a marker for a set of striatal efferent fibers. Neuroscience 1988;27:799.

39. Chai SY, Mendelsohn FAO, Paxinos G. Angiotensin converting enzyme in rat brain visualized by quantitative in vitro autoradiography. Neuroscience 1987;20:615.

40. Chai SY, Mckinley MJ, Paxinos G, et al. Angiotensin converting enzyme in the monkey (*macaca fascicularis*) brain visualized by in vitro autoradiography. Neuroscience 1991; 42:483.

41. Yamada H, Fabris B, Allen AM, et al. Localization of angiotensin converting enzyme in rat heart. Circ Res 1991;68:141.

42. Sun Y, Weber KT. Tissue angiotensin converting enzyme (TACE) and myocardial remodeling after infarction. Abstract of the 15th International Society of Hypertension. Melbourne. March 1994:S187.

43. Hubert C, Houot AM, Corvol P, et al. Structure of the Angiotensin I-converting enzyme gene. Two alternate promoters correspond to evolutionary steps of a duplicated gene. J Biol Chem 1991;266:15377.

44. Testut P, Soubrier F, Corvol P, et al. Functional analysis of the somatic angiotensin I converting enzyme promoter. Biochem J 1993;293:843.

45. Goraya TY, Kessler SP, Kumar RS, et al. Identification of positive and negative transcriptional regulatory elements of the rabbit angiotensin-converting enzyme gene. Nucl Acids Res 1994;22:1194.

46. Sibony M, Gasc J-M, Soubrier F, et al. Gene expression and tissue localization of the two isoforms of angiotensin I converting enzyme. Hypertension 1993;21:827.

47. Kumar RS, Thekumkara TJ, Sen G. The mRNAs encoding the two angiotensin-converting isozymes are transcribed from the same gene by a tissue-specific choice of alternative transcription initiation sites. J Biol Chem 1991;266:3854.

48. Langford KG, Shai SY, Howard TE, et al. Transgenic mice demonstrate a testis-specific promoter for angiotensin-converting enzyme. J Biol Chem 1991;266:15559.

49. Howard T, Balogh R, Overbeek P, et al. Sperm-specific expression of angiotensin-converting enzyme (ACE) is mediated by a 91-base-pair promoter containing a CRE-like element. Mol Cell Biol 1993;13:1.

50. Turner AJ, Hryszko J, Hooper NM, et al. Purification and characterization of a peptidyl dipeptidase resembling angiotensin converting enzyme from the electric organ of torpedo marmorata. J Neurochem 1987; 48:910.

51. Lamango N, Isaac RE. Identification of an ACE-like peptidyl dipeptidase activity in the housefly, Musca domestica. Biochem Soc Trans 1993;21:245.

52. Cornell MJ, Coates D, Isaac RE. Characteristics of putative Drosophila angiotensin converting enzyme cDNA clones. Biochem Soc Trans 1993;21:243.

53. Krulewitz AK, Fanburg BL. Stimulation of bovine endothelial cell angiotensin converting enzyme activity by cAMP related agents. J Cell Physiol 1986;129:147.

54. Dasarathy Y, Fanburg BL. Involvement of second messenger systems in stimulation of angiotensin converting enzyme of bovine endothelial cells. J Cell Physiol 1991;148: 327.

55. Krulewitz AH, Baur WE, Fanburg BL. Hormonal influence on endothelial cell angiotensin-converting enzyme activity. Am J Physiol 1984;247:C163.

56. Friedland J, Setton C, Silverstein E. Angiotensin converting enzyme induction by steroids in rabbit alveolar macrophages in culture. Science 1977;197:64.

57. Yotsumoto H, Imai Y, Kuzuyu N, et al. Increased levels of serum angiotensin converting enzyme activity in hyperthyroidism. Ann Intern Med 1982;96:326.

58. Kokubu TE, Ueda E, Ono M, et al. Effects of captopril (SQ14,255) on the renin-angiotensin-aldosterone system in normal rats. Eur J Pharmacol 1980;62:269.

59. Fyhrquist F, Florslund T, Tikkanen I, et al. Induction of angiotensin-converting enzyme in rat lung with captopril (SQ 14225). Eur J Pharmacol 1980;67:473.

60. Larochelle P, Genest J, Kuchel O, et al. Effect of captopril (SQ14225) on blood pressure, plasma renin activity and angiotensin I converting enzyme activity. Can Med Assoc J 1979;121:309.

61. Fyhrquist F, Hortling L, Gronhagen-Riska C. Induction of angiotensin I-converting enzyme by captopril in cultured human endothelial cells. J Clin Endocrinol Metab 1982; 55:783.

62. King SJ, Oparil S. Converting-enzyme inhibitors increase converting-enzyme mRNA and activity in endothelial cells. Am J Physiol 1992;263:C743.

63. Schunkert H, Ingelfinger JR, Hirsch AT, et al. Feedback regulation of angiotensin converting enzyme activity and mRNA levels by angiotensin II. Circ Res 1993;72:312.

64. Schunkert H, Dzau VJ, Tang SS, et al. Increased rat cardiac angiotensin converting enzyme activity and mRNA expression in pressure overload left ventricular hypertrophy. J Clin Invest 1990;86:1913.

65. Hirsch AT, Talsness CE, Schunkert H, et al. Tissue-specific activation of cardiac angiotensin converting enzyme in experimental heart failure. Circ Res 1991;69:475.

66. Shiota N, Miyazaki Mokunishi H. Increase

of angiotensin converting enzyme gene expression in the hypertensive aorta. Hypertension 1992;20:168.

67. Alhenc-Gelas F, Richard J, Courbon D, et al. Distribution of plasma angiotensin I-converting enzyme levels in healthy men; relationship to environmental and hormonal parameters. J Lab Clin Med 1991;117:33.

68. Cambien F, Alhenc-Gelas F, Herbeth B, et al. Familial resemblance of plasma angiotensin-converting enzyme level: the Nancy Study. Am J Hum Genet 1988;43:774.

69. Rigat B, Hubert C, Alhenc-Gelas F, et al. An insertion/deletion polymorphism in the angiotensin I-converting enzyme gene accounting for half the variance of serum enzyme levels. J Clin Invest 1990;86:1343.

70. Rigat B, Hubert C, Corvol P, et al. PCR detection of the insertion/deletion polymorphism of the human angiotensin converting enzyme gene (DCP 1) (dipeptidyl carboxypeptidase 1). Nucl Acids Res 1992;20:1433.

71. Tiret L, Rigat B, Visvikis S, et al. Evidence from combined segregation and linkage analysis, that a variant of the angiotensin I-converting enzyme (ACE) gene controls plasma ACE levels. Am J Hum Genet 1992;51:197.

72. Hilbert P, Lindpaintner K, Beckmann J, et al. Chromosomal mapping of two genetic loci associated with blood pressure regulation in hereditary hypertensive rats. Nature 1991;353:521.

73. Jacob HJ, Lindpaintner K, Lincoln SE, et al. Genetic mapping of a gene causing hypertension in the stroke-prone spontaneously hypertensive rat. Cell 1991;67:213.

74. Deng Y, Rapp JP. Cosegregation of blood pressure with angiotensin converting enzyme and atrial natriuretic peptide receptor genes using Dahl salt-sensitive rats. Nature Genet 192;1:267.

75. Jeunemaitre X, Lifton R, Hunt SC, et al. Absence of linkage between the angiotensin converting enzyme locus and human essential hypertension. Nature Genet 1992;1:72.

76. Harrap SB, Davidson HR, Connor JM, et al. The angiotensin I-converting enzyme gene and predisposition to high blood pressure. Hypertension 1993;21:455.

77. Zee RYL, Lou YK, Griffiths LR, et al. Association of a polymorphism of the angiotensin I-converting enzyme gene with essential hypertension. Biochem Biophys Res Commun 1992;184:9.

78. Morris BJ, Zee RYL, Ying L-H, et al. Independent, marked associations of alleles of the insulin receptor and dipeptidyl carboxypeptidase I genes with essential hypertension. Clin Sci 1993;85:189.

79. Higashimori K, Zhao Y, Higaki J, et al. Association analysis of a polymorphism of the angiotensin converting enzyme gene with essential hypertension in the japanese population. Biochem Biophys Res Comm 1993;2:399.

80. Ross R. The pathogenesis of atherosclerosis: a perspective for the 1990s. Nature 1993;362:801.

81. Chiu AT, Roscoe WA, McCall DE, et al. Angiotensin II-1 receptors mediate both vasoconstrictor and hypertrophic responses in rat aortic smooth muscle cells. Receptor 1991;1:133.

82. Powell JS, Clozel JP, Miller RKM, et al. Inhibitors of angiotensin-converting enzyme prevent myointimal proliferation after vascular injury. Science 1989;245:186.

83. Cambien F, Poirier O, Lecerf L, et al. Deletion polymorphism in the gene for angiotensin-converting enzyme is a potent risk factor for myocardial infarction. Nature 1992;359:641.

84. Bohn M, Berge KE, Bakken A, et al. Insertion/deletion (I/D) polymorphism at the locus for angiotensin I-converting enzyme and parental history of myocardial infarction. Clin Genet 1993;44:298.

85. Tiret L, Kee F, Poirier O, et al. Deletion polymorphism in angiotensin-converting enzyme gene associated with parental history of myocardial infarction. Lancet 1993;341:991.

86. Bohn M, Berge KE, Bakken A, et al. Insertion/deletion (I/D) polymorphism at the locus for angiotensin I-converting enzyme and myocardial infarction. Clin Genet 1993;44:292.

87. Ruiz J, Blanch H, Cohen N, et al. Insertion/deletion polymorphism of the angiotensin-converting enzyme gene is strongly associated with coronary heart disease in non-insulin-dependent diabetes mellitus. Proc Natl Acad Sci USA 1994;91:3662.

88. Evans AE, Poirier O, Kee F, et al. Polymorphism of the angiotensin-converting enzyme gene in subjects who die from coronary heart disease. Q J Med 1994;87:211.

89. Marian AJ, Yu QT, Workman R, et al. Angiotensin-converting enzyme polymorphism in hypertrophic cardiomyopathy and sudden cardiac death. Lancet 1993;342:1085.

90. Raynolds MV, Bristow MR, Bush EW, et al. Angiotensin-converting enzyme DD genotype in patients with ischemic or idiopathic

dilated cardiomyopathy. Lancet 1993;342: 1073.

91. Ohishi M, Fujii K, Minamino T, et al. A potent genetic risk factor for restenosis. Nature Genet 1993;5:324.

92. Schunkert H, Hans-Werner H, Holmer SR, et al. Association between a deletion polymorphism of the angiotensin-converting-enzyme gene and left ventricular hypertrophy. N Engl J Med 1994;330:1634.

93. Furuya K, Yamaguchi E, Hirabayashi T, et al. Angiotensin I-converting enzyme gene polymorphism and susceptibility to cough. Lancet 1994;343:354.

94. Danser AHJ, Koning MMG, Admiraal PJJ, et al. Metabolism of angiotensin I by different tissues in the intact animal. Am J Physiol 1992;263:H418.

95. Moncada RS, Palmer RMJ. Generation of prostacyclin and endothelium-derived relaxing factor from endothelial cells. Biology and pathology of platelet-vessel wall interactions. 1986;6:289.

96. Aceto JF, Baker KM. [Sar[1]]angiotensin II receptor-mediated stimulation of protein synthesis in chick heart cells. Am J Physiol 1990;258:H806.

97. Baker KM, Johns DW, Vaughan EDJ, et al. Antihypertensive effects of angiotensin blockade: saralasin versus captopril. Clin Exp Hypertens 1980;2:947.

98. Sadoshima J-I, Xu Y, Slayter HS, et al. Autocrine release of angiotensin II mediates stretch-induced hypertrophy of cardiac myocytes in vitro. Cell 1993;75:977.

99. Houghton JL, Carr AA, Prisant LM, et al. Morphologic, hemodynamic and coronary perfusion characteristics in severe left ventricular hypertrophy secondary to systemic hypertension and evidence for non atherosclerotic myocardial ischemia. Am J Cardiol 1992;69:219.

100. Polese A, DeCesare N, Montorsi P, et al. Upward shift of the lower range of coronary flow autoregulation in hypertensive patients with hypertrophy of the left ventricle. Circulation 1991;83:845.

101. Eberli FR, Apstein CS, Ngoy S, et al. Exacerbation of left ventricular ischemic diastolic dysfunction by pressure-overload hypertrophy. Modification by specific inhibition of cardiac angiotensin converting enzyme. Circ Res 1992;70:931.

Chapter 22

Regulation of Fibrillar Collagen Gene Expression

Ramareddy V. Guntaka, Ph.D., Attila Kovacs, M.D.,
Jagan C. Kandala, Ph.D., Karl T. Weber, M.D.

Introduction

Extracellular matrix (ECM), composed of a mixture of several macromolecules which include collagen, elastin, proteoglycans, and adhesive glycoproteins surrounding individual cells, confers structural integrity to the tissue and governs attachment, growth, and differentiation of cells. Only a few decades ago ECM was considered inert merely providing scaffolding support to the tissue, but in the last decade, it became obvious that ECM is a dynamic entity engaged in an active role in information exchange between cells. Many of the physiological processes observed in tissue culture appear to be quite different from their natural state, i.e., when cells are separated by ECM.[1-3]

Collagen is the principal constituent of the ECM of almost all tissues and is the most abundant protein in the animal kingdom. While in many tissues like bone, skin, tendon, etc., collagens constitute a major proportion, they are also widely distributed in all other tissues. Collagens are involved in the maintenance of the structural integrity of the tissues and impart strength to the skin, tendons, cartilage and bone. In a number of human diseases, abnormal accumulation of collagens, particularly types I and III, result in fibrosis that adversely affects the normal function of the tissue. While aberrant deposition can lead to the malfunction of the tissue, formation of fibrous tissue is a normal physiological process during wound healing and in various reparative processes. Collagen fibers, which impart tensile strength to the connective tissue everywhere in the body, become less extensible during aging, resulting in sagging skin and impairment of functions in several major organs, including the heart, kidneys, lungs, and blood vessels.

Collagen molecules, especially types I, II, III, V, and XI are aligned into fibers and hence these are called fibrillar collagens. Collagens are triple helix forming molecules generated from individual procollagen subunits upon removal of NH_2 and COOH-end propeptides. Although about 30 distinct polypeptide chains exist, most of the work on the genetic organization and regulation has been carried out with the fibril forming type I collagen. Here we outline the mechanism of regulation of fibrillar collagen gene expression, especially the *cis*-acting elements and various transcription factors interacting with these *cis*-acting elements in modulating collagen gene expression. Finally, an attempt is made to understand the role of renin-angiotensin-aldosterone-system (RAAS) and various cytokines in controlling collagen gene expression and the physiological significance of collagen deposition (fibrosis) in cardiovascular diseases, with particular reference to the heart. We are aware that the literature on the latter is scanty and whatever information available is far from complete and precludes drawing of definitive conclusions.

From Weber KT, MD *Wound Healing in Cardiovascular Disease*, Armonk, NY, Futura Publishing Company Inc., © 1995.

Collagen Gene Organization

Nineteen collagen types containing about 30 distinct polypeptide chains have been identified to date and most of these genes have been localized to at least 12 different chromosomes.[4] Based on the formation of supramolecular structures, the collagens are divided into fibril forming or fibrillar collagens and nonfibrillar collagens. Since types I and III collagens are recognized as the predominant species involved in maintaining the structural organization of tissues of various organs, including the heart, and because of the importance of these types in wound healing, we will focus on the genetic organization and regulation of expression of these two types of collagens.

Collagens are triple helical structures formed from three polypeptide chains with a characteristic gly-X-Y repeat sequence. The polypeptides are remarkably constant in their size, approximately 1014 to 1029 amino acids in length, with nontriple helix forming amino- and carboxyl-ends and triple helix forming central domain. Type I collagen is the most abundant and is the best characterized fibrillar collagen that consists of three polypeptides. The triple helical domain consists of 23 exons of the size of 54 bp, 8 exons of 108 bp, one exon of 162 bp, and 5 exons each of 45 bp and 99 bp. In addition, the amino- and carboxyl-end propeptides are encoded by joining exons (reviewed in ref. 5).

Type I collagens are heterotrimers formed from two α_1 (I) chains and one α_2 (I) chain, and type III collagens are formed by trimerization of three identical α_1 (III) chains. In the former, the two α_1 (I) and α_2 (I) chains are present in any cell at a stoichiometric ratio of 2:1 and the rate of synthesis of type I and type III procollagens are approximately 6:1 (reviewed in ref. 6). The genes encoding these chains are co-ordinately regulated, and this appears to be mainly at the transcriptional level.

Transcription of Collagen Genes

In some tissues, like skin, bone, and tendons, the proportion of collagen components is more than 70% to 80% of the total ECM, whereas in others, such as myocardium, collagens comprise less than <10% of the ECM. In several disease states with extensive fibrosis (scleroderma, cirrhosis, and keloids) the levels of collagen molecules dramatically increase, whereas in several types of tumors, these levels fall significantly below control levels suggesting that tissue-specific factors, which are subject to changes by external signals, govern relative expression of these genes. Although our primary interest is in the regulation of collagen gene expression in wound healing of cardiovascular diseases, we have to rely on a large body of information available on collagen gene regulation in normal fibroblasts, in order to draw some valid conclusions about the changes in diseased state, as there is very little information available in the literature on this topic. A vast knowledge base is available on the molecular mechanisms of cardiac growth and hypertrophy, but the literature on the effect of various growth factors and cytokines on collagen mRNA synthesis and turnover is limited. Here we attempt to summarize the progress on the regulatory elements of the collagen promoter and various transacting factors that interact with these elements and govern transcription of collagen types I and III genes.

The α_1 (I) collagen genes of human and mouse were the first genes to be isolated and characterized in detail.[5-7]. Recent advances on yeast artificial chromosomes (YACs) provided a valuable technique to introduce large sized DNA molecules into cells. Using YAC system, it became possible to transfer purified 150-Kb YAC, encompassing the mouse α_1 (I) gene very efficiently into embryonic stem cells and these transfectants were then used to produce chimeric founder mice.[8] Two different assays indicated that the transgene was expressed at levels comparable to the endogenous collagen gene suggesting that all the cis-acting elements involved in tissue-specific expression reside within this 150-Kb. Other experiments showed that the 2000–bp sequence upstream from the transcription start site is sufficient for tissue-specific pattern of α_2 (I) collagen gene.[9] Further deletion analysis has revealed that as few as 300-bp upstream of the start of transcription are sufficient to confer tissue-specific expression. Cell-specific transcription of human pro-α_2 (I) collagen gene has been mapped to the 3.5-Kb upstream element.[10] Additional deletion experiments narrowed the active segment to a sequence between -376 and -108.[10] In contrast, similar analysis has indicated that the same region in pro-α_1 (I) gene failed to express in a cell-specific manner.[10] Similar analysis of human α_1 (I) collagen gene with transgenic mice indicated that the 2.3-Kb 5'-flanking sequence, with or without the first intron, confers tissue-specificity whereas the 0.44-Kb 5'-flanking sequence was inadequate suggesting that the sequence between 2.3-Kb and 0.44 Kb contains the tissue-specific cis-acting regulatory elements.[11] Even the 2.3 Kb 5'-flanking sequence appeared to be devoid of some elements for muscle-specific expression as the transgene failed to express at levels comparable to the endogenous gene, pointing to the requirement of additional regions for α_1 (I) gene expression in muscle. Nevertheless, these studies have identified a minimum upstream sequence required for efficient tissue-specific expression of type I collagen genes and that for each gene the location of these controlling elements may vary. Based on this knowledge, we have proceeded to describe in certain detail the regulatory sequences and their cognate transcription factors that are essential for optimal expression of types I and III collagen genes as well as the mechanism of up or down regulation in various diseased states. In addition, we make an attempt to review the pertinent literature on the mechanism of signal transduction in response to various oncogenes and the role of phosphorylation in collagen gene expression.

Promoter Elements

a. CCAAT Sequence and CCAAT Binding Factors

One of the earliest observations with cloned collagen genes was the identification of an inverted CCAAT box required for transcriptional activation.[5] In most of the genes, the CCAAT sequence is usually present around -80 to -120 bp upstream of the transcription start site in an orientation that is the same as the direction of transcription, i.e., the same polarity as that of transcribing strand. However, in several other genes, including collagen genes, this sequence is present in the direction opposite of transcription, i.e., in the negative or nonsense strand (Figure 1, I-CAT). There are two such sequence motifs in α_1 (I) collagen gene, one located at -96 to -100 and the other around -122 to -126, whereas in α_2 (I) of mouse it is present around -80 to -84[5] (Figure 1). That this sequence is essential for collagen gene expression has been shown by mutational analysis.[12] Point mutations in this pentanucleotide of the α_2 (I) promoter greatly reduced the promoter activity, strongly suggesting that its function is required for collagen gene expression.

The factors binding to this canonical sequence have been purified, cloned, and sequenced. One factor, termed CBF (CCAAT binding factor) consists of a heterodimer of two distinct subunits A and B.[13,14] The A subunit is a polypeptide chain of 207 amino acids (aa) while the B subunit has 341 aa, but neither subunit can alone bind to the CCAAT sequence. An analogous protein from yeast, HAP, containing three subunits, HAP2, HAP3, and HAP4, was found to bind to the CCAAT sequence. The subunits A and B share extensive amino acid sequence homology with subunits HAP3 and HAP2, respectively, suggesting conservation of this protein throughout evolution.[13]

Two other DNA binding proteins, C/EBP and CTF/NF1,[15,16] also recognize DNA sequences that contain the CCAAT box, but they fail to activate transcription from the α_2 (I) promoter.[13] CBF, on the other hand, in its native form, stimulates transcription from both the $\alpha 1$ (I) and α_2 (I) collagen promoters and also from other promoters containing inverted CCAAT box, such as Rous sarcoma virus LTR.[17,18] The differences in binding of these factors appear to be due to nucleotides flanking CCAAT box or the interaction with other transcription factors. Interestingly, the binding site for NF-1 contains the CCAAT and the adjacent 12-bp GCrich direct repeat that are preserved in mice, rats, and humans (Figure 1). Another remarkable feature in type I collagen genes

RAT α1 (I) COLLAGEN UPSTREAM SEQUENCE

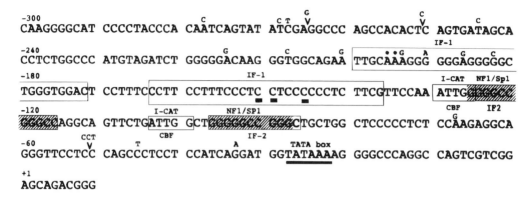

Figure 1. Upstream Regulatory Sequence of Rat α1 Collagen Gene. Small letters above the main sequence denote changes in the mouse α1 collagen gene. The sequence motifs to which various transcription factors bind, are shown in open or shaded boxes. The role of these factors is discussed in the text. I-CAT indicate the CCAAT box, which is present in an orientation against the direction of transcription. +1 indicates the transcription start site, and the negative numbers denote the nucleotide numbers of the upstream sequence. •• above the letters indicate deletions.

is the presence of a conserved Sp1 factor binding site (GGGGCGGG) which also overlaps with the NF-1 binding site.[19] Overexpression of Sp1 inhibits α1 (I) promoter activity in NIH-3T3 cells whereas overexpression of NF-1 stimulates, indicating that the interaction of these factors to their cognate sequences is mutually exclusive in that binding of one transcription factor to α1 (I) promoter at the overlapping site prevents binding of the other trans-activating factor. Any agonist which increases one factor, such as NF1, relays signal for transactivation of only those genes responsive to NF1. Presence of cis-acting sequences does not necessarily mean that specific factors bind to these elements and activate or repress transcription. For instance, as alluded to above, the transcription factor CTF/NF1 does not interact efficiently with the CCAAT at −84 but effectively binds to a CCAA sequence motif located around −300 and mediates the activation of α2 (I) promoter by transforming growth factor-β (TGF-β).[20] Therefore, it is important to recognize that depending on the signal transduction pathway, specific and subtle interactions of transcription factors can selectively activate only a subset of the responsive genes and the choice of these interactions determine the cell- and tissue-specific expression of various genes.

Another negative cis-element has been identified in the α1 (I) collagen promoter. A 12-bp Grich sequence that is repeated twice and is located immediately 3' end to the ATTGG (inverted CCAAT box) (Figure 1, 1-CAT) constitutes this element.[21] A metalloprotein factor that requires zinc cations for efficient binding has been purified from mouse lymphocytes.[21] Two well-characterized transcription factors Sp1 and NF1, have been shown to interact with the 12-bp cis-element. However, it has been unambiguously demonstrated that mutations in the Sp1 binding site failed to eliminate binding to IF2 strongly suggesting that although both Sp1 and IF2 bind to identical or similar sequences, they are different proteins.[21] Similarly, NF1 also interacts with the same 12-bp Grich motif, yet it is quite distinct and appear to be reciprocally regulated. Taken together, these data would suggest that depending on the tissue and cell type, and depending on the environment, i.e., the presence of angiotensin II (angII), hormones, cytokines, and their receptors, different pathways leading to activation of transcription of collagen genes, may be utilized, and these subtle interactions may have profound effects in controlling fibrosis.

b. Polypyrimidine and Polypurine Sequences and Transcription Factors Specific for these Regions

Functional dissection of mouse $\alpha 1$ (I) collagen promoter indicated that the 220-bp 5' flanking sequence displays strong promoter activity both in in vitro transcription assays and in in vivo transfection experiments.[17] This region contains two unusually long stretches of exclusively pyrimidines or purines, and this arrangement of polypyrimidine and polypurine tracts is highly conserved between mouse and man implying an important function for these sequences.[22–24] A 35-bp tract of C/T residues (-172 to -138), which is virtually identical between mouse and rat $\alpha 1$ (I) upstream sequence (Figure 1), appears to act as a negative regulator of transcription as minor deletions of as few as 3 bp results in elevated expression of the reporter gene.[25] A factor, IF1, binds to this sequence. Interestingly, the same factor also interacts with a further upstream purine rich sequence (-194 to -168). This is somewhat surprising in that the -194 to -168 polypurine stretch is almost complementary to the adjacent (-172 to -138) 3'-polypyrimidine tract and has the potential to form a cruciform structure. The inhibitory factor interacting with these sequences may likely form homo- or heterodimers and bind asymmetrically to this structure.

In this connection, it is noteworthy to point out that factors in rat cardiac fibroblast (RCF) nuclear extracts form complexes with double-stranded oligonucleotides corresponding to these two regions (-198 to -173 and -170 to -141) and that the interaction between the -170 to -141 oligonucleotide, and nuclear factors, which is augmented by the presence of cold $-198/-173$ oligonucleotide but not vice versa, suggests that more than one factor interacts with the linked polypurine-polypyrimidine sequences (Kovacs et al, unpublished observations). Further, we have shown that a triple helix forming oligonucleotide actually inhibits binding of factors in RCF and HeLa cell nuclear extracts to these sequences and also suppresses transcription from $\alpha 1$ (I) collagen promoter (Kovacs et al, unpub-

lished observations). This is somewhat unexpected in light of the negative regulation by IF-1 because we expect enhanced synthesis of α_1 (I) promoted transcript rather than inhibition. These differences could be reconciled if we assume that different cell-specific factors, upon forming appropriate complexes, could potentially elevate or inhibit collagen gene transcription. More experiments need to be performed to understand interactions between various cellular factors and α_1 (I) collagen promoter in different cell types.

Besides these factors and their interacting *cis*-elements in α_1 (I) collagen 5'-flanking sequences, another negative regulator has been mapped to sequences between -361 to -339.[26] All these *cis*-acting regulatory elements above appear to be in the region that is sensitive to DNaseI, S1 nuclease, and restriction enzyme digestions. Sensitivity to these enzymes has been correlated with transcriptional activity of the promoter[27] and the isolation and characterization of transcription factors that recognize sequences within this exposed chromatin region suggest that these factors play a major role in the regulation of collagen gene expression.

Similar mutational analysis with mouse α_2 (I) has also revealed the presence of at least three different upstream elements, one in the CCAAT motif (-80 to -84), the second element around -250, and a third element between -315 and -295 which binds to the NF1.[12] Except for the inverted CCAAT box, there is no similarity between these *cis*-acting sequences and those present in α_1 (I) gene. In spite of the lack of these related regulatory elements, both genes are co-ordinately regulated to produce a 2:1 ratio of transcripts. It should be extremely interesting and important to identify common transcription activation factors so that modulation of type I collagen gene expression could be studied.

Information on the regulatory sequences and the tissue-specific factors that recognize these motifs in α_1 (III) collagen 5'-flanking sequences is scanty. One factor, resembling AP1, has been found to interact with a sequence around -150.[28] The intensively characterized heterodimeric CBF, which avidly binds to the CCAAT box and activates transcription from α_1 (I) promoter, did not bind to α_1 (III) promoter, although both types I and III collagen genes are co-expressed in a number of tissues except in bone.

It should be pointed out that in spite of the fact that the biochemistry of collagen molecules is quite advanced, mechanisms involved in the regulation of collagen gene expression are poorly understood. Identification of factors involved in this regulation and their tissue distribution should enable us to develop drugs that inhibit abnormal accumulation of collagen in ECM in diseases like cirrhosis and in cardiovascular disease states like atherosclerosis, left ventricular hypertrophy (LVH), and heart failure where fibrosis can adversely alter organ function.

c. Regulatory Elements in the first Intron of Type I Collagen Gene

The region from +221 to +1607 constitutes the first intron of the human α_1 (I) collagen gene is highly conserved between rodent and human genes.[29] However, there is very little homology in the first intron between the α_1 (I) and α_2 (I) collagen genes of humans.[30] Although controversial, several lines of evidence indicates that the first intron contains cis-acting elements capable of modulating transcription, both positively and negatively (reviewed in ref. 31). The intron also contains the consensus sequences for transcription factors AP1 and Sp1. In the first intron of human α_1 (I) gene, the positively acting element has been mapped to a region between +292 and +670.[32] The AP1 factor appears to bind to a sequence within this segment as mutations which inhibited the binding of AP1 to its cognate sequence also blocked the enhancer activity of this fragment. Further deletion analysis, coupled with DNaseI protection assays, have identified this sequence to be between +590 and +615. Interestingly, this sequence acted as a positive element in some cells and as a negative regulator in other cells.[33] In the mouse α_2 (I) collagen gene, a Sp1 factor or a Sp1-like protein binds to a sequence in the intron and deletion of this sequence abolished factor binding in vitro and de-

creased its enhancer activity in vivo.[34] Taken together, these results indicate the existence of both positively and negatively regulating elements in the first intron of α_1 (I) and α_2 (I) collagen genes and depending on the type of cell, the presence of different transacting factors govern expression of these genes. The fact that a functional AP1 site is present in these type I collagen genes suggest that signal transduction occurs via the early response genes, c-fos and c-jun.

That the intron does contain cis-acting sequences that determine tissue-specific expression of α_1 (I) gene has been shown in transgenic mice in which the murine leukemia provirus was inserted in the first intron. In these mice (MOV13), provirus insertion inactivated the $\alpha1$ gene in fibroblasts and other mesenchymal tissues,[35,36] but not in odontoblasts and osteoblasts.[37] These results suggest that interaction of tissue-specific factors with various cis-acting elements, determine expression of different collagen genes.

Mutations in Types I and III Collagen Genes

Mutations in collagen genes have been identified in several diseases. These include osteogenesis imperfecta (OI), Ehlers-Danlos syndrome (EDS), Marfan Syndrome, osteoporosis, and aortic aneurysms (reviewed in ref. 4). More than 120 mutations in α_1 (I), α_2 (I) and α_1 (III) genes of collagen molecules have been characterized.[4,38] A vast majority of these mutations were found in patients with OI, which affect bones, skin, ligaments, and tendons. A predominant number of mutations are base substitutions that convert a glycine codon to other amino acids, which can result in abnormal posttranslational processing and triple helix formation. In some other OI patients, insertions and deletions as well as defects in RNA splicing were detected.[38] Some of the most interesting mutations have been identified in variants of EDS. A mutation in one allele of α_2(I) gene results in the accumulation of α_2 chains in which N-propeptide remained attached to the triple helical protein in EDS-VII B, whereas in EDS-VII A the N-propeptide remained attached in α_1 (I) collagen gene due to the loss of N-proteinase cleavage site. These mutations result in generalized laxity and fragility of the skin.[39]

Very few mutations have been identified or described that cause abnormalities in the cardiovascular system. One mutation in type III collagen gene, occurring in patients with EDS-IV that cause aortic aneurysms resulting in aortic rupture, has been discovered. This mutation was a substitution of A for G in the intron 20 of the α_1 (III) gene that caused aberrant splicing of RNA.[40] In one member of a family with aortic aneurysms, without connective tissue diseases, a substitution of arginine for glycine at 619 was found.[40] In Marfan syndrome, a mutation at position 618 resulted in a change from arginine to glutamine in the α_2 (I) gene causes cardiovascular (e.g., aortic aneurysms and rupture, mitral valve prolapse) and skeletal deformities.[41] Further experiments with transgenic mice indicated that the same mutation caused progressive dilatation of aorta. These results attest to the importance of collagen in maintaining the integrity of cardiovascular structure and any defect that causes abnormal processing of the collagen molecules can result in the disruption of structure and function of tissue.

Inducers of Collagen Gene Transcription

Endothelins

Endothelins (ETs) are vasoconstrictive peptides of 21 amino acids (aa) produced by endothelial cells. They bind to specific receptors and induce a variety of genes, including the early response genes, c-fos and c-myc, in fibroblasts, smooth muscle cells and epithelial cells.[42] Two types of ET receptors, ET_A and ET_B, have been identified, cloned, and characterized. The receptors for these peptides are G-protein-coupled molecules with seven transmembrane domains.[43,44] Upon binding to distinct receptors, ETs trigger a cascade of events, including activation of phospholipase C (PLC) via a pertussis toxin-insensitive G-protein.[45] Phospholipase C rapidly induces production of inositol 1,4,5-trisphosphate (IP3) and

diacylglycerol (DAG) from phosphatidylinositol 4,5-bisphosphate (PIP-2). The formation of IP3 mobilizes Ca^{++} and the DAG activates protein kinase C (PKC). In addition to activation of these signaling pathway components, endothelins also rapidly stimulate protein tyrosine kinases (PTKs)[46] and mitogen activated protein kinases in mesangial cells.[47] Rapid phosphorylation of various cellular substrates from 70 to 220 kDa by PTKs may have important ramifications in the transduction of signals from cytoplasm to nucleus and activation of the early response genes, c-fos and c-myc.

Since in cultured mesangial cells, ET induces c-fos expression via PKC, it is likely that AP-1 transcription factors in conjunction with mitogen-activated protein kinases augment expression of several target genes and cause cell proliferation. Although no information is available on the ET-induced expression of collagen genes in cardiovascular diseases, the presence of AP-I site in the $\alpha1$ (I) collagen gene first intron suggests that ET may stimulate synthesis of type I collagen in interstitial fibroblasts of myocardium through AP-1, leading to interstitial fibrosis. Experiments from our laboratory have demonstrated that adult rat cardiac fibroblasts possess both ET_A and ET_B receptors[48] and that ET augments expression of types I and III collagen mRNAs in cultured rat cardiac fibroblasts (RCF). However, this ET response appears to decline in serially passaged RCF (Kovacs et al, unpublished data).

Angiotensin II

Ample evidence indicates that the renin-angiotensin-aldosterone system (RAAS) is an important determinant of cardiovascular homeostasis.[49,50] The existence and functional importance of local tissue RAS, besides the classic circulating RAS, is well documented. The presence of intracardiac RAS has been demonstrated by directly detecting angiotensinogen and renin mRNA using dot-blot and Northern hybridization.[51–54] Angiotensin II (AngII), which regulates blood pressure and salt retention is an octapeptide hormone, generated from angiotensinogen in a two-step cleavage reaction. In the first step, the aspartyl protease renin cleaves angiotensinogen to a decapeptide angiotensin I, which is subsequently cleaved by angiotensin converting enzyme (ACE) to the active octapeptide angiotensin II (reviewed in ref. 49).

Receptors for AngII are found in the myocardium of almost all species examined. Both high affinity and low affinity receptors have been detected in the myocardium, as well as on coronary vessels, in human hearts and a number of factors modulate expression of these receptors.[55] Several studies have suggested that among these factors AngII may be a critical factor in mediating cardiac hypertrophy and fibrosis.[56] Animal studies demonstrated that inhibition of ACE prevented left ventricular hypertrophy and fibrosis and normal deposition of collagen in cardiovascular tissues.[57–59] Using an AT_1 receptor antagonist fibrosis remote to site of an infarction could be prevented.[60]

AngII induces hypertrophic response on cardiac myocytes and fibroblasts primarily through AT_1 receptors. AngII rapidly induces many early response genes (*c-fos, c-jun, junB, Egr1* and *c-myc*)[61] which in turn activate α-actin and growth factors. In neonatal rat cardiac fibroblasts, AngII is mitogenic, which may be partly responsible for cardiac hypertrophy and ventricular fibrosis. At least in neonatal cardiac myocyte cell culture, it has been shown that stretch-induced AngII released by cardiac myocytes and that this local AngII may act as an initial mediator of stretch-induced hypertrophic response.[62] Since AngII increases types I and III collagen gene expression, it is possible that any hormone or cytokine that elevate local AngII could potentially cause interstitial fibrosis.

AngII stimulation induces several genes within 15 minutes of binding to G-protein-coupled receptors and activating PLC, PLD, PLA2, and protein tyrosine kinases. PLC activation liberates IP3 which then mobilizes Ca^{2+} from storage sites. Depending on the cell type, AngII could activate PKC, as well as adenylate cyclase. One of the consequences of AngII on fibroblasts is the induction of collagen mRNA synthesis. Unfortunately, the mechanism of activation of collagen genes by AngII is not known. The fact that AngII induces rapid changes in phosphorylation of several cellular proteins suggest that the effects of AngII could be mediated by changes in the phosphorylation status of transcription factors or in the translocation of these factors from cytoplasm to nucleus. We have observed that in cultured rat cardiac fibroblasts AngII increases collagen synthesis as measured by ^{3}H-proline incorporation[56] and by direct analysis of α_1 (I) mRNA using Northern blots (Kovacs et al., unpublished results). Aldosterone (ALDO) also appears to enhance collagen synthesis in RCF, but this effect seems to be more pronounced in early passage RCF (Zhou et al, unpublished results). We have also found that staurosporine which inhibits PKC and genistein which inhibits PTK, dramatically decrease the AngII-induced collagen mRNA transcription in rat cardiac fibroblasts (unpublished results). Whether heart interstitial fibroblasts contribute to the AngII-induced remodeling of the cardiac interstitium by regulating the expression of collagen genes in a variety of pathological conditions remain to be explored.

Aldosterone

Complex pathophysiological mechanisms link elevations in plasma hormones of the RAAS with the abnormal fibrous tissue found in the cardiovascular system. Compelling evidence indicates that perivascular fibrosis is more correlated with mineralocorticoid excess rather than by hemodynamic conditions.[64–67]

Cytokines

Several different cytokines, such as transforming growth factor β (TGF-β), interleukin-1 (IL-1), tumor necrosis factor-α (TNF-α), and interferon-γ, (IFN-γ), modulate type I collagen gene expression in a variety of cells. These act by augmenting the rate of transcription and/or increasing or decreasing the stability of mRNAs. Many of these effects have been described in detail in an excellent review[31] and therefore will not be covered here.

Inhibitors of Collagen Gene Transcription-Oncogenes

While it has been shown that many cytokines augment expression of collagen genes, some like IL-1 and γINF, as well as certain oncogene products, inhibit collagen mRNA synthesis. Several studies have demonstrated increased expression of collagen mRNA synthesis in cultured cells by TGF-β, and TNF-α, but IL-1 has been shown to decrease transcription of α_1 (I) and α_2 (I) genes in murine ostoblastic cell lines (reviewed in ref. 31). With only a few exceptions, the most consistent inhibition of type I collagen gene expression, primarily at the level of transcription, was observed with oncogenes. A decrease in the amount of collagen in the extracellular matrix and an increase in the production of collagenases and metalloproteinases enhance the proclivity of transformed cell to penetrate and metastasize to distant areas in the organ or in the body.

A large number of physical, and chemical, and biological agents transform animal cells. Production of collagen is subject to modulation in transformed cells. One of the best studied down-regulator of collagen mRNA synthesis is the Rous sarcoma virus (RSV) encoded v-src oncogene.[68] Transformation of chick embryo fibroblasts and skin fibroblasts by RSV down-regulates α_1 (I) collagen synthesis and in some cases fibronectin synthesis, whereas transformation of vertebral chondrocytes resulted in down-regulation of α_2 (I) collagen synthesis.[68-74] Studies with RSV containing mutations in the src gene clearly indicated that the src gene product is involved in the suppression of collagen gene transcription.[68] It has been shown that the mutant used in these studies has an arginine (residue 416) changed to histidine[75,76] and this amino acid substitution greatly diminished the catalytic activity of the tyrosine kinase encoded by pp60v-src. These results strongly suggest that phosphorylation of tyrosine residues in target protein(s), possibly transcription factors or some accessory proteins that stimulate or interact with transcription factors, represses transcription of type I collagen genes. How-

ever, the mechanism remains to be elucidated.

Fibroblasts bind to the extracellular matrix molecules, fibronectin and vitronectin via the β subunit of integrin and this interaction causes phosphorylation of focal adhesion kinase (FAK) by v-src protein tyrosine kinase. The FAK in turn phosphorylates src homology 2 (SH2)-containing proteins, including paxillin and tensin.[77-79] This association between src and FAK probably sends a signal to the nucleus through serine-threonine kinases which phosphorylate transcription factors involved in transcription of collagen genes. Since collagen is a major constituent of ECM, binding of the fibroblast to the ECM might convey the signal to phosphorylate factors that are involved in the repression of transcription of fibrillar collagen genes.

It has been shown that ras, an oncogene coding for the GTPase involved in signal transduction, and mos, a serine-threonine kinase also inhibit transcription of type I collagen genes, suggesting that external stimuli activate signal transduction pathway mediated by ras with a potential downstream mediator mos or other serine hreonine kinases (e.g., raf) and activate or repress collagen gene transcription. In this context, the work of Slack et al.[80] is most significant, in that they have clearly demonstrated dramatic reduction of type I collagen synthesis in rodent cells transformed by N-ras and Ha-ras oncogenes. Further, Slack et al. have shown that oncogenic ras regulates the type I collagen genes at both transcriptional and posttranscriptional levels, which may be mediated by sequences located within the body of the gene itself or in the distal 3'-flanking region. It should be pointed out that although down-regulation of type I collagen gene is quite common in ras-transformed cell lines, overexpression of ras itself is not sufficient to inhibit collagen-specific mRNA synthesis in a different cell line.[81] Taken together, we can conclude that depending on the cell line, and depending on the signal transduction pathway, different oncogenes elicit their effects on various target genes in a diverse manner.

In addition to v-src and N-ras or Ha-ras, other oncogenes like c-myc, v-mos, and v-fos have been shown to suppress either α1 (I) or α2 (I) gene transcription.[81–83] C-*myc* gene product, a DNA binding protein, cooperates with *ras* in tumorigenic conversion of primary rat embryo fibroblasts.[84] Moreover, as c-*myc* appears to be a downstream mediator of *ras*-induced transformation pathway, it is likely that suppression of collagen gene transcription by c-*myc* and v-*ras* may affect the same signal transduction pathway. On the other hand, V-*mos*, a serine threonine kinase, might inhibit collagen gene transcription by specific phosphorylation of transcription factors.

The question remains whether transformation of fibroblasts *per se* suppresses collagen gene transcription. Available data generally supports this notion. In several revertants, suppression of collagen gene transcription has not been relieved. In other words, reversion of the transformed phenotype to a normal phenotype does not automatically restore normal levels of collagen mRNA, suggesting that whatever the mode of inhibition of collagen gene transcription by oncogenes, in the vast majority of cases, this repressive effect is maintained.

Concluding Remarks

Reparative processes in cardiovascular disease include the inflammatory response during which neutrophils secrete a variety of cytokines and hormones that activate fibroblasts to secrete extracellular matrix proteins, including collagens. Local RAAS is activated as a result of which AngII is released. This autocrine AngII release from cardiac myocytes may then act on myofibroblasts and induce a cascade of events involving rapid phosphorylation of target proteins, and signal transducing molecules, including proto-oncogenes, resulting in the modification of transcription factors that induce or suppress genes that are involved in hypertrophy and fibrosis. As the old adage goes "all roads lead to Rome" irrespective of the initial signaling pathways that are responsive to external stimuli, the final outcome is the transcription of cellular genes required in reparative processes, wound healing, and structural remodeling of the tissue.

In several prevalent diseases, like heart failure, and cirrhosis, fibrosis due to abnormal deposition of collagen is the principal cause of tissue dysfunction and poor patient prognosis. Understanding these critical regulatory events is of utmost importance. Identification and characterization of tissue-specific transcription factors that are subject to activation or repression of gene transcription by peptide hormone-like AngII and identification of *cis*-acting elements in the target genes, should make it possible to develop specific inhibitors.

Although the genes for a large number of collagen molecules have been cloned and sequenced, characterization of the *cis*-regulatory elements and *trans*acting factors is still in its infancy. Much of the work cited in this chapter has raised more questions than it has provided answers regarding the complexity of regulatory mechanisms. A vast body of information has been obtained from cells cultured in vitro and therefore these results should be regarded as tentative until reproduced in vivo under more natural conditions, as well as pathological states. This is especially true for a cell like the interstitial fibroblast which in its natural state has tremendous clonal diversity and functional heterogeneity that can be influenced by other types of cells like myocytes as well as by the ECM itself. With the advent of modern recombinant DNA techniques coupled with gene transfer methodology, it should be possible to address issues with precision concerning fibrosis in various disease states and the role of systemic and local RAAS in these processes.

References

1. Hay ED. Collagen and other matrix glycoproteins in embryogenesis. In: Hays ED, ed. Cell Biology of Extracellular Matrix. 2nd ed. New York, NY: Plenum Press, 1991:419–462.
2. Woessner JF Jr. Introduction to serial reviews: the extracellular matrix. FASEB J 1993;7:735–736.
3. Lin CQ, Bissell MJ. Multi-faceted regulation of cell differentiation by extracellular matrix. FASEB J 1993;7:737–743.
4. Kivirikko KI. Collagens and their abnormalities in a wide spectrum of diseases. Ann Med 1993;25:113–126.
5. Vuorio E, de Crombrugghe B. The family of

collagen genes. Annu Rev Biochem 1990;59: 837–172.

6. Uitto J, Chu M-L. Regulation of collagen gene expression in human skin fibroblasts and its alterations in diseases. In: Olsen BR, Nimni ME, eds. Collagen. Vol. IV. Molecular Biology. Boca Raton, Fla.: CRC Press, 1989: 109–123.

7. Ramirez F. Organization and evolution of the fibrillar collagen genes. In: Olsen BR, Nimni ME, eds. Collagen. V. IV. Molecular Biology. Boca Raton, Fla.: CRC Press, 1989: 21–30.

8. Strauss WM, Dausman J, Beard C, et al. Germ line transmission of a yeast artificial chromosome spanning the murine α_1(I) collagen locus. Science 1993;259:1904–1907.

9. Goldberg H, Helaakoski T, Garrett LA, et al. Tissue-specific expression of the mouse α2 (I) collagen promoter. Studies in transgenic mice and in tissue culture cells. J Biol Chem 1992;267:19622–19630.

10. Boast S, Su MW, Ramirez F, et al. Functional analysis of cis-acting DNA sequences controlling transcription of the human type I collagen genes. J Biol Chem 1990;265: 13351–13356.

11. Slack JL, Liska DJ, Bornstein P. An upstream regulatory region mediates high-level, tissue-specific expression of the human α1(I) collagen gene in transgenic mice. Mol Cell Biol 1991;11:2066–2074.

12. Karsenty G, Golumbek P, de Crombrugghe B. Point mutations and small substitution mutations in three different upstream elements inhibit the activity of the mouse α2(I) collagen promoter. J Biol Chem 1988;263: 13909–13915.

13. Maity SN, Vuorio T, de Crombrugghe B. The B subunit of a rat heteromeric CCAAT-binding transcription factor shows a striking sequence identity with the yeast Hap2 transcription factor. Proc Natl Acad Sci USA 1990;87:5378–5382.

14. Vuorio T, Maity SN, de Crombrugghe B. Purification and molecular cloning of the "A" chain of a rat heterotrimeric CCAAT-binding protein. J Biol Chem 1990;265: 22480–22486.

15. Landschulz WH, Johnson PF, McKnight SL. The leucine zipper: a hypothetical structure common to a new class of DNA binding proteins. Science 1988;240:1759–1764.

16. Santoro C, Mermod N, Andrews PC, et al. A family of human CCAAT-box-binding proteins active in transcription and DNA replication: cloning and expression of multiple cDNAs. Nature 1988;334:218–224.

17. Maity SN, Golumbek PT, Karsenty G, et al. Selective activation of transcription by a novel CCAAT binding factor. Science 1988; 241:582–585.

18. Hatamochi A, Golumbek PT, Van Schaftingen E, et al. A CCAAT DNA binding factor consisting of two different components that are both required for DNA binding. J Biol Chem 1988;263:5940–5947.

19. Nehls MC, Grapilon ML, Brenner DA. NF-I/ Sp1 switch elements regulate collagen α1(I) gene expression. DNA Cell Biol 1992;11: 443–452.

20. Rossi P, Karsenty G, Robert AB, et al. A nuclear factor 1 binding site mediates the transcriptional activation of a type I collagen promoter by transforming growth factor-β. Cell 1988;52:405–414.

21. Karsenty G, Ravazzolo R, de Crombrugghe B. Purification and functional characterization of a DNA-binding protein that interacts with a negative element in the mouse α1(I) collagen promoter. J Biol Chem 1991;266: 24842–2448.

22. Harbers K, Kuehn M, Delius H, et al. Insertion of retrovirus into the first intron of α1(I) collagen gene leads to embryonic lethal mutation in mice. Proc Natl Acad Sci USA 1984; 81:1504–1508.

23. Lichtler A, Stover ML, Angilly J, et al. Isolation and characterization of the Rat α1(I) collagen promoter: regulation by 1,25-dihydroxyvitamin D. J Biol Chem 1989;264: 3072–3077.

24. Chu ML, de Wet W, Bernard M, et al. Fine structural analysis of the human pro-α1(I) collagen gene. Promoter structure, AluI repeats, and polymorphic transcripts. J Biol Chem 1985;260:2315–2320.

25. Karsenty G, de Crombrugghe B. Two different negative and one positive regulatory factors interact with a short promoter segment of the α1 (I) collagen gene. J Biol Chem 1990; 265:9934–9942.

26. Ravazzolo R, Karsenty G, de Crombrugghe B. A fibroblast-specific factor binds to an upstream negative control element in the promoter of the mouse α1(I) collagen gene. J Biol Chem 1991;266:7382–7387.

27. Liau G, Szapary D, Setoyama C, et al. Restriction enzyme digestions identify discrete domains in the chromatin around the promoter of the mouse α_2(I) collagen gene. J Biol Chem 1986;261:11362–11368.

28. Ruteshouser EC, de Crombrugghe B. Characterization of two distinct positive cis-acting elements in the mouse α1(III) collagen promoter. J Biol Chem 1989;264:13740–13744.

29. Bornstein P, Sage H. Regulation of collagen gene expression. Prog Nucleic Acid Res Mol Biol 1989;37:67–106.

30. Sherwood AL, Bornstein P. Transcriptional control of the α1(I) collagen gene involves orientation- and position-specific intronic sequences. Biochem J 1990;265:895–897.

31. Slack JL, Liska DJ, Bornstein P. Regulation of expression of the Type I collagen genes. Am J Med Gen 1993;45:140–151.

32. Liska DJ, Slack JL, Bornstein P. A highly conserved intronic sequence is involved in transcriptional regulation of the α1(I) collagen gene. Cell Regul 1990;1:487–498.

33. Katai H, Stephenson JD, Simkevich CP, et al. An AP-1–like motif in the first intron of human proα1(I) collagen gene is a critical determinant of its transcriptional activity. Mol Cell Biochem 1992;118:119–129.

34. Pogulis RJ, Freytag SO. Contribution of specific cis-acting elements to activity of the mouse pro-α2(I) collagen enhancer. J Biol Chem 1993;268:2493–2499.

35. Schnieke A, Harbers K, Jaenisch R. Embryonic lethal mutation in mice induced by retrovirus insertion into the α1(I) collagen gene. Nature 1983;304:315–320.

36. Hartung S, Jaenisch R, Breindl M. Retrovirus insertion inactivates mouse α1(I) collagen gene by blocking initiation of transcription. Nature 1986;320:365–367.

37. Schwarz M, Harbers K, Kratochwil K. Transcription of a mutant collagen I gene is a cell type and stage-specific marker for odontoblast and osteoblast differentiation. Development 1990;108:717–726.

38. Kuivaniemi H, Tromp G, Prockop DJ. Mutations in collagen genes: causes of rare and some common diseases in humans. FASEB J 1991;5:2052–2060.

39. Chiodo AA, Hockey A, Cole WG. A base substitution at the splice acceptor site of intron 5 of the COL1A2 gene activates a cryptic splice site within exon 6 and generates abnormal type I procollagen in a patient with Ehlers-Danlos syndrome type VII. J Biol Chem 1992;267:6361–6369.

40. Kontusaari S, Tromp G, Kuivaniemi H, et al. Inheritance of an RNA splicing mutation ($G^{+1 \text{ IVS20}}$) in the type III procollagen gene (COL3A1) in a family having aortic aneurysms and easy bruisability: phenotypic overlap between familial arterial aneurysms and Ehlers-Danlos syndrome type IV. Am J Hum Genet 1990;47:112–120.

41. Phillips CL, Shrago-Howe AW, Pinnell SR, et al. A substitution at a non-glycine position in the triple-helical domain of proα2(I) collagen chains present in an individual with a variant of the Marfan syndrome. J Clin Invest 1990;86:1723–1728.

42. Masaki T. Endothelins: homeostatic and compensatory actions in the circulatory and endocrine systems. Endocr Rev 1993;14:256–268.

43. Arai H, Hori S, Aramori I, et al. Cloning and expression of a cDNA encoding an endothelin receptor. Nature 1990;348:730–732.

44. Sakurai T, Yanagisawa M, Takuwa Y, et al. Cloning of a cDNA encoding a non-isopeptide-selective subtype of the endothelin receptor. Nature 1990;348:732–735.

45. Takuwa Y, Kasuya Y, Takuwa N, et al. Endothelin receptor is coupled to phospholipase C via a pertussin toxin insensitive guanine vascular smooth muscle cells. J Clin Invest 1990;85:653–658.

46. Force T, Kyriakis JM, Avruch J, et al. Endothelin, vasopressin and angiotensin II enhance tyrosine phosphorylation by protein kinase C-dependent and independent pathways in glomerular mesangial cells. J Biol Chem 1991;266:6650–6656.

47. Wang Y, Simonson MS, Pouyssegur J, et al. Endothelin rapidly stimulates mitogen-activated protein kinase activity in rat mesangial cells. Biochem J 1992;287:589–594.

48. Katwa LC, Guarda E, Weber KT. Endothelin receptors in cultured adult rat cardiac fibroblasts. Cardiovasc Res 1993;27:2125–2129.

49. Lindpaintner K, Ganten D. The cardiac renin-angiotensin system: an appraisal of present experimental and clinical evidence. Circ Res 1991;68:905–921.

50. Baker KM, Booz GW, Dostal DE. Cardiac actions of angiotensin II: role of an intracardiac renin-angiotensin system. Annu Rev Physiol 1992;54:227–241.

51. Kunapuli SP, Kumar A. Molecular cloning of human angiotensinogen cDNA and evidence for the presence of its mRNA in rat heart. Circ Res 1987;60:786–790.

52. Dostal DE, Rothblum KN, Chernin MI, et al. Intracardiac detection of angiotensinogen and renin: a localized renin-angiotensin system in neonatal rat heart. Am J Physiol 1992;263:C838-C850.

53. Campbell DJ, Habener JF. Cellular localization of angiotensinogen gene expression in brown adipose tissue and mesentery: quantification of messenger ribonucleic acid abundance using hybridization in situ. Endocrinology 1987;121:1616–1626.

54. Cassis LA, Lynch KR, Peach MJ. Localization

of angiotensinogen messenger RNA in rat aorta. Circ Res 1988;62:1259–1262.

55. Sun Y, Diaz-Arias AA, Weber KT. Angiotensin-converting enzyme, bradykinin and angiotensin II receptor binding in rat skin, tendon and heart valves: an in vitro quantitative autoradiographic study. J Lab Clin Med 1994;123:372–377.

56. Weber KT, Brilla CG. Pathological hypertrophy and cardiac interstitium: fibrosis and renin-angiotensin-aldosterone system. Circulation 1991;83:1849–1865.

57. Beinlich CJ, White GJ, Baker KM, et al. Angiotensin II and left ventricular growth in newborn pig heart. J Mol Cell Cardiol 1991;23:1031–1038.

58. Keeley FW, Elmoselhi A, Leenan FHH. Enalapril suppresses normal accumulation of elastin and collagen in cardiovascular tissues of growing rats. Am J Physiol 1992;262:H1013-H10121.

59. Makino N, Matsui H, Masutomo K, et al. Effect of angiotensin converting enzyme inhibitor on regression in cardiac hypertrophy. Mol Cell Biochem 1993;119:23–28.

60. Smits JFM, van Krimpen C, Schoemaker RG, et al. Angiotensin II receptor blockade after myocardial infarction in rats: effects on hemodynamics, myocardial DNA synthesis, and interstitial collagen content. J Cardiovasc Pharmacol 1992;20:772–778.

61. Sadoshima J, Izumo S. Mechanical stretch rapidly activates multiple signal transduction pathways in cardiac myocytes: potential involvement of an autocrine/paracrine mechanism. EMBO J 1993;12:1681–1692.

62. Sadoshima J, Xu Y, Slayter HS, et al. Autocrine release of angiotensin II mediates stretch-induced hypertrophy of cardiac myocytes in vitro. Cell 1993;75:977–984.

63. Brilla CG, Weber KT. Mineralocorticoid excess, dietary sodium and myocardial fibrosis. J Lab Clin Med 1992;120:893–901.

64. Doering CW, Jalil JE, Janicki JS, et al. Collagen network remodeling and diastolic stiffness of the rat left ventricle with pressure overload hypertrophy. Cardiovasc Res 1988;22:686–695.

65. Jalil JE, Doering CW, Janicki JS, et al. Fibrillar collagen and myocardial stiffness in the intact hypertrophied rat left ventricle. Circ Res 1989;64:1041–1050.

66. Weber KT, Brilla CG, Campbell SE, Zhou G, Matsubara L, Guarda E. Pathologic hypertrophy with fibrosis: the structural basis for myocardial failure. Blood Pressure 1992;1:75–85.

67. Brilla CG, Matsubara LS, Weber KT. Anti-aldosterone treatment and the prevention of myocardial fibrosis in primary and secondary hyperaldosteronism. J Mol Cell Cardiol 1993;25:563–575.

68. Allebach E, Boettiger D, Pacifici M, et al. Control of Types I and II collagen and fibronectin gene expression in chondrocytes delineated by viral transformation. Mol Cell Biol 1985;5:1002–1008.

69. Kamine J, Rubin H. Coordinate control of collagen synthesis and cell growth in chick embryo fibroblasts and the effect of viral transformation on collagen synthesis. J Cell Physiol 1977;92:1–22.

70. Sandmeyer S, Bornstein P. Declining procollagen mRNA sequences in chick embryo fibroblasts infected with Rous sarcoma virus. J Biol Chem 1979;254:4950–4953.

71. Parry G, Soo W-J, Bissell MJ. The uncoupled regulation of fibronectin and collagen synthesis in Rous sarcoma virus transformed avian tendon cells. J Biol Chem 1979;254:11763–11766.

72. Sandmeyer S, Gallis B, Bornstein P. Coordinate transcriptional regulation of type I procollagen genes by Rous sarcoma virus. J Biol Chem 1981;26:5022–5028.

73. Adams SL, Boettiger D, Focht RJ, et al. Regulation of the synthesis of extra cellular matrix components in chondroblasts transformed by a temperature-sensitive mutant of Rous sarcoma virus. Cell 1982;30:373–384.

74. Pacifici M, Boettiger D, Roby K, et al. Transformation of chondroblasts by Rous sarcoma virus and synthesis of sulfated proteoglycan matrix. Cell 1977;11:891–899.

75. Welham MJ, Wyke JA. A single point mutation has pleiotropic effects on pp60v-src function. J of Virol 1988;62:1898–1906.

76. Parsons JT, Weber MJ. Genetics of src: structure and functional organization of a protein tyrosine kinase. Curr Topics Microbiol Immunol 1989;147:79–125.

77. Hildebrand JD, Schaller MD, Parsons JT. Identification of sequences required for the efficient localization of the focal adhesion kinase, pp125[FAK], to cellular focal adhesions. J Cell Biol 1993;123:993–1005.

78. Guan J-L, Shalloway D. Regulation of focal adhesion-associated protein tyrosine kinase by both cellular adhesion and oncogenic transformation. Nature 1992;358:690–692.

79. Lipfert L, Haimovich B, Schaller MD, et al. Integrin-dependent phosphorylation and activation of the protein tyrosine kinase

pp125^{FAK} in platelets. J Cell Biol 1992;119: 905–912.

80. Slack JL, Parker MI, Robinson VR, et al. Regulation of collagen I gene expression by *ras*. Mol Cell Biol 1992;12:4714–4723.

81. Hoemann CD, Zarbl H. Use of revertant cell lines to identify targets of v-fos transformation-specific alterations in gene expression. Cell Growth Differ 1990;1:581–590.

82. Yang BS, Geddes TJ, Pogulis RJ, et al. Transcriptional suppression of cellular gene expression by c-myc. Mol Cell Biol 1991;11: 2291–2295.

83. Schmidt A, Setoyama C, deCrombrugghe B. V-mos transformation regulates the expression of the α2(I) collagen promoter introduced in NIH 3T3 cells. Nature 1985;314: 286–289.

84. Land H, Parada LF, Weinberg RA. Tumorigenic conversion of primary embryo fibroblasts requires at least two cooperating oncogenes. Nature 1983;304:596–602.

Chapter 23

In Search of Common Ground

Karl T. Weber, M.D.

Introduction

Organs are composed of parenchyma and stroma. Parenchyma refers to highly differentiated cells that impart very specific functions and morphologically distinctive features to an organ. These very specialized cells, however, have lost their functional and phenotypic diversity. Stroma is located between individual or groups of parenchymal cells (see Figure 1) and therefore considered an extracellular matrix that includes: (1) structural proteins, collagen, and elastin; (2) carbohydrates bound to proteins and termed glycosaminoglycans and proteoglycans; (3) undifferentiated, pluripotent cells (e.g., fibroblasts and macrophages), having considerable phenotypic and functional diversity; (4) vessels that transport arterial and venous blood and lymph; and (5) tissue fluid, which is in dynamic equilibrium with lymph. Tissue fluid contains signals that govern stromal and/or parenchymal cell function and phenotypic transformation. These signals gain access to the interstitium from any one of several sources, including plasma, parenchyma, fibroblasts, macrophages, adrenergic nerve endings or cells that invade the extracellular space from the circulation (e.g., inflammatory cells). The extracellular matrix has broad ranging functions that regulate cell migration, differentiation, and gene expression.[1,2]

The time is propitious to search for common pathophysiological mechanisms of disease—*the common ground*. The direc-tion that such a research enterprise should take becomes apparent when addressing several fundamental questions. *What characteristic of tissue is common to most organs?* Stroma and its pluripotent mesenchymal cells and tissue fluid. At the organ level, stroma therefore represents the common ground. At the cellular level, the common ground includes fibroblasts and their repertoire of extensive clonal heterogeneity that provides fibroblast-like cells with a wide range of functions and properties, including considerable diversity with respect to structural protein synthesis, expression of receptors, response to regulatory molecules, rates of cell turnover, and distinctive morphological features.[3–5] In the heart, for example, different clonal subsets appear to contribute to fibroplastic and fibrogenic responses and subsequent fibrous tissue remodeling.[6] At the molecular level the common ground for stroma includes genes that govern the phenotypic expression and behavior of interstitial cells involved in tissue repair and their subsequent expression of fibronectin and types I and III collagen genes.

What property of stroma is common to vascularized tissue? Wound healing with its inflammatory and reparative components. In reaching for the common ground found in stroma and expressed within the paradigm of inflammation and healing, it is necessary to integrate each of these levels of biological organization. This could be achieved by working from a candidate gene upward in search of its importance in diseased organs. Molecular biologists might favor this ap-

[1] This work was supported in part by NIH Grant R01-HL-31701.

From Weber KT, MD *Wound Healing in Cardiovascular Disease*, Armonk, NY, Futura Publishing Company Inc., © 1995.

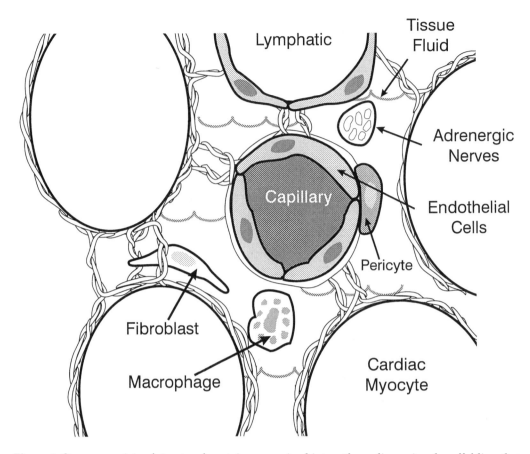

Figure 1. Stroma consists of structural proteins, organized into a three-dimensional scaffolding that supports parenchymal cells and the vasculature. It likewise houses pluripotent cells of mesenchymal organ, including fibroblasts and macrophages, that are bathed by a tissue fluid common to the interstitial space of the organ.

proach. For a clinician and integrative biologist, like myself, it is more appropriate to first examine the inflammation healing paradigm at the organ and then cellular level, finally sharpening one's focus further to identify candidate genes that govern the behavior of interstitial cells and turnover of structural proteins in a particular disease state.

The perspective provided herein takes this latter viewpoint. It will address the importance of aberrations in stroma formation and factors that contribute to its disproportionate or pathological accumulation. The heart is specifically targeted for discussion. Three broad topics are considered: (1) stromal growth relative to parenchyma; (2) cells involved in stromal formation; and (3) candidate genes that govern stromal structure.

Stromal Growth Relative to Parenchyma

Adaptive and Pathological Remodeling

Myocardial growth, expressed as an increase in ventricular mass, is determined primarily by the growth of cardiac myocytes. Cardiac myocytes represent but one-third of all cells that compose the myocardium. Their size, however, accounts for two-thirds of its structural space. Parenchymal growth must be accompanied by stromal growth if tissue homogeneity is to be preserved and ventricular hypertrophy to prove an adaptive response (Figure 2). Collagen turnover, involving steady state synthesis and degradation, is the major deter-

PATTERNS OF TISSUE GROWTH
Parenchyma and Stroma

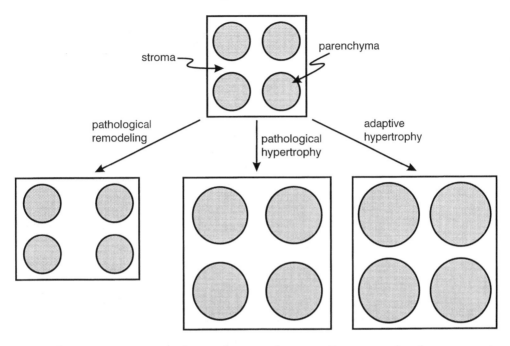

Figure 2. Organs are composed of parenchyma and stroma. Organ growth, when expressed as proportionate growth of parenchyma and stroma, leads to an adaptive hypertrophy. Disproportionate stromal growth, relative to parenchyma growth, leads to pathological hypertrophy. Stromal growth in the absence of parenchymal growth accounts for a pathological remodeling of the organ. Reproduced from Weber KT. Stroma and the search for common ground. *Cardiavasc Res* 1995;29: 330–335.

minant of stromal growth. The normal regulation of collagen turnover guarantees that collagen concentration in the hypertrophied myocardium remains within normal limits under a variety of conditions. Collagen synthesis has to exceed its degradation if collagen concentration is to remain normal in the now hypertrophied myocardium; had it not, collagen concentration, relative to hypertrophied myocytes, would have fallen. Collagen content (concentration × ventricular mass) is increased in the hypertrophied ventricle. For example, with the hypertrophy that accompanies the stretch of myocardium due to ventricular volume overload (e.g., secondary to isotonic exercise training, atrial septal defect, arteriovenous fistula, or chronic anemia), collagen concentration remains normal while collagen content is in-

creased.[7] Collagen concentration of the hypertrophied myocardium remains normal with the pressure overload hypertrophy associated with infrarenal aortic banding[8]; collagen content is again increased. Thus, hemodynamic factors dictate ventricular loading and thereby govern myocyte growth. Myocardial stretch and force generation likewise appear to contribute to an appropriate increase in collagen content in a manner that resembles stress-mediated collagen formation in bone. Reversal of these underlying experimental conditions is associated with both a regression of myocardial mass and stroma so that tissue structure remains homogenous.

Disproportionate stromal growth, relative to cardiac myocytes, accounts for an inappropriate increase in myocardial collagen concentration and is defined as fibrosis. The abnormal accumulation of fibrous tissue creates a pathological remodeling of the myocardium. When disproportionate stromal growth occurs in the setting of cardiac myocyte growth it accounts for pathological ventricular hypertrophy (Figure 2). This is found in the pressure overloaded, hypertrophied left ventricle in hypertensive heart disease. However, the disproportionate growth of stroma is not due to hypertension. This is further underscored by the appearance of fibrosis in the normotensive, nonhypertrophied right ventricle in hypertensive heart disease. In the absence of myocyte growth, disproportionate accumulation of stroma produces a pathological remodeling of tissue (Figure 2). A generalized growth of stroma is found in other organs (e.g., pancreas) in hypertensive cardiovascular disease—organs which are not hypertrophied—indicating that parenchymal cell growth need not dictate collagen turnover.

Role of Hemodynamic and Hormonal Factors

The importance of hemodynamic factors on myocyte growth has been addressed (vida supra). In rats, a chronic excess of either thyroid hormone or growth hormone likewise promotes myocyte hypertrophy in the absence of altered myocyte loading. In either of these experimental models, however, an abnormal increase in myocardial collagen concentration has not been seen.[9,10] Chemical mediators of stromal formation have been largely neglected. Emerging evidence would support a role for certain cytokines (e.g., transforming growth factor-β (TGF)-β_1) and hormones. Cytokines have been the subject of several recent reviews[11-13] to which the interested reader is referred. Herein, the less well-recognized role of hormones will be considered.

A chronic inappropriate (relative to dietary sodium) excess of either circulating angiotensin II (AngII) or aldosterone (ALDO), effector hormones of the renin-angiotensin-aldosterone system (RAAS), can lead to generalized perivascular fibrosis of systemic and coronary arterioles. In man, this has been seen with renin-dependent hy-

peraldosteronism, such as unilateral renal ischemia or Bartter's syndrome, and in non-renin-dependent mineralocorticoid excess, such as adrenal adenoma, 11β-hydroxylase deficiency, or anabolic steroid use that produces chronic elevations in either ALDO or deoxycorticosterone, respectively.[14]

These clinical observations have been extended using various experimental conditions in previously normal rats.[14,15] A perivascular fibrosis of intramyocardial coronary arteries, involving the right and left ventricles, has been observed in the following animal models: bilateral and unilateral renal ischemia, where both circulating AngII and ALDO are increased; in rats given AngII by implanted minipump, where both AngII and ALDO are increased in plasma; in uninephrectomized rats on a high sodium diet that were also receiving either ALDO, deoxycorticosterone acetate, or androgens; and where plasma AngII alone was suppressed or both AngII and ALDO were suppressed.[7] They further emphasize that AngII and mineralocorticoids are each contributory and likely involve different mechanisms. In using various pharmacological agents the importance of these circulating hormones of the RAAS on fibrosis was further demonstrated. By interfering with AngII generation or occupying ALDO receptors, the role of these hormones in promoting fibrosis was addressed. This included: rats with unilateral renal ischemia that received captopril[16]; rats with suprarenal aortic banding that received an antihypertensive or non-antihypertensive dose of ramipril[15]; and uninephrectomized rats that received ALDO and the ALDO receptor antagonist spironolactone in a large or small dose that did or did not prevent hypertension.[17] In each model, perivascular fibrosis of intramural vessels was not seen. A separate role for AngII and ALDO was suggested in studies that demonstrated a difference in the temporal sequence to the appearance of perivascular fibrosis when each hormone was administered.[18] In previously normal rats receiving AngII by implanted minipump, a perivascular fibrosis of intramyocardial coronary arteries and arterioles and microscopic scarring was seen in each ventricle as early as day 14. These reactive and reparative fibrous tissue responses became progressively more advanced at 4 and 6 weeks of AngII administration. In contrast, ALDO treatment by implanted minipump in uninephrectomized rats on a high sodium diet elicited a similar perivascular fibrosis and microscopic scarring, but only after 4 weeks of administration. Each became progressively more advanced at 6 weeks. The nature of the pathophysiological response and cellular response therefore would appear to be distinct in each case.

In the case of AngII treatment, the perivascular fibrosis has been linked to enhanced coronary vascular permeability to macromolecules (e.g., albumin and fibronectin).[19–21] Whether AngII itself or other vasoactive substances released in response to AngII administration enhances permeability remains to be defined. Myocyte necrosis accompanies elevations in plasma AngII and has been related to catecholamine release from the adrenal medulla.[21] Coronary hyperpermeability is not seen with ALDO administration,[20] and therefore the mechanism involved in its leading to a perivascular fibrosis remains uncertain. Spironolactone, an ALDO receptor antagonist, is able to prevent perivascular fibrosis in rats receiving ALDO.[22] On the other hand, myocyte necrosis with subsequent scarring, is related to myocardial potassium depletion in the setting of chronic mineralocorticoid excess and can be prevented by spironolactone,[22] the potassium-sparing diuretic amiloride,[23] or dietary KCl supplementation.[24] Amiloride did not prevent the perivascular fibrosis associated with chronic ALDO administration. A role for magnesium deficiency in promoting cardiac myocyte necrosis[25] in the setting of chronic ALDO treatment cannot be discounted.

Myocardial fibrosis is not seen in uninephrectomized rats on a high sodium diet alone or when receiving ALDO while on a low sodium diet. Thus, chronic inappropriate (relative to sodium intake) elevations in either AngII and/or mineralocorticoids are associated with a reactive fibrous tissue response of intramural arteries. This suggests that these hormones may be mediators of wound healing and when present in inappropriate quantities in the circulation for any length of time fibrous tissue accumulation appears in the heart and systemic arterioles.

Stroma and Tissue Repair

The stromal composition of the myocardium is increased as a natural response to tissue repair. A reparative fibrosis, for example, occurs in response to parenchymal cell necrosis while a reactive fibrosis accompanies tissue irritation or the interruption of tissue by foreign material. These responses are contained to the site of necrosis or foreign material (e.g., silk suture), provided the degree of parenchymal and microvascular damage is minor and regulatory signals are limited to involved tissue. On the other hand, an entire organ may be involved in the disproportionate accumulation of stroma. This occurs following transmural myocardial infarction, where a reparative fibrosis appears at the site of necrosis in the infarcted ventricle and is accompanied by a reactive fibrosis in the noninfarcted ventricle and interventricular septum. Albeit of uncertain pathophysiological origins, the formation of stroma at remote sites could be explained by a dispersion of fibrogenic signals within tissue fluid of the interstitial space that is common to both ventricles and septum. These signals, however, do not reach the circulation to promote an unwanted tissue repair response in other organs. When fibrogenic signals gain access to the circulation, as exemplified for chronic elevations in plasma AngII or mineralocorticoids, the heart and systemic organs are involved in an unwanted accumulation of stroma—a wound healing response gone awry.

Cells Involved in the Regulation of Stromal Formation

The sound experimental basis for the functional heterogeneity of fibroblasts provides a new and exciting springboard for experiments designed to probe the mechanisms of human fibrotic disorders. The amplification of a subset of fibroblasts by selective informational molecules . . . provides a mechanism for the control of connective tissue synthesis and deposition.[26]

Fibroblast-like Cells

Fibroblasts are pivotal to tissue repair. Like endothelial cells, vascular smooth muscle cells, pericytes, and adipocytes, fibroblasts are derived from mesenchyme. Fibroblasts found in adult tissues retain pluripotentiality and accordingly exhibit marked diversity in their functions, a trait presumptively related to distinct phenotypic subtypes.[3-5] Phenotypic interconversion can also occur between these cells of mesenchymal origin, as evidenced by ALDO-mediated transformation of fibroblast-like cells into adipocytes.[27]

Between tissues and within a given tissue, fibroblasts demonstrate extensive clonal heterogeneity not unlike hemopoietic cells. For example, fibroblast-like cells appear at the site of cardiac myocyte necrosis and repair several days after myocardial infarction due to coronary artery ligation or freeze-thaw injury.[6,28] These cells are larger than the usual fibroblast, have a prominent nucleus and endoplasmic reticulum, and in addition have acquired α-smooth muscle actin microfilaments during phenotypic transformation from presumably quiescent fibroblasts of the interstitium and/or pericytes that normally reside in the adventitia of the intramural coronary vasculature. These actin filaments contribute to the ability of these cells to contract.[29] Contractile fibroblasts involved in tissue repair are termed *myofibroblasts*.[30] The contraction of granulation tissue is thought to be related to the contractility of these cells and their having cell to cell and cell to stroma connections. Such remodeling of granulation tissue, however, does not occur until several weeks after its formation. It accounts for a reduction in the volume of infarcted myocardium, infarct thickness, and the retraction of scar tissue.[31-33] Cells taken from granulation tissue at 21 and 28 days are able to contract collagen gels to a greater extent than cells isolated after 7 and 14 days.[34] In the heart, signals responsible for the phenotypic transformation into myofibroblasts and which regulate their contractility are uncertain. These signals may differ between the heart and other organs, but to my way of thinking this is only likely to be the case under special circumstances. Such signals could be derived from the circulation, fibroblasts themselves, neighboring endothelial cells, platelets, or inflammatory cells. Transforming growth factor-β_1 has been implicated in evoking this response in other tissues.[11,35-38]

Using a monoclonal antibody to recognize additional antigenic determinants of these cells, Sun et al.[28] found that myofibroblasts located at diverse sites of fibrous tissue formation in the heart contain angiotensin converting enzyme (ACE). It is tempting to speculate that the appearance of ACE in these cells serves to regulate local concentrations of AngII and BK—peptides that contribute to the healing response and growth factor expression (vide infra). At sites of tissue repair, myofibroblasts express the transcript for type I collagen,[28] the major fibrillar collagen found in scar tissue in the heart.[39-41] Cultured myofibroblasts predominantly secrete the procollagen for type I collagen.[42]

Myofibroblasts, which play a central role in connective tissue formation and matrix remodeling, are gradually reduced in number at the site of repair.[6,28,43] Their rate of disappearance, however, appears to be different.[6] Fibrocytes, smaller fibroblasts with less prominent organelles and without α-smooth muscle actin filaments, remain. The disappearance of some myofibroblasts may be secondary to programmed cell death (apoptosis) in a fashion similar to hemopoietic cells; inhibitory factors could also be involved. Marked ACE binding, however, remains at fibrous tissue sites for prolonged periods.[28] ACE binding has been observed as long as 6 months postinfarction (Y. Sun, personal communication). ACE-positive myofibroblasts are also found at sites of reactive fibrosis remote to infarction. This includes the endocardial fibrosis of the interventricular septum and perivascular fibrosis of intramural vessels found in the right ventricle. Signals derived from necrotic myocytes and which may traverse the common interstitial space may or may not be a requisite for their appearance. Myofibroblasts are seen with the pericardial fibrosis that follows pericardiotomy without infarction and the foreign-body fibrosis that accompanies placement of a silk ligature around the left coronary artery without infarction. Because myofibroblasts were found in sham-operated animals without infarction at sites of pericardial and foreign-body fibrosis suggests signals derived from necrotic myocytes are not involved in these responses.[28] Irrespective of the location or nature of the inciting stimulus to connective tissue formation in the heart, myofibroblasts are the dominant cell involved in stromal formation in each of these diverse pathological conditions. The functional and/or morphological diversity to these α-smooth muscle-actin containing cells, such as that seen in other expressions of fibrous tissue formation,[4] remains to be ascertained.

Other fibroblast-like cells that also contain α-smooth muscle actin and ACE are found within the connective tissue of the adventitia surrounding intramyocardial coronary arteries. They are referred to as *pericytes*. Whether these cells contribute to the remote perivascular fibrosis that involves intramural coronary arteries of the right ventricle postinfarction is unknown. They could also contribute to the perivascular fibrosis of these vessels that appears in both right and left ventricles in association with chronic elevations in circulating AngII.[18] This latter fibrous tissue response is initiated in response to the escape of plasma macromolecules (e.g., fibronectin) into the perivascular space.[19] This sets into motion the subsequent appearance of fibroblast-like cells that express type I collagen mRNA[19] and ultimately accounts for the perivascular accumulation of fibrillar collagen.[44]

Because of their α-smooth muscle actin microfilaments, pericytes have contractile properties.[45–49] Pericyte contraction is induced by AngII, bradykinin (BK), and prostaglandins (PG), substances found in tissue fluid. A hemangiopericytoma of the kidney can present as a renin-producing neoplasm.[50]

Heart valve leaflets are composed largely of connective tissue and collagen turnover here is normally high. Within the interior of the leaflet are *valvular interstitial cells*. These fibroblast-like cells are normal residents of leaflet tissue. They contain α-smooth muscle actin filaments and demon-

strate marked ACE binding. Unlike vascular smooth muscle cells and some myofibroblasts, valvular interstitial cells do not have desmin (A. Ratajska, personal communication). Preliminary data (L. Katwa, unpublished findings) indicate these cells are able to generate AngII presumably as a result of protease cleavage of requisite angiotensinogen precursor and ACE activity, components whose RNA transcripts have been found in these cells. Valvular interstitial cells also contain mRNA for type I collagen. AngII stimulates collagen synthesis in these cells via AT_1 receptor binding suggesting an autocrine role for this peptide in collagen turnover. Filip et al.[51] have found that cultured valvular interstitial cells contract in response to AngII.

Thus, the phenotypically transformed fibroblast with α-smooth muscle actin, ACE, and type I collagen mRNA predominate at normal and pathological sites of high collagen turnover. This includes a nonpermanent resident cell, the myofibroblast, and permanent resident pericytes and valvular interstitial cells. Signal(s) involved in the expansion of the myofibroblast clonal subset in the myocardium is uncertain. In both growing and quiescent human skin fibroblasts, TGF-β_1 stimulates the appearance of α-smooth muscle actin protein and its mRNA expression.[35] Subcutaneous administration of TGF-β_1 leads to the appearance of myofibroblasts within granulation tissue and which is not seen with the similar administration of PDGF or TNF-α. The control of connective tissue formation and its remodeling under normal or pathological conditions, therefore appears to depend on the relative proportions of this fibroblast-like phenotype and its diverse functions. Cultured myofibroblasts, pericytes, and valvular interstitial cells offer unique models with which to address issues of signal generation and collagen turnover at sites of repair. The role of fibrocytes would appear to be more related to normal daily turnover of collagen in the myocardium—a dynamic process in its own right.[52]

Metabolic Activity of Fibroblast-like Cells

The clonal subset of fibroblasts found at sites of high collagen turnover, exemplified by myofibroblasts, pericytes, and valvular interstitial cells, have functions quite distinct from fibrocytes. They are a major determinant of connective tissue repair and therefore are of considerable interest. Regulation of wound healing by locally generated signals guarantees that wounds are confined to injured tissue. For example, cytokine expression is contained within sites of injury. What regulates cytokine expression is less well understood. Parenchymal cell necrosis may be important,[53] but is not a requisite to all fibrous tissue reactions. An attractive concept would be to suggest that fibroblast-like cells have an intrinsic ability to generate their own signals (e.g., AngII, TGF-β_1, BK, and PGE$_2$) which in an autocrine and paracrine manner regulate collagen turnover. This possibility was addressed in Chapter 1. Mounting evidence would indicate this is the case. AngII induces the expression of TGF-β_1 mRNA in cultured neonatal rat cardiac fibroblasts.[54] Fibroblasts are known to produce PGE$_2$, particularly in response to BK stimulation.[55,56]

Regulation of Fibroblast-like Cell Collagen Turnover

The contractile behavior of α-smooth muscle-actin containing fibroblast-like cells has already drawn attention to the potential role of locally generated hormones (e.g., AngII, BK, and PG) in scar tissue remodeling. These substances serve as chemical mediators of inflammation. Through a biological economy of action such peptides appear to likewise contribute to connective tissue repair at normal sites, such as valve leaflets and vascular adventitia, as well as at sites of fibrous tissue formation. This involves valvular interstitial cells, pericytes, and myofibroblasts, respectively. Is there evidence that this might be the case? A cautious affirmative would appear to be emerging.

Receptors for AngII and BK have been identified in intact heart valves[57] and cultured valvular interstitial cells[58]; in each case they are predominantly of the AT$_1$ and BK$_2$ subtypes. The synthesis of type I collagen by valvular interstitial cells is promoted by AT$_1$ receptor-ligand binding.[58] BK and

PGE$_2$, on the other hand, have an inhibitory effect on collagen synthesis in these cells (Katwa et al., unpublished observations) suggesting AngII, BK, and PGE$_2$ may contribute in a reciprocal manner to the regulation of connective tissue formation. Whether this would also be the case for myofibroblasts and pericytes remains to be determined. In like manner, the contribution of cytokines, or growth factors, to collagen turnover in these fibroblast-like cells is uncertain. Evidence is at hand that such regulatory peptides regulate fibroblastic cell phenotype[4,35,37,38] and cell contraction.[34]

Candidate Genes that Govern Stromal Structures

The question of how much functional and positional information is encoded in the primary sequence of genes and how much the environment influences gene expression . . . is central to life science research in many fields.[1]

It would appear evident that stroma and its pluripotent fibroblast-like cells represent the common ground involved in tissue repair—a fundamental property of vascularized tissues. It no longer is tenable to consider stroma inert. Quite to the contrary, it is a dynamic metabolic entity involved in peptide and cytokine generation which in an autocrine/paracrine manner regulate fibrillar collagen formation at sites of tissue repair.

Fibroblast-like cells have an extensive repertoire—expressed as phenotypic and functional diversity. This includes diversity in cell turnover rates, expression of specific cell surface receptors, and morphological features. A discussion of these topics can be found elsewhere.[3-5] Alpha smooth muscle actin, ACE-containing fibroblast-like cells involved in collagen turnover, and extracellular matrix remodeling include: myofibroblasts, at sites of pathological fibrous tissue formation; pericytes, within the adventitia of aorta, intramyocardial coronary arteries, and arterioles; and valvular interstitial cells of heart valve leaflets. Gene(s) that regulate phenotypic conversion from quiescent phenotype to metabolically active fibroblast-like cells is an important direction for future research.

Hormone (e.g., AngII) and growth factor (e.g., TGF-β_1) generation may be important in regulating the phenotypic conversion and functional diversity of fibroblast-like cells. The presence of ACE in these cells is integral to modulating local hormone concentrations that regulate cell phenotype and collagen synthesis and degradation. Understanding the regulation of the ACE gene, that governs tissue expression of this carboxypeptidase, as well as the TGF-β_1 gene is of fundamental importance. Boluyt et al.[59] have reported that the transition from stable left ventricular hypertrophy to a state of congestive heart failure in spontaneously hypertensive rats is associated with an increase in fibronectin and fibrillar collagen mRNA expression in association with the appearance of interstitial fibrosis. This transcriptional regulation of structural protein deposition was accompanied by an increase in TGF-β_1 mRNA expression. The mechanism(s) responsible for the increased expression of types I and III collagens, fibronectin, and TGF-β_1 mRNAs is uncertain and may be linked to one another.

Guntaka et al. have suggested (see Chapter 22), "all roads lead to Rome," wherein the regulation of types I and III fibrillar collagen genes is the finally common denominator to tissue repair. Do locally produced peptides (e.g., AngII) or polypeptides (e.g., TGF-β_1) regulate collagen synthesis and degradation in intact tissues, and are these transcriptional and/or posttranslational events? The expression of collagen genes is likely governed by tissue-specific factors interacting with cognate cis-acting elements in fibroblast DNA. The role of cis-acting DNA sequences in the regulatory region of type I collagen gene involved with hormone-activated factors needs to be identified as do transcription factors that interact with cis-acting elements. Is the metabolic activity of stroma independent of cytokines and parenchyma? Not likely. Cytokines and growth factors are recognized important mediators of the various phases of the inflammation healing paradigm. TGF-β_1, for example, contributes to the following: macrophage and fibroblast chemotaxis; fibroblast proliferation and phenotypic transformation; stimulation of collagen synthesis; and scar tissue remodeling.[11-13] On days

1 and 2 following coronary artery ligation in the rat, TGF-β_1 mRNA is expressed in infarcted tissue.[53,60] In cultured human cardiac fibroblasts this growth factor increases the expression of type I collagen mRNA and TIMP mRNA severalfold.[61] A potential association between TGF-β_1 and AngII in intact tissue remains to be examined. In cultured neonatal rat cardiac fibroblasts, AngII has been found to augment the expression of TGF-β_1 gene via AT_1 receptor binding.[54]

These studies, while focusing on the heart and its stroma, likely apply to other organs and their capacity for tissue repair. In solving these questions, fundamental aspects of wound healing and fibrogenesis may emerge. Answers can be used to advantage in developing strategies that prevent unwanted fibrous tissue accumulation or which promote fibrosis when it is needed.

References

1. Bissell MJ, Hall HG, Parry G. How does the extracellular matrix direct gene expression? J Theor Biol 1982;99:31–68.
2. Caplan AI. The extracellular matrix is instructive. Bioessays 1986;5:129–132.
3. McCulloch CAG, Bordin S. Role of fibroblast subpopulations in periodontal physiology and pathology. J Periodont Res 1991;26:144–154.
4. Sappino AP, Schürch W, Gabbiani G. Differentiation repertoire of fibroblastic cells: expression of cytoskeletal proteins as marker of phenotypic modulations. Lab Invest 1990;63:144–161.
5. Schor SL, Schor AM. Clonal heterogeneity in fibroblast phenotype: implications for the control of epithelial-mesenchymal interactions. Bioessays 1987;7:200–204.
6. Vracko R, Thorning D. Contractile cells in rat myocardial scar tissue. Lab Invest 1991;65:214–227.
7. Weber KT, Brilla CG, Campbell SE, Zhou G, Matsubara L, Guarda E. Pathologic hypertrophy with fibrosis: the structural basis for myocardial failure. Blood Pressure 1992;1:75–85.
8. Brilla CG, Pick R, Tan LB, et al. Remodeling of the rat right and left ventricle in experimental hypertension. Circ Res 1990;67:1355–1364.
9. Holubarsch C, Holubarsch T, Jacob R, et al. Thiedemann K. Passive elastic properties of

myocardium in different models and stages of hypertrophy: a study comparing mechanical, chemical and morphometric parameters. In: Alpert NR, ed. Myocardial Hypertrophy and Failure. New York, NY: Raven Press, 1983:323–336. (Katz AM, ed. Perspectives in Cardiovascular Research; vol 7).

10. Gilbert PL, Siegel RJ, Melmed S, et al. Cardiac morphology in rats with growth hormone-producing tumours. J Mol Cell Cardiol 1985;17:805–811.

11. Bennett NT, Schultz GS. Growth factors and wound healing: biochemical properties of growth factors and their receptors. Am J Surg 1993;165:728–737.

12. Bennett NT, Schultz GS. Growth factors and wound healing: part II. Role in normal and chronic wound healing. Am J Surg 1993;166: 74–81.

13. Lawrence WT, Diegelmann RF. Growth factors in wound healing. Clin Dermatol 1994; 12:157–169.

14. Weber KT, Sun Y, Campbell SE, et al. Chronic mineralocorticoid excess and cardiovascular remodeling. Steroids 1995;60: 125–132.

15. Linz W, Schaper J, Wiemer G, et al. Ramipril prevents left ventricular hypertrophy with myocardial fibrosis without blood pressure reduction: a one year study in rats. Br J Pharmacol 1992;107:970–975.

16. Jalil JE, Janicki JS, Pick R, Weber KT. Coronary vascular remodeling and myocardial fibrosis in the rat with renovascular hypertension: response to captopril. Am J Hypertens 1991;4:51–55.

17. Brilla CG, Matsubara LS, Weber KT. Anti-aldosterone treatment and the prevention of myocardial fibrosis in primary and secondary hyperaldosteronism. J Mol Cell Cardiol 1993;25:563–575.

18. Sun Y, Ratajska A, Zhou G, Weber KT. Angiotensin converting enzyme and myocardial fibrosis in the rat receiving angiotensin II or aldosterone. J Lab Clin Med 1993;122: 395–403.

19. Ratajska A, Campbell SE, Cleutjens JPM, Weber KT. Angiotensin II and structural remodeling of coronary vessels in rats. J Lab Clin Med 1994;124:408–415.

20. Reddy HK, Campbell SE, Janicki JS, Zhou G, Weber KT. Coronary microvascular fluid flux and permeability: influence of angiotensin II, aldosterone and acute arterial hypertension. J Lab Clin Med 1993;121:510–521.

21. Ratajska A, Campbell SE, Sun Y, Weber KT. Angiotenin II associated cardiac myocyte necrosis: role of adrenal catecholamines. Cardiovasc Res 1994;28:684–690.

22. Brilla CG, Weber KT. Reactive and reparative myocardial fibrosis in arterial hypertension in the rat. Cardiovasc Res 1992;26: 671–677.

23. Campbell SE, Janicki JS, Matsubara BB, Weber KT. Myocardial fibrosis in the rat with mineralocorticoid excess: prevention of scarring by amiloride. Am J Hypertens 1993; 6:487–495.

24. Darrow DC, Miller HC. The production of cardiac lesions by repeated injections of desoxycorticosterone acetate. J Clin Invest 1942; 21:601–611.

25. Weglicki WB, Mak IT, Phillips PM. Blockade of cardiac inflammation in Mg^{2+} deficiency by substance P receptor inhibition. Circ Res 1994;74:1009–1013.

26. LeRoy EC. Collagen deposition in autoimmune diseases: the expanding role of the fibroblast in human fibrotic disease. In: Evered D, Whelan J, eds. Fibrosis. London: Pitman, 1985:196–207.Ciba Foundation Symposium.

27. Rondinone CM, Rodbard D, Baker ME. Aldosterone stimulated differentiation of mouse 3T3-L1 cells into adipocytes. Endocrinology 1993;132:2421–2426.

28. Sun Y, Cleutjens JPM, Diaz-Arias AA, Weber KT. Cardiac angiotensin converting enzyme and myocardial fibrosis in the rat. Cardiovasc Res 1994;28:1423–1432.

29. Gabbiani G, Hirschel BJ, Ryan GB, et al. Granulation tissue as a contractile organ. A study of structure and function. J Exp Med 1972;135:719–734.

30. Gabbiani G. The myofibroblast: a key cell for wound healing and fibrocontractive diseases. In: Deyl Z, Adam M, eds. Connective Tissue Research: Chemistry, Biology, and Physiology. New York, NY: Liss, 1981: 183–194.

31. Fishbein MC, Maclean D, Maroko PR. Experimental myocardial infarction in the rat. Am J Pathol 1978;90:57–70.

32. Jugdutt BI, Amy RWM. Healing after myocardial infarction in the dog: changes in infarct hydroxyproline and topography. J Am Coll Cardiol 1986;7:91–102.

33. Jugdutt BI. Left ventricular rupture threshold during the healing phase after myocardial infarction in the dog. Can J Physiol Pharmacol 1987;65:307–316.

34. Finesmith TH, Broadley KN, Davidson JM. Fibroblasts from wounds of different stages of repair vary in their ability to contract a collagen gel in response to growth factors. J Cell Physiol 1990;144:99–107.

35. Desmoulière A, Geinoz A, Gabbiani F, et al. Transforming growth factor-β_1 induces α-

smooth muscle actin expression in granulation tissue myofibroblasts and in quiescent and growing cultured fibroblasts. J Cell Biol 1993;122:103–111.

36. Bruijn JA, Roos A, de Geus B, et al. Transforming growth factor-β and the glomerular extracellular matrix in renal pathology. J Lab Clin Med 1994;123:34–47.

37. Ronnov-Jessen L, Petersen OW. Induction of α-smooth muscle actin by transforming growth factor-β_1 in quiescent human breast gland fibroblasts. Implications for myofibroblast generation in breast neoplasia. Lab Invest 1993;68:696–707.

38. Vyalov SL, Gabbiani G, Kapanci Y. Rat alveolar myofibroblasts acquire α-smooth muscle actin expression during bleomycin-induced pulmonary fibrosis. Am J Pathol 1993; 143:1754–1765.

39. Bishop J, Greenbaum J, Gibson D, et al. Enhanced deposition of predominantly type I collagen in myocardial disease. J Mol Cell Cardiol 1990;22:1157–1165.

40. Weber KT, Janicki JS, Shroff SG, et al. Collagen remodeling of the pressure-overloaded, hypertrophied nonhuman primate myocardium. Circ Res 1988;62:757–765.

41. Mukherjee D, Sen S. Collagen phenotypes during development and regression of myocardial hypertrophy in spontaneously hypertensive rats. Circ Res 1990;67:1474–80.

42. Oda D, Gown AM, Vande Berg JS, et al. The fibroblast-like nature of myofibroblasts. Exp Mol Pathol 1988;49:316–329.

43. Darby I, Skalli O, Gabbiani G. α-Smooth muscle actin is transiently expressed by myofibroblasts during experimental wound healing. Lab Invest 1990;63:21–29.

44. Chapman D, Weber KT, Eghbali M. Regulation of fibrillar collagen types I and III and basement membrane type IV collagen gene expression in pressure overloaded rat myocardium. Circ Res 1990;67:787–794.

45. Sims DE. The pericyte—a review. Tissue Cell 1986;18:153–174.

46. Tilton RG, Kilo C, Williamson JR, et al. Differences in pericyte contractile function in rat cardiac and skeletal muscle microvasculature. Microvasc Res 1979;18:336–352.

47. Crocker DJ, Murad TM, Geer JC. Role of the pericyte in wound healing. An ultrastructural study. Exp Mol Pathol 1970;13:51–65.

48. Arora PD, McCulloch CAG. Dependence of collagen remodelling on α-smooth muscle actin expression by fibroblasts. J Cell Physiol 1994;159:161–175.

49. Miller FN, Sims DE. Contractile elements in the regulation of macromolecular permeability. Fed Proc 1986;45:84–88.

50. Pedrinelli R, Graziadei L, Taddei S, et al. A renin-secreting tumor. Nephron 1987;46: 380–385.

51. Filip DA, Radu A, Simionescu M. Interstitial cells of the heart valves possess characteristics similar to smooth muscle cells. Circ Res 1986;59:310–320.

52. Laurent GJ. Dynamic state of collagen: pathways of collagen degradation in vivo and their possible role in regulation of collagen mass. Am J Physiol 1987;252:C1-C9.

53. Thompson NL, Bazoberry F, Speir EH, et al. Transforming growth factor beta-1 in acute myocardial infarction in rats. Growth Factors 1988;1:91–99.

54. Sadoshima J, Izumo S. Molecular characterization of angiotensin II-induced hypertrophy of cardiac myocytes and hyperplasia of cardiac fibroblasts. Critical role of the AT_1 receptor subtype. Circ Res 1993;73:413–423.

55. Diaz A, Munoz E, Johnston R, Korn JH, Jimenez SA. Regulation of human lung fibroblast α1(I) procollagen gene expression by tumor necrosis factor α, interleukin-1β, and prostaglandin E_2. J Biol Chem 1993;268: 10364–10371.

56. Evers AS, Murphree S, Saffitz JE, et al. Effects of endogenously produced leukotrienes, thromboxane, and prostaglandins on coronary vascular resistance in rabbit myocardial infarction. J Clin Invest 1985;75:992–999.

57. Sun Y, Diaz-Arias AA, Weber KT. Angiotensin-converting enzyme, bradykinin and angiotensin II receptor binding in rat skin, tendon and heart valves: an in vitro quantitative autoradiographic study. J Lab Clin Med 1994;123:372–377.

58. Katwa LC, Ratajska A, Cleutjens JPM, et al. Angiotensin converting enzyme and kininase II-like activities in cultured valvular interstitial cells of the rat heart. Cardiovasc Res 1995;29:57–64.

59. Boluyt MO, O'Neill L, Meredith AL, et al. Alterations in cardiac gene expression during the transition from stable hypertrophy to heart failure. Marked upregulation of genes encoding extracellular matrix components. Circ Res 1994;75:23–32.

60. Casscells W, Bazoberry F, Speir E, et al. Transforming growth factor-β_1 in normal heart and in myocardial infarction. Ann NY Acad Sci 1990;593:148–160.

61. Chua CC, Chua BHL, Zhao ZY, et al. Effect of growth factors on collagen metabolism in cultured human heart fibroblasts. Connect Tissue Res 1991;26:271–281.

Index